Helping
Children with Autism
Learn

Helping Children with Autism Learn

TREATMENT APPROACHES FOR PARENTS AND PROFESSIONALS

Bryna Siegel, Ph.D.

OXFORD
UNIVERSITY PRESS
2003

OXFORD
UNIVERSITY PRESS

Oxford New York
Auckland   Bangkok Buenos Aires Cape Town
Chennai Dar es Salaam Delhi Hong Kong Istanbul Karachi Kolkata
Kuala Lumpur Madrid   Melbourne Mexico City Mumbai Nairobi
Sao Paulo Shanghai Taipei Tokyo Toronto

Siegel, Bryna.
Helping children with autism learn : treatment approaches for parents and professionals/
Bryna Siegel.
p. cm.
Includes bibliographical references and index.
ISBN 0-19-513811-2 (hardcover : alk. paper)
1. Autistic children—Education. 2. Learning disabilities—Treatment.
3. Communicative disorders in children—Treatment. I. Title.
LC4717 .S54 2003
371.94—dc21
2002151673

ISBN 0-19-513811-2

3 5 7 9 8 6 4 2

Book design by planettheo.com

Printed in the United States of America
on acid-free paper

To My Beginning:
My Mother

To My Foundation:
David

And for those for Whom I do My Work:
All the Families of Children with Autism

CONTENTS

ACKNOWLEDGMENTS

In the eight years since the publication of *The World of the Autistic Child: Understanding and Treating Autistic Spectrum Disorders,* my view of autism has been expanded and enriched by many opportunities I've had to travel and speak to groups of parents and educational, medical, and mental health professionals. I've been honored to have the chance to share ideas with teachers and their paraprofessional aides, speech and language therapists and occupational therapists, school and clinical psychologists, child psychiatrists and pediatricians, social workers, and infant educators. We live in a fortunate society indeed, where so many people can be dedicated to helping children who are among the hardest to reach. I've been touched by everyone who is trying to help. I've had the chance to see numerous schools—many, many classrooms—and to watch teachers, therapists, and tutors doing all sorts of work. I've seen and heard great ideas for treatment programs and seen some incredibly gifted teachers and therapists in action.

I'm a pragmatist. If I see something that works, I pass it on. If something works because it makes sense, that's good. I've never been much attracted to things that aren't common sense. That's why I prefer to rely on science when it's available. The best research results almost always make common sense once they are discovered. In this book I have had to rely a lot on what I've experienced, somewhat on theory, and to a lesser extent (because there isn't much) on evidence-based research. I have tried to gather together all these ways of understanding autism to convey an understanding of the disorder that is recognizable and coherent to my research colleagues but, more important, so that the information is usable for the folks doing the hard work—those spending day after day with the children with autism and trying to raise them in as the best way possible.

My work is made possible by several people. First of all, my husband, David Bradlow, tolerates the large space in my life that autism can occupy. He is an incredible sounding board when I need to talk over ideas. He has an accute ear and an articulate voice. He brings a fresh perspective when I am bogged down with how to explain something.

My life at work is made possible by those who work with me, support me, and endure my comings and goings and my inability to keep up with my voice mail and e-mail, and to consistently complete written patient evaluations in a timely fashion. The first person I must thank is Cathy Hayer who has served as the Autism Clinic Coordinator and my research collaborator for four years. Cathy and now, Michelle Ficcaglia, run the clinic day-to-day, making it possible for me to lecture and write. Bernice Musante, my administrative assistant for ten years, and Glen Elliott, Director of The Children's Center at the University of California, San Francisco, have each in their own way made the completion of this book possible. Also invaluable to the process of running the Autism Clinic and completing research studies are clinic and research volunteers—the stalwarts over the period of this writing being Jen Herbert and Juanita Traver, Lyre Caruz, Cindy Arnold, Van Kober, Heather Erba, Nicki Pelette, Melanie Callen, Lyn Shapiro, Michael Mace, and Alina Brotea. Stories on these pages and other adventures in the Autism Clinic come also from Autism Clinic child psychiatrists—Roger Wu, Brian Zimnitsky, and years of child psychiatry fellows who have bravely served.

Other research collaborators have been dear friends and have helped sustain all the different directions my autism work goes—Adriana Schuler with whom I have worked on treatment outcomes, Nicole Gage with whom I've worked on studies of the brain, and the late Lisa Capps with whom I worked on the effects of autism on the family. I also acknowledge the friends I've made who work with children with autism every day and who continue to strive to build better programs for them:in the San Francisco Bay Area—Hilary Baldi; in Orange County—Andrea Walker; in Hawaii—Jenny Wells, Alida Gandy, Barbara Ward and Char Tarr; in Las Vegas—Jan Crandy; and in the California Central Valley—Howard Cohen, to name just a few. I want to acknowledge the role of special education attorneys with whom I often work—Kathryn Dobel, Michael Zatopa, Sandra Woliver, Diane Finkelstein and Stan Levin. Litigation, often painful, occasionally misguided, serves a very important role in moving services forward for children with autism by propelling research, practice, and treatment together, albeit at times on a bit of a collision course.

Finally, I acknowledge and thank all the mothers, fathers, and children who come my way. No one asks to become a parent of a child with autism. The way you all rise to the occasion contains a message of love and forbearance from which the whole world can take a lesson.

Bryna Siegel
San Francisco
September 2002

FOREWORD

HELPING CHILDREN WITH AUTISM LEARN

The syndrome we know as autism has been the subject of continuous interest on the part of researchers and clinicians from the time of first description by Leo Kanner sixty years ago. As a disorder which affects the most fundamental aspects of social development autism has posed important challenges—for theories of child development, brain development, and education. Essentially every possible approach has been used in trying to understand this disorder and related conditions. Over the past sixty years research findings have enriched not only the field of autism but the broader field of developmental psychopathology. Attempts to understand why children with autism have problems with relating to others, expressing and recognizing emotions, sharing an interest with other people, falling in love and empathizing with others, and in using and understand language to communication have enriched our theories of the whole set of abilities and motivations that allow a child to become a family member and social being.

This volume builds on the tremendous project that has been made over the past decade. This author synthesizes her research work with her extensive clinical experience with children with autism. Principles and findings from this experience are used to illustrate aspects of intervention. The effort to understand the nature of learning challenges in autism and to address them is critically needed. As this volume indicate these learning styles are the adaptations that children with autism use in an attempt to compensate for their difficulties—an awareness of these styles is essential as the starting point for intervention.

This book will be of great interest to teachers, parents, and clinicians in their efforts to facilitate the learning of the child with autism. It draws on the large, and increasing, body of work generated in recent years. It is important to emphasize that because of its many implications for children's development autism has served to shape the multi-disciplinary approach to developmental disabilities and this volume will facilitate the efforts of all those who work with autistic children and their families.

Over the past sixty years, particularly over the last decade, the impact of a child with autism on family life has undergone a sea-change as appropriate services have become more available. The attempt to ease the burden on families has been facilitated by research findings on early identification and intervention which make such a difference for many children with the condition. As the recent National Research Council Report (2001) emphasizes early identification and intervention can make a tremendous difference in the lives of children with autism. At the same time it is important to realize that legitimate differences in approach exist and these differences can add to the burden of parents as well as to clinicians. This volume provides a synthesis of clinical experience and research which can help guide intervention. It will be of great value to teachers and professionals as well as parents. It will help teachers be more effective in the classroom and parents more effective as advocates. Legitimate debate will, of course, continue to exist and concepts will be refined as research moves forward. The present volume provides us with an invaluable synthesis of the current state of knowledge and will help us be more effective as we develop interventions for children with autism.

Fred R. Volkmar MD
Yale University
New Haven, CT

National Research, C. (2001). *Educating Young Children with Autism.* Washington, D.C., National Academy Press.

". . . Let him step to the music he hears, however measured or far away."

—*Henry David Thoreau*

Defining the Issues

The purpose of this book is to guide teachers, therapists, and parents who are directing the development of children with autistic spectrum disorders. This book is about how these children with different forms of autism learn. It is also about how to teach children with autism—based on how they can best learn. Autism is a "spectrum disorder," meaning that it manifests itself differently in each child. Like a row of dominoes, if an early aspect of development is affected in a particular case of autism, other later-emerging aspects of development will be affected too. As a result, each case of autism presents a slightly different profile of learning abilities and learning disabilities. Each learning ability and each learning disability may influence how a particular child with autism may or may not learn something the way other children without autism may learn that same thing. These autism-specific learning barriers are referred to in this book as *autistic learning disabilities*. The autism-specific learning strengths are referred to as *autistic learning styles*.

We are at a very difficult point in autism treatment. We have very good descriptions of autistic spectrum disorders. We have better and increasingly early diagnosis. We have a mandate for early treatment. We have good empirical research that describes specific symptoms and specific ways in which skill acquisition for children with autism may be deficient. We do not, however, have very much empirical, truly scientific, treatment outcome research. Testing a new treatment for autism is not as simple as testing a new drug where one group gets the new drug, and the other group gets the placebo or "old" drug. Unlike a drug treatment trial, treatment for autism is not like just swallowing a pill: In an educational or behavioral treatment research study, it would be almost impossible to control whether certain parents might also naturally be doing other very helpful things, or even pursuing additional simultaneous treatments. Then, there are the problems of treatment fidelity— controlling things like whether each child in a study is getting a good teacher or therapist or a less talented one. Under those circumstances, there would be no way to know whether the parents' own added treatments or the main treatment being studied was the more powerful, or even if different simulta- neous treatments helped (or hindered) one another in some synergistic way. Emotionally, it's another story still: First and foremost, parents will always feel they can't afford *not* to treat autism in their child using whatever method has the loudest rooting section at the moment. Many parents, understandably, are unwilling even to be part of studies that compare treatments, lest the treatment passed over be their child's "silver bullet."

So as a professional, what do you recommend? As a parent, what do you select? Who do you listen to? The bottom line is that the very little scientific outcome research that exists is not enough to tell us for sure what to do for each case of autism. Instead, in designing autism treatment, we must often rely on theory, which is a second, and in some ways less ideal, source of information to select and individualize treatments. A third source of information about treatment comes from the clinical experience of those who have closely studied or worked with children with autistic spectrum disorders over time, and have had an opportunity to see what has helped some improve a great deal, and others improve less. It is harder to evaluate information from clinical claims since some come from those who are very experienced with autism, but others come from "johnny-come-latelys" who feel they may have come across a remarkably effective treatment based on one or a handful of cases. In addition, with the advent of the Internet, parents, and sometimes even professionals, rely on a fourth, even less solid, source of data—personal or anecdotal reports that may be tied to no widely accepted scientific studies, little or no theory or preexisting theory, and little or no long-term clinical experience.

Treatment research in autism has been dealt a really unkind blow by those only interested in a cure, a medical cure, for autism. Undoubtedly, wanting a cure is a more noble ambition than being satisfied with palliation, which is what treatments from the fields of education and psychology are all about. However, even most researchers working on "cure" research would be the first to admit that any breakthroughs are not as likely to "cure" those children now autistic as to prevent future cases.

We need good solid plans to help the children who have autism now. There are some, like myself, who believe that on the path of palliation, there is much to be learned about expression of the disorder and that this knowledge will be needed to trace back to the core neurobehavioral, neurocognitive, and neurogenetic factors that shape the autistic spectrum disorders.

LOOKING AT AUTISM IN A NEW WAY

The picture of autism treatment is further complicated by the fact that there are very different perspectives from which to view treatment: developmental, behavioral, educational, cognitive, and medical. These perspectives overlap, but each emphasizes different things. Practitioners from these different perspectives often don't understand one another's vocabularies. It is like blind men feeling the elephant from different parts of the animal and getting very different impressions of the creature. What we will do here is cross disciplinary boundaries and integrate different perspectives by stripping away terminology that delineates and separates perspectives and instead focus on the mechanics of what to do to carry out treatment, based on research, theory, and clinical experience.

In the last 15 years, treatment for autism has mushroomed, but so has the chaos about how to carry out treatment. Parents often feel they must adopt one treatment perspective and go with it: They fear that questioning a practitioner in any way may be seen as possibly disloyal, and if they really question any aspect of their child's treatment, they may be cast out from those treatment services and their child relegated to some horribly long waiting list for alternative services that might not be as good or might not come to pass at all. Parents feel panicked once the child is diagnosed and just want to get started on treatment right away. Parents of recently diagnosed children may be told by parents of older children "You have to do 'X'! You have to start now!" Such advice is given altruistically, but there can be pitfalls: First, the parents of a newly diagnosed child have no way of knowing just how much "X" is helping the older child, and whether some other things might not have helped him just as much—or more. Second, those giving the advice logically believe that what they have selected is best, but can have no way of knowing whether another child will respond the same way. Advice of other parents is invaluable but is just one tool that should be considered in making treatment decisions. Perspectives from experienced diagnosticians and therapists, as well as readings, should also be weighed to consider all the factors that define a child with autism's individual learning style.

My first goal in this book is to be practical. I try to speak of theory in terms of examples. I hope the theory and research upon which I rely and refer is made clear, but is not so omnipresent as to obfuscate. A chapter-by-chapter annotated bibliography cites exemplary research and reviews that lead back to the primary sources that informed this writing and is intended mainly for making this book useful as a teaching text, without the whole book being plodding or pedantic. My second goal in writing this book was to make a conceptual contribution that would support integrating developmental, behavioral, educational, and medical research and theory. It is based on three principles: First, autism is a spectrum disorder; there are innumerable combinations of possible symptoms. Second, when we treat autism, we treat the individual symptoms of autism, not the diagnosis. Third, each symptom of autism is dependent in its expression and possible amelioration on which other symptoms are also present. In this way, symptoms can be seen as forming from a matrix of ability and disability. Each symptom connotes a learning weakness and requires a survey of an individual child's particular strengths (non-symptom areas, if you will) to determine what possible remedial strategies are most likely to be effective.

Autism as a Learning Disability. This conceptualization of learning weaknesses and strengths is core to the whole field of learning disabilities and to compensatory educational approaches. For this reason, I've come to see autism as a learning disability syndrome, with each symptom connoting a related cluster of learning weakness or an area of "autism-specific learning disability."

Using autistic learning disabilities as the organizing construct, it is possible to reconceptualize treatment for autism: The first step is to inventory a particular child's autistic learning disabilities. The second step is to examine existing treatment strategies and treatment programs and systematically ask what each has to offer in the way of compensation with respect to a specific autistic learning disability. The third step is to put the first two steps together—taking the list of treatments that may be relevant to a particular child's specific profile of autistic learning disabilities and then figuring out how, within this child's matrix of abilities and disabilities, to select treatment components that will address each weakness using strategies that utilize the child's relative strengths. In this way, a very specific set of treatment needs can be formulated and a very individualized treatment plan developed.

Reconceptualizing autism as a learning disability syndrome is intended to help break disciplinary barriers. Sometimes parts of the behavioral model for treating autism will be used, sometimes not. Sometimes, a more educational model will fit, sometimes a more social-developmental model. By philosophically adhering to just one treatment or another you will surely treat some, maybe even most, symptoms in a particular case of autism. However, each child should be treated for all his or her symptoms of autism, and this systematic approach, reconceptualizing each symptom as a learning disability, assures that each sign is addressed.

TEACHING TO AUTISTIC LEARNING STYLES

All children learn as they grow, and children with autistic spectrum disorders are no different; they also learn as they grow. This book is about both sides of this process, teaching and learning. The first part of the teaching and learning process is the adult's side of the story, the teaching. Whether the adult is the parent, the teacher, or both, that adult's job is to act in the child's best interests. What we assume every adult wants is to help a child fulfill his or her potential. In the best of circumstances, children enjoy learning.

Of course, there is no way for children to know what they don't know (but need to learn—like talking), so sometimes children are initially less than overjoyed at the lessons we give them. This is one of the many things that make teaching or parenting a challenging experience. The adult's mandate is to find the best way to teach a child—so that the child learns efficiently and learning becomes a rewarding experience that the child seeks to continue.

The second part of the teaching-learning process is the child's side of the story—learning. The child's learning capacity, whether he or she is autistic or not, is defined by the child's "hardware," (essentially, the child's brain) which is the repository of the child's strengths and weaknesses. The hardware can be "programmed" for optimal performance, and it is the adult's responsibility to identify these strengths and weaknesses so that targeted treatment can be efficiently carried out. The identification process consists of understanding how a particular child with autism is different from typically developing children and from other learners with autism. Then, the adult, as teacher, needs to learn what different teaching strategies have to offer for a child's particular profile of strengths and weaknesses.

Both sides of the teaching-learning process need to be understood to tell the full story of how best a child with autism can learn. The experiences the adult gives the child can change the child's behavior, and even change the child's brain. However, no child is a lump of clay that is infinitely malleable. There will always be something that even a very high functioning child with autism can't do (perhaps understanding how it can be hurtful to tell his grandmother that she's fat), just like there are always things that a very smart child without autism may not be able to do (like playing major league baseball or the violin).

The Holy Grail. The best of everything: the best treatment, the best teachers, the best medicines—as much as is needed, as early as possible—still may not yield all the hoped for results when it comes to autism treatment. Parents need to know this as they start seeking treatments. They need to be reminded of it as treatment proceeds. Part of any treatment's success is recognizing what the child has accomplished. Parents also need to learn when to give their child's teacher a pat on the back when a job has been done well, even if there is still work to do. Likewise, parents sometimes need a pat on the back from teachers; it is parents who reinforce and round out what is learned in school and treatment. Finally, parents need to pat one another on the back once in a while; autism treatment is a Sisyphean struggle. It can help to remind one another how the cup is half full, not half empty.

There will always be things that the child brings (or can't bring) to his own treatment: A big part of treatment response is the result of which treatments are given. However, another part of the treatment response is what the child brings to the table: his innate capacities. Both parents and teachers need to be able to recognize and respect the child when he is working as hard as he can and accomplishing as much as he can. Both teachers and parents need to learn how to recognize when a child is doing his best. We all want the child to learn more but also to be happy, not perpetually anxious or stressed.

In the last 25 years, there has been tremendous progress in how children with autism are treated. A number of methods for teaching children with autism have been devised, tested, and used. But, parents and teachers often become mired in controversy about what should be done—which method to use, how closely the teaching must adhere to the principles of the original method, where teaching should take place, how individualized the instruction should be, how much instruction there should be, who should teach, which peers belong or don't belong in the child's classroom, and so on.

I'll give you the answer to all of these questions now: There *is no one answer.* There is no one *right* answer. Every child is educationally and biologically unique and will need something slightly different. The challenge is to understand the range of differences that make up what are called the autistic spectrum disorders and then to understand the individual differences that can be described in terms of slightly different profiles of strengths and weaknesses. The design of truly individual treatment plans that exploit strengths and compensate for weaknesses begins with a detailed understanding of how learning is different for children with autism than for those without autism and how learning is different among different children with autism.

WHAT'S IN THIS BOOK

Is this a book just about autism? Is it about PDD or PDD,NOS too? Is this a book that will be helpful in planning for a child with Asperger's syndrome? In this book, the focus will be on the symptoms that comprise the autistic spectrum much more than any one autistic spectrum diagnosis or other. The approach here is that when we treat autism, we treat symptoms, not a diagnosis: Children with diagnoses of PDD (i.e., pervasive developmental disorder) and PDD,NOS (pervasive developmental disorder, not otherwise specified) have the same symptoms as children with autism—but they are fewer and, sometimes, less marked. Similarly, children with Asperger's have many of the same symptoms, too, but they usually have better language skills in certain ways. That's why the term autistic spectrum disorders is sometimes used to refer to all of these diagnoses collectively. No matter where in the autistic spectrum you focus, the same issues about conducting assessments, selecting treatment methods, and changing treatments pertain.

First, we will look at where symptoms of autism and autistic learning disabilities have their roots. Second, we will explicitly define autistic learning disabilities and explain how they map onto the diagnostic signs of autistic spectrum disorders. Third, we will review model educational methods and programs for autism and develop an understanding of how each may or may not address each area of autistic learning disability. The book is therefore divided into three parts: Part I begins with three chapters that define the things that make for the unique learning differences of those with autism. Chapter 1 reviews our best, current understanding of the origins of autism. While we still do not know exactly what parts of the brain may be affected in each child, or exactly what role is played by genetics, a current understanding of work in those areas is laid out. Chapter 2 presents a model for understanding how neurodevelopmental weakness in basic aspects of perception and information processing can come together and form a matrix of abilities and disabilities that begin to form the symptoms of autism. Chapter 3 will then describe how these autistic learning disabilities can be derived from a "map" of the diagnostic symptoms of autism and what each autistic learning disability means for what a child may or may not perceive or accurately process.

The second part of the book focuses on strategies for addressing autistic learning disabilities. The first chapter in this section, chapter 4, is about social autistic learning disabilities, the problems children with autistic spectrum disorders have in reading social information. This chapter defines these problems and gives approaches for increasing social interaction, especially with peers. Chapter 5 is the first of three on communication, defining autistic learning disabilities related to the understanding of communicative affect such as facial expression and body language, as well as spoken language. Chapter 6 focuses on communication-based autistic learning disabilities and approaches that can be helpful in overcoming and compensating for missed verbal and nonverbal communicative "signals" with emphasis on how to carry out interventions with the preverbal or nonverbal child. Chapter 7 also focuses on treatment of communication-based autistic learning disabilities but concentrates on treatments for the verbal child. Chapter 8 details how learning is often altered for children with autistic spectrum disorders because of the uneven ways they process information from various sensory "channels," and, subsequently, how this influences their actions with objects, and especially play with toys. Chapter 9 covers many of the adaptive deficits most common to autistic children and how they can be addressed with modifications to motivational strategies, which can enhance the effectiveness of more conventional behavioral strategies as they are used for children who are not autistic. The second part of the book concludes by describing the Autistic Learning Disabilities and Autistic Learning Styles Inventory (ALDI). The ALDI is designed as a way of organizing observations about learning difficulties and learning strengths in a particular child in preparation for selecting methods of teaching and teaching content.

The third part of the book covers model methodologies for teaching children with autism and some model programs that utilize these methods. At this point in the book, the reader will have a solid understanding of how to construct an autistic learning disabilities profile of any particular child and can read this section with an eye to how a particular child may benefit from all or part of the features that a particular teaching method may offer. Chapter 10 describes the use of the applied behavior analysis discrete trial training approach, including an analysis of how it addresses specific autistic learning disabilities and takes advantage of commonly encountered autistic learning strengths. Chapter 11 describes the TEACCH curriculum, another widespread approach for teaching children with autism and tells how it addresses specific autistic learning disabilities and takes advantage of commonly encountered autistic learning strengths. Chapter 12 analyzes inclusive and integration-based educational approaches in which children with autism are included in general education programs alone, or with other special education students. Chapter 13 provides a "travelogue" of model programs around the United States as a way of describing how autism-specific curricula look when all the ideas that have been discussed are implemented in a model or particularly exemplary class. The final chapter of this section, chapter 14, deals with using the information that has been provided to innovate more individualized treatments—putting the 'I' back in IEP.

A Word Is a Word. Throughout this book, an effort is made to use the most accurate and gentle disability-sensitive terminology grammatically possible. Many statements refer to those with autistic spectrum disorders, which means broadly any person with a diagnosis that falls under the DSM-IV classification of "Pervasive Developmental Disorder." I find the term "pervasive developmental disorder" often somewhat inaccurate and ungentle, and I avoid it where possible. I prefer the term "autistic spectrum disorders" (or ASD) because it more accurately reflects our knowledge about the causes and relationships among different and related diagnostic labels such as autistic disorder, PDD,NOS and Asperger's disorder. At times, the term "autism" may be used as a shorthand for restating "autistic spectrum disorders," and it is often preferred to an abbreviation like ASD which at times, sounds clinical. Also, it can be agreed that is more respectful to refer to a child as an individual with autism—rather than saying an autistic child—though sometimes the latter is almost impossible to avoid grammatically.

This book is also a book mainly about children. Much of what is said does pertain to adults with autism, too—and where relevant, I try to give examples of adults as well as children. Mostly, I refer to the child with autism as "he"— since most readers will have mostly males in mind (since autism is four to five times more prevalent in males). While parents and teachers are clearly both male and female, I more often refer to the helping adult as she—at times for clarity of pronoun use between child and teacher or parent, and also because most teachers of children with autism are women, and in many families, the majority of parenting activities fall to mothers, and this is important to acknowledge.

Finally, this book is intended as much for teachers and other professionals as it is for parents. Hardly anybody I know who spends much of the day with children with autism is likely to stay awake in the evening to read a really boring but informative book on autism. I assume that I can open more people to new ideas about autism by writing in a conversational narrative manner rather than writing as I do for a journal or professional volume. This book falls into a relatively new category of work being referred to as "translational research"— taking theory and empirical studies from scientific publications and making the content into "news you can use." At the end of the book is an annotated bibliography of further readings that provide references to the primary sources as well as key research reviews I've used—pour yourself a cup of coffee (or two), and delve into them when you need to know more!

PART I

The Fundamentals of Autistic Learning Styles

Part I is designed to give you a sense of what makes the autistic spectrum disorders distinct from other neurodevelopmental problems. At its core, autism is a disorder in the capacity for social understanding. Along with this, there come to be certain ways that the child with autism also has difficulties with language and how he processes the information coming from the senses. First, in chapter 1, we'll review ideas about how a child might develop autism. Chapter 2 introduces a way of understanding how various inborn problems in receiving and processing social, linguistic, and sensory information combine to form the characteristic symptoms we recognize as autism. Then in chapter 3, the idea of regarding these symptoms as autistic learning disabilities will be introduced. In this way, the stage is set for understanding each of autism's hallmark symptoms in terms of their possible causes, their implications for learning, and then, in Part II of the book, the treatments for each of these autistic learning disabilities.

CHAPTER ONE

Understanding the Origins of Autism and Its Meaning for Development

In this chapter we will begin by exploring the fundamentals of how children with autistic spectrum disorders can be developmentally different from others. One of the first things that I find parents of children with autism grappling to understand is the fact that their children's brains are developing differently. At first this can sound scary and absolute in a nihilistic way. But, really, it isn't. All brains are different, just the way everyone's face is a little different. Infant faces look more similar to one another than 40-year-old faces do because experience and learning are reflected in one's face. The same process occurs with the brain. Infants are born with different potentials for development: It is not a coincidence that Picasso's father was a painter, and Mozart's father was a musician. Children with autism also inherit some predilections from their parents, but some of these things can also direct development in the characteristic ways that we've come to call "autism." In order to understand these things that direct development in characteristically autistic ways, it can be helpful to start at the beginning of development and review what we have come to understand so far about how autism comes to be expressed in a particular child.

ARE THERE MORE CHILDREN WITH AUTISM?

I am often asked whether there is more autism than there used to be—obviously a good and interesting question. The answer is unclear for several reasons. One observation, which has nothing to do with the biology of the disorder, is that there is clearly more public awareness and education about autism. Overall, our society is more open about disability. There is less social stigma attached to "autism" than to some other disability "labels" (like mental retardation) and, in many places, there are more entitlements associated with autism as a category of disability. Autism, in particular, seems to have accumulated a certain mystique—from Dustin Hoffman's *Rain Man* to the *New York Times*'s running a Sunday magazine article on the alleged miracles of facilitated communication or Asperger's disorder as "Little Professor syndrome," or *Wired* magazine's speculating that there may be more autism in Silicon Valley due to the "Geek syndrome."

The Impact of Changing Diagnostic Categories on Prevalence. Another reason there may seem to be a rising incidence of autistic spectrum disorders is that autism is unquestionably being more widely diagnosed than it was ten or 15 years ago. One reason is that the official criteria used to diagnose it (called the DSM—the *Diagnostic and Statistical Manual of Mental Disorders*, published by the American Psychiatric Association) have been revised again and again, each time including more children or more diagnostic categories as part of the autistic spectrum. In 1987 there was a shift from the DSM-III (the third edition) diagnostic criteria to the DSM-III-R (the revised third edition) criteria. In 1994 there was a second shift, from DSM-III-R to DSM-IV. At the time of this first shift, about a third more children became diagnosable with autistic spectrum disorders. These included many children who earlier would have been diagnosed as having mental retardation "with autistic features," as well as children with a number of normal intellectual abilities but with some "autistic-like" use of language, and poor play and social skills. It took a while for the shifts adopted in DSM-III-R and DSM-IV to be recognized by the wider community of clinicians who diagnose autism. In 1994 DSM-IV added the diagnostic label of Asperger's disorder (more widely referred to as Asperger's syndrome) for the first time. This resulted in many individuals being newly diagnosed as now falling within the autistic spectrum, including many older children, teens, and even adults who previously had been awkwardly diagnosed as having schizoid or schizotypal personality, as well as many individuals with language disorders and social awkwardness. (Of course, this does not mean that anyone with these difficulties really has Asperger's instead.) Many clinicians are still coming to understand Asperger's syndrome, and the label is not yet used consistently. Even in the primary research, there are debates about what Asperger's syndrome is and what "high-functioning autism" is—and whether it is important to draw a distinction. Undoubtedly, the diagnostic category of Asperger's disorder will undergo further refinements in future DSMs.

It has long been recognized that many siblings of children with autism had language difficulties. Over the years, it also became clear that many siblings with these language difficulties had some social awkwardness as well. Initially, it was suspected that the social awkwardness might be due solely to communication difficulties. But, even with language therapy and improvements in speech proficiency, many of these children remained socially maladroit. Increasingly, these siblings of children with autism are diagnosed as having PDD,NOS, high-functioning autism, or even Asperger's syndrome, as our awareness of inheritance of autistic traits has grown clearer.

Arguably, this shift to diagnosing more individuals with some kind of autistic spectrum disorder is generally a positive one because it acknowledges that many children have "features" of autism, and with the "label" of autistic spectrum disorder, pervasive developmental disorder, or Asperger's disorder, they might gain better access to services designed to target these autistic symptoms.

The Impact of Earlier Diagnoses on Prevalence. More children with signs of autism are being diagnosed earlier as early diagnosis instruments improve. We now have a better understanding of the importance of earlier interventions, and so it has become a conservative clinical practice to diagnose and treat autism early rather than taking a wait-and-see approach. This practice is largely a very positive one that is long overdue. However, we may be diagnosing children with much milder and subtler difficulties that, untreated, *might* have fully or partially been resolved just by particularly attentive care to a child who seemed especially shy or slow to talk. This is *not* to be taken to mean that the wait-and-see approach is preferred. It is very unlikely to hurt any child to receive some enriched stimulation in the form of an early intervention program or the increased parental awareness of developmental milestones that come with participating in such programs. In the context of the present discussion, it does suggest that perhaps we now have "more" young children with autism because subtle and wider-ranging forms of early developmental delays are being labeled as a form of an autistic spectrum disorder. (We will discuss this issue more fully later on, in the context of designing and initiating early intervention programs.)

The Impact of Service Delivery Entitlements on the Prevalence of Autism. Another factor in assigning a diagnosis of autism is what effect it has on the provision of services. Many developmental disabilities program directors and special education administrators can tell you that the percentage of their budget apportioned to clients or pupils with autism is on the rise. All other things being equal, it is probably safe to say that any increases in expenditures are likely to be stressful to an administrator. One way that many agencies have tried to close the floodgates on demand for autism services is to draw a distinction between autism (autistic disorder) and other pervasive developmental disorders (like PDD,NOS and Asperger's). As a result, some diagnosticians, aware of how the diagnosis of PDD,NOS or Asperger's may limit access to services, may prefer to assign the diagnosis of autistic disorder or be asked to do so by savvy parents or their advocates. This presents a complex set of issues that certainly needs to be thoroughly considered and discussed. We will discuss them in the next chapter as the concept of autistic learning disabilities is discussed. Suffice it to say for now that the issue of where to draw the boundaries in diagnosis has likely contributed to the documented rise in the diagnosis of autistic spectrum disorders.

Biological Risk Factors. Finally, there may be more cases of autism resulting from biological factors: Some of the pre- and perinatal risk factors we will discuss later may be contributing to autism, but comprehensive studies of these possible risks have not been carried out and would be difficult to do with all necessary controls. Similarly, the more speculative hypotheses generated mainly by grassroots concerns about geographical "clusters," environmental toxins, vaccines, and so on may eventually prove to account for some cases, or raise the likelihood of autism in certain genetically or otherwise neurodevelopmentally vulnerable individuals, though there is no solid evidence as of yet that any such factors are proven risks.

WHAT DO WE KNOW ABOUT THE CAUSES OF AUTISM?

Most parents don't have much reason to know a lot about autism until they become concerned that their child may have it. Then, they want to know everything. Even many special education teachers, speech and language pathologists, and occupational therapists encountering children with autism for the first time might know little about autism if it was not part of their coursework or was not encountered in their training or teaching internships. No parent starts out an expert. Each child is different, and that means that professionals must hone their expertise as they undertake to treat each new child.

For both parents and teachers, the first question is "What are we going to do to help this child?" The answer to that question is sufficiently long and so complex that it will fill this book. It has filled many books. But, in the beginning, when the child is first diagnosed, all parents ask: "What caused *my* child to have autism?" Somehow this question seems to need some answering as part of comprehending the diagnosis and then getting on with what needs to be done about it. In any one case of autism, we can make some guesses as to what the greatest risk factors were. We will be discussing these. However, there is a lot we still don't know about the causes of autism, and a great deal of speculation. It's human nature to want to have an explanation, an answer to "Why me?" or "Why my child?" when an event as profound as the diagnosis of autism befalls a family. It is the domain of some researchers, particularly those studying genes and what different genes do in developing the brain. What seems clear from research so far is that you can get to be autistic in many ways. But, the important thing to know is that no matter how a particular child might have come to have autism, treatment proceeds from understanding the child's problem from ways he is best able to learn. So, the focus here is on understanding what exactly is wrong with what the child knows or doesn't know, how the child behaves, and how to alter it.

What "Cause" Means for Understanding Treatment. There are a couple of levels at which one can talk about "causes" of autism. The first level involves some innately atypical processes (such as genetic differences) that grow a brain that is physically different in certain ways. The second level involves how experience may "write" on a brain that is physically different. We will talk about both kinds of causes. Discussing the first level of cause may help you understand how a particular child became autistic. Discussing the second level of cause is intended to help you to understand how brain development and learning experiences influence each other. Understanding this second level of cause can be useful in understanding how different kinds of interventions may work, or if interventions don't work, why it is that they may not be working.

First of all, the use of the word "cause" must be carefully qualified: Over the years, there have been a number of correlational studies about causes of autism, which is the first step in understanding the true cause of something. A correlation means that two things go together, like cigarette smoking and lung cancer. A correlational study, however, does not tell us "how" or "why." How do cigarettes make a lung grow cancer cells? Why doesn't everyone who smokes get lung cancer? The real "causes" are the biological factors that trigger a strong risk for the disease when one is exposed to cigarette smoke, or cause chemical changes in the lungs when one is exposed to smoke, so some might say that the cause is not the cigarettes themselves. When the risk is high enough, as it is with cigarette smoking and lung cancer, we tend to think of the former "causing" the latter. But not all correlations are as strong as smoking and lung cancer.

What we know about the causes of autism, at this point, is all correlational, and many of the correlations are rather weak—some are just theories formed from a series of case observations rather than from an objective comparison of large groups of children exposed to some possible "cause". But we do know some things about the "causes" (that is, strong correlations) of autism. The strongest evidence supports genetic causes, even though almost everyone would agree that not every case of autism is genetically caused. There is some evidence supporting prenatal (occurring during pregnancy) and perinatal (occurring during birth) causes. Evidence for these causes is much weaker than for genetic causes and falls into the category of "risk factors," meaning that there are events that seem to make autism more likely, probably when other things (like genetic factors) are also non-optimal. There is absolutely no evidence that psychological trauma either to the mother during or after pregnancy, or to the child can cause autism. Autism does not appear to be caused by any illnesses, accidents, or injuries. There are isolated cases of autism being attributed to such causes, but the appearance of signs of autism in these cases often just happens to coincide with these supposedly causative events.

Sometimes autism is blamed on things that are common, like infant vaccinations or a mother's yeast infection. This is about as logical as saying that autism is caused by drinking orange juice, something that almost everyone does. To qualify as a bona fide "probable cause," it is helpful to have a scientifically reasonable theory about how one thing would cause another. To properly study such theories—vaccines for example—one must find children who were vaccinated and compare them to children of the same age and sex who were not vaccinated, then examine the rates of autism. This would be hard to do in the United States today because so many children are vaccinated, but a more recent study done in the United Kingdom compared children who were not vaccinated (before the MMR (measles, mumps, rubella) vaccine was introduced) with those who were vaccinated, and no difference in the rate of autism was found. Similarly, retrospective statistics for U.S. samples have led the American Academy of Pediatrics, the National Institutes of Health, the Institute of Medicine, and the World Health Organization all to conclude that vaccines do not cause autism. The "probable cause" finger was pointed at thimerisol, a mercury-containing preservative in vaccines. However, the kind of mercury in vaccines is different from the "bad" mercury in contaminated foods. Mercury is a chemical element, like hydrogen or nitrogen—which might be bad for you, too—and, like them, it needs to be studied in the form of the specific compound being indited. This kind of logic is important to consider because of the correlation-does-not-prove-causation problem: It has been known for a while—from before there was an MMR vaccine or the number of vaccines children receive today—that about a third of children with autism start to develop language and then lose it, right around 18-32 months, the age when so many vaccines are being given.

GENETICS AND AUTISM

What's a Genotype? The most important, and informative, likely cause of autism is genetics. The study of genes that may cause a disorder is the study of that disorder's *genotype*. There are a few basic ways to look at the genetics of autism. First, there are genetic abnormalities. These can consist of either inherited abnormalities that have been passed to the child from either a parent or more distant relative, or a genetic abnormality that is not inherited, a genetic mutation, which is a more random, one-time event. Examples of known inherited genetic abnormalities would be developmental disorders like Fragile-X syndrome, or medical conditions like cystic fibrosis or sickle cell anemia. Examples of developmental disorders that represent genetic mutations would include Down's syndrome (also known as trisomy 21), and more recently, Retts syndrome, the latter of which, at times, shares features with autism. So, there likely are cases of autism caused by inherited gene mutations as well as cases caused by one-time gene mutations. Evidence from certain kinds of studies of large groups, "segregation analyses," have suggested that autism is not likely caused by one gene, but by several genes coming together in the genetic make-up of one particular child. Since no child in a family gets all the same genes (except identical twins) not all the siblings will have autism.

One other thing we know about the genetics of autism is that 10 to 25 percent of siblings of children with an autistic spectrum disorder have a minor to marked language-based difficulty (that is, the child may have something as minor as a speech impediment that requires six months of speech therapy at the start of kindergarten, or as significant as a need to remain through all of elementary school in a special-education class for communicatively impaired children). This may mean that these children got some, but not all, of the genes involved in their sibling's autism. Some of these siblings may have minor social difficulties as well. It may be that it is more common to see half-siblings with just a language difficulty (that is, just certain of the genes), though there are no good statistics on just how common this might be.

It is also important to think of autism genes as autism "risk" genes since at least some of these genes probably don't cause autism all of the time, but only when they are activated by certain other things, like events of the pregnancy and birth, which we will discuss separately later on. The idea of multiple "risk" genes is one reason it is likely that most children with a genetic cause for their autism are getting contributing genes from both parents, because while half-siblings are quite common these days, half-siblings who both have autism are certainly nowhere near as common as full siblings who both have autism. This is pretty good news for parents of autistic children who remarry and want more children.

There seem to be different "strains" of autistic spectrum disorders, with some families having members who have language problems (as described above), other families having members with obsessive traits, and still other families having lots of relatives with depression and anxiety disorders. Some families seem to have more than their share of relatives with unknown forms of mental retardation or developmental disability, and some of these families may actually have relatives with autism that have never been diagnosed because of where the child lives, or because the relative is still too young, or so old that "no one knew in those days."

The bottom line is that these autism-risk genes contain some of the many, many instructions that make the brain. If some of the instructions are wrong, whether it is because the child inherited the wrong information (a gene mutation) or there are no instructions (a gene deletion), the brain develops in a way that is slightly different and can make for an autistic spectrum disorder.

What's a Phenotype?   However, the story of genetics and autism is more complicated than the one just told. As more families with multiple children with autism have been studied, it has become clearer that the affected children have a condition that may result from a heavier dose of something that one, or even both, parents may have, but that in the parent's case doesn't cause a "disorder." A *phenotype* is how the *genotype* is expressed, how severe the autism is. Just having a particular gene mutation doesn't tell us whether that gene will produce a notable problem. It probably depends on many things, like how optimal other growth and environmental factors are and what other gene mutations are present. There is evidence that in some cases, partial or very mild forms of autism exist in parents and other close relatives. There is a term for this—"the broader autism phenotype." Think of it as the oak tree from which the acorn has fallen. The little "acorns," the children with autism, either have this heavier dose, or have multiple doses from different genetic factors (probably coming from both parents) that together make for an autistic spectrum disorder. These genetic factors in isolation might be quite adaptive—such as a parent who is a successful physicist or computer programmer, or who works at any job that requires a high level of attention to detail. The same mental talents that help the parent succeed may also turn out to be a relative advantage for the family member with autism. The area(s) of strength, however, may be less readily brought into play for the person with autism because he is likely contending with other, simultaneous social difficulties related to having a full-blown case of autism. These can include difficulties in abstracting the main point of a situation, prioritizing needed tasks, or understanding what others expect of him—all workplace skills that any physicist or computer programmer needs. Autism may also manifest itself in a sometimes adaptive trait that is so strongly expressed that it becomes dysfunctional: Think, for example, of the difference between a "neat freak" who is a highly valued office manager, and a person with obsessive compulsive disorder who feels she must wash her hands ten times in a row any time she may have touched a surface with germs on it. The office manager may have the "broader

phenotype" for autism; her child with autism may compulsively align Matchbox
cars that only he can reposition.

The Likelihood of Having a Second Child with Autism. The most convincing
evidence that autism is strongly genetic comes from studies of siblings. We know
that if a family has one *boy* with autism, the likelihood that the next child will
be born with autism is about three percent. If the first child with autism is a *girl,*
the possibility that another child will be autistic is as high as 12 percent. This is
to say that autism seems about four times as likely to have been genetically caused
in the smaller number of girls who have it. However, overall, autism is four to
five times more common in boys than in girls. Families with two children with
autism are not uncommon. Often, the second child is conceived or born before
the first child is diagnosed. A much smaller number of families end up with three
autistic spectrum children: If a family has two children with autistic spectrum
disorders, the risk that a third child will have an autistic spectrum disorder is
about one in three.

Much less is known about the exact probability of having a child with autism
if one of the parents has an autistic brother or sister, or if there is a niece or
nephew of either parent who has autism. It is usually felt that such families run
a somewhat higher risk than the numbers just cited. One of the reasons that
autism is increasingly thought of as a "spectrum" disorder is that when autism
runs in a family, it is not likely the same autistic spectrum disorder in everyone.
Because many genes are probably involved, different children along the autistic
spectrum probably have different combinations of these genes, as well as having
differences among them from having the various genes more or less strongly
expressed.

Taking Family History into Account. If you have one child who is autistic, but
none of the 25 kids of your five brothers and sisters and none of the 16 kids of
your spouse's six brothers and sisters have a child who is remotely autistic, your
risk of having another child with autism is probably *less* than three percent. On
the other hand, if you're an engineer who has only one sister and her only son
is autistic, and your husband, a software developer has only one brother and he's
an odd duck with no friends and two master's degrees who works a night shift
somewhere, your risk is probably *higher* than three percent to have another

autistic child. This is not to say that there is anything genetically risky about engineers or software developers, but one person's talent may, when combined with some other less useful genes, become a profile of splintered abilities that presents as an autistic spectrum disorder.

Not only does it seem that the phenotype can vary from parent to child, and mean the difference between talent and disability, it can likely also vary among multiple autistic children in one family. When more than one child in the family has an autistic spectrum disorder, there are often different diagnoses along the autistic spectrum represented—such as one child with autism, one with PDD,NOS, and one with Asperger's syndrome. One family with three children illustrates this well: I first met them when their boys were five years, three years, and 13 months old. The middle brother, who was clearly autistic, had been diagnosed first—just before they came to me the first time. After the parents had learned what autism was, they began to realize that their five-year-old shared many of the same characteristics, although he could talk well. It turned out that he had Asperger's syndrome. As the hours of the five-year-old's diagnostic visit went on, I became increasingly concerned about the 13-month-old: He didn't play with toys, he didn't babble much or respond to language, and he hit his mother in the chest without so much as a "So there!" look in the eye when she wouldn't nurse him on demand. At 17 months of age, he was seen again and diagnosed with autism, and at age three was better described as having PDD,NOS. At age four, there were still some mild language problems, but socially was doing as well—or even a little better than—his now eight-year-old brother with Asperger's. The "good news" from these clinical observations as well as what has already been said about our understanding of genetics is that if one child with autism is quite severely affected, it will not necessarily mean that the next child with autism will also be severely affected. Among families with three children in the autistic spectrum, I can think of several in which there is one with "classical" autism, one with PDD, and one with Asperger's syndrome. Sometimes, just one has an autistic spectrum disorder, but other siblings have symptoms of what can be better described as social anxiety or a language disorder.

The Story with Twins. The most dramatic evidence that genetics plays a role in many cases of autism comes from what we know about identical twins (children having the same genes): In 90 to 95 percent of cases, if one identical twin has autism, so does the other. This is strong evidence indeed for a genetic cause for autism. What is interesting is what we also learn about a disorder's being "genetic": When identical twins both have autism, they are never autistic in exactly the same way. One may be more cognitively impaired than the other; one may be more obsessively internalizing while the other is more aggressively avoidant. Some differences, such as which twin has more cognitive impairment, may appear to be related to which twin had the harder time at birth. Other times, we are probably simply observing the results of individual variation in how fully a gene's instructions are being carried out in the making of the brain. But what about the five to ten percent of identical twins in which one is not on the autistic spectrum? In the only identical twins I've seen in which only one had autism, the one with autism, sadly, died of a brain tumor when he was six. His symptoms of autism may have been of a non-genetic type in the first place and related to whatever led to the brain tumor, which may be why his identical twin was unaffected. It has also been suggested that when identical twins are not both autistic, it may be because they were among the rarer identical twins who developed in different amniotic sacs with different placentas, suggesting that the identical genetics might have to interact in identical prenatal environments to result in autism.

In nonidentical, fraternal twins, who are no more closely related genetically than other siblings (that is, they have about 50 percent of the genes in common), the likelihood of both having a form of autism is between five and 15 percent—a bit higher than for siblings that didn't share a pregnancy. This suggests that the slightly higher rate of autism in nonidentical twins may be due to some kind of additional compromise that came from sharing the same pregnancy—even though fraternal twins have different placentas and different amniotic sacs. Just looking at statistics like these helps us to begin to appreciate the complex relationship that likely exists between genes and events of pregnancy and birth, both of which certainly play some role in how genetic predispositions get expressed.

PRE- AND PERINATAL RISK FACTORS AND AUTISM

Possible Triggers for Genetic Risk

When genetic research on autism began in the late 1960s, there was the implied belief that there must be an autism gene. After all, why else would identical twins almost always both have autism, and nonidentical twins almost never both have autism? This gave way to the assumption that there were likely several autism genes because there were so many differences in the way autism occurred, and that autism was, in fact, a syndrome. By the early 1990s the focus began to shift to an understanding that these genes were "vulnerability" genes, or "risk" genes, as we have discussed.

As we've also just discussed, there was an increasing awareness of phenotypic variation, the idea that the same autism genes did not come out looking exactly the same in identical twins. One identical twin might be affected more severely than the other or have different specific symptoms. Another observation was that the autistic child's weakness and strengths might be mirrored in a parent with a milder, similar, but non-handicapping intellectual profile (what was referred to as the "broader phenotype"). So the question was: What could trigger vulnerability? What would make the affected genes active? What would it take to trigger developmental circumstances significant enough that the child had a diagnosable condition? The answer to all of these questions is that we do not yet know for sure, but we are starting to find some clues.

Epidemiology and Prenatal Screening. Epidemiology is the study of the prevalence of a disease or disorder in a population of people. We know from epidemiological studies of autism that it occurs at approximately the same rates in different countries and in different ethnic and racial groups. Wherever it is studied, autism occurs four to five times more frequently in boys than in girls. This finding is part of what helps us know that there is no single autism "gene" that occurs mostly in one ethnic group the way Tay-Sachs disease affects people of Jewish descent, and sickle cell anemia affects people of African descent. This kind of finding raises the probability that something has gone wrong either with a gene itself or with how that gene gets expressed (meaning whether or not the gene is able to carry out its instructions properly).

Another epidemiological fact about autistic spectrum disorders is that the full syndrome of autism co-occurs with some degree of mental retardation about 70 percent of the time. Of the 30 percent of children whose overall intellectual function is in the average (not retarded) range, two-thirds have significantly more impairment in language abilities, so that language skills may be in the borderline or mildly mentally retarded range even though overall IQ is pulled into the average range by significantly better "performance" or non-language intellectual abilities. The fact that mental retardation and autism are overlapping rather than independent phenomena corresponds closely to what is known about how a number of possible risk factors sometimes seen in autism (which will be enumerated later) are not unique to autism or to mental retardation, but may occur in cases of either or both.

Many parents as well as teachers and therapists may be under the impression that prenatal screening using blood tests or amniocentesis are ways of learning whether a child will be autistic or mentally retarded. In fact, tests like an amniocentesis, an AFP (alpha-fetal protein) screen, or a Fragile–X screen are not indemnifications against developmental disability in the baby. A clean bill of health on an amniocentesis rules out common known causes for a number of forms of mental retardation and heritable genetic diseases for about a third of cases eventually diagnosed with some form of developmental disorder (including autism) that is presumed to be of genetic origin. Presently, there are no known markers for autism that are clinically useful, though many researchers are working toward this important goal.

Parental Age. Another clue about the causes of autism is that risk of a neurodevelopmental disorder (not just autism but also mental retardation and most syndromes resulting from known genetic anomalies) is higher for children born to older mothers. "Older" in this context generally means older than 35, with risk rising gradually for about five years, and more sharply between 40 and 45 years of age. A small amount of newer research suggests that there may be similar risks associated for older fathers, even after the mother's age is taken into account. The risk seems a little higher for older mothers having a first baby, especially if the first baby is a boy (since most developmental disorders, not just autism, occur in boys). Generally, the risk associated with age is understood to be related to the aging of the mother's eggs in her ovaries. It does not seem related to whether she is a worn-down, worn-out forty-year-old rather than one who goes to the gym daily and bikes 50 miles on the weekend. More autism from older mothers supports the reasoning of those who might hypothesize that there is something wrong with the genetic material. Also, there is no reason to believe that one theory may cancel another out: In some cases, genetic material may be compromised by a mother's or father's age; in another, damage to the same genes might be due to some outside agent. In fact, multiple risk factors might have to be present.

Fertility Treatments. A related issue concerns babies born after the mother was treated for infertility. At this stage there seem to be no studies of the rates of developmental disability in children born to women who got pregnant through the use of ovulation-stimulating drugs and/or in vitro fertilization methods ("test tube" babies). Fertility specialists consider a live birth with no obvious physical defects a success and seem to stop keeping records at that point. There are no really good numbers for how many babies with autistic spectrum disorders are born as a result of these kinds of procedures, so it is impossible to say for sure whether these procedures add to the risk of a baby's having a developmental disability. Obviously, women who undergo fertility treatments include those who have habitually miscarried or have had other prolonged problems getting or staying pregnant. This is at least partly related to being an older mother or an older, first-time mother, which, as discussed, is already known to add to risk. Fertility procedures also result in twins and other multiple births more often than getting pregnant the old-fashioned way—and twins and multiple births also experience higher rates of developmental problems. One recent study, however, suggested an additional effect on the rate of developmental disabilities. It suggested that more-educated mothers have a higher risk of having a baby with developmental disabilities. One possible explanation for this is that more-educated mothers are more likely to use fertility-enhancing procedures—as these methods are seldom paid for by medical insurance and are likely not as well understood among less sophisticated consumers of medical services. I found myself worrying about this with one family, an "older" mother and father, who had two children with autism—both from the same in vitro fertilization—with the second child having been a frozen-embryo conceived from the same in vitro fertilization as his older brother. This kind of case might indicate that not just genes, but possibly some event in the very early development of the embryo, might also play a role in the expression of autism.

When a woman's body does not seem to want to maintain a healthy pregnancy on its own, it may be a sign that all is not well with the raw material (the eggs) or with the integrity of the prenatal environment. One hopes that more studies will address this in the future. For now though, we have no solid reason to believe that fertility procedures alone are a singular causative factor in autism.

PREGNANCY RISKS

Earlier research on the etiology of autism explored seemingly obvious connections between birth trauma and autism, or between a risky pregnancy and autism. That research, which generally wasn't able to control for presence or absence of different kinds of autistic symptoms or even subtypes of autism, wasn't tremendously informative. But the research did seem to support a few findings. Prenatal and perinatal suboptimality (risky events) did appear related to how much mental retardation accompanied the autism. The more compromised of twins usually had more severe problems, for example, and the more risk factors, the more likely that one of the children would be multihandicapped.

As just discussed, the genetic makeup of the baby is determined at conception and it is believed that, in most cases, it is not altered after that. This means that prenatal development might be pretty normal, prior to some sort of prenatal "insult." However, we know that there is no such thing as an autism "insult." No one risky thing that might happen in pregnancy consistently leads to autism. Instead, the greater the number of risky events, the greater the likelihood that something will be wrong with the baby. It is important to understand that there is no point at which we can be sure that a baby has been exposed to so many risks that he will certainly have lasting developmental problems. However, there is a continuous rise in the likelihood of permanent damage with an increase in the number of risk factors. Pre- and perinatal risk factors are broadly seen as increasing the risk that autism will be expressed, but not as being sufficient to lead to autism specifically: So, for example, preemies are not significantly more likely to be autistic, though they are more likely than others to have developmental problems. Again, this kind of observation supports the idea that some predisposition to becoming autistic has to be triggered. This takes us back to the idea that there is some genetic vulnerability that is inherited, anomalous, or both, that has to be there in order for the pre- or perinatal event to produce autism. This picture is complicated by the fact that there is substantial evidence that genetics alone can be responsible for autism, even if the pregnancy and delivery were "picture perfect," as is often the case.

There may also be suboptimal pregnancy events that a mother is not aware of but that increase the risk that her child will be autistic, if the child carries the genetic vulnerability. Some people have suggested that these might include toxins in the environment, such as in the food, water, or the place in which the family resides. It is important to note that no relationship between any specific toxin and autism has ever been proven conclusively. It is possible that a teratogen (poison) that might cause a number of neurodevelopmental disorders, not just autism, might be expressed as autism in a family particularly (genetically) vulnerable to autistic spectrum disorders. The father of one family with three children in the autistic spectrum (two autistic, one with Asperger's) told me that they live in a new subdivision built on what was once farmland and that is near the former sites of a glass factory and a well-known military weapons depot. The mother then told me that she worries about where they live because the special-education bus is filled within a couple blocks of their home, with her children as well as children with other learning problems. At first, this story sounded horrifying. On closer questioning, however, it turns out that the family moved to this home early in the pregnancy with their second child. They know that some of the other special-education children were conceived in this subdivision, but others were not. If I were to make an educated guess, I would say that this family is at greater genetic risk than most to have another autistic child, and that, possibly, environmental factors were the "trigger" for two of their three boys. Such stories have to be interpreted very cautiously because, while they are scary, there is no real evidence about what is buried in their soil, what teratogens the children may have come in contact with, where their water comes from—or any other things that one would need to be known to begin a systematic, scientific investigation of such a story.

Other studies that have been made of so-called clusters—whole communities in which there is a lot of autism and some environmental risk factor—have not produced particularly clear findings about what causes autism. In one case, many of the children were not autistic, though many had other mild-to-severe developmental concerns. In another study, there were an unusual number of children with autism, but the number was the same whether or not the children were born in that town, which suggests that findings might be tied to diagnosis issues and not necessarily to environmental toxins.

Another kind of pregnancy insult that seems to increase at least somewhat the chances of a child's being autistic is the use of psychotropic substances that cross the blood-brain barrier. Most women take prenatal vitamins and swear off anything that might be vaguely detrimental to their baby, including alcohol, cigarettes, and even caffeine. Over-the-counter medicines as well as commonly prescribed antibiotics are usually avoided too. In fact, many mothers tell me that they started taking prenatal vitamins as soon as they began to try to get pregnant! There are those who worry that the half bottle of champagne they split with their husband the night they likely conceived caused the autism, or that a night of Montezuma's Revenge in Mazatlán during the seventh month of pregnancy caused the autism. There is no reason to believe that isolated events such as these are damaging, even when there are other vulnerabilities, or we'd likely have a lot more autistic and developmentally disabled children.

Then there are others who decide it's OK to be pregnant even though they are prescribed a major antipsychotic, mood stabilizer, or other heavy-hitting psychoactive medication. There certainly are ways of managing these medications with the pregnancy in mind though, in some cases, not getting pregnant might be the best alternative. There is clearly added risk in certain cases, but again there probably need to be other factors present to trigger autism. It is particularly difficult to disentangle the cause of a child's disability when the mother's psychiatric disorder, for which she is taking medication, has a genetic basis (such as major depression), and this disorder may contribute to the genetic "cocktail" that produces a disorder in the child that might include symptoms of both depression and autism.

The mothers I have never really understood are those who use street drugs during their pregnancies. I recall one mother who was let out of prison a bit early so that she could attend her three-year-old severely retarded autistic daughter's evaluation at my clinic. While giving the history of her pregnancy she cried crocodile tears as she told me that she would have given up crack and heroin if only someone had told her that they could harm her baby. At the end of the morning she asked if I thought her taking drugs while she was pregnant caused her baby's problems. I said, "Yes, I think so."   Like other risks, using certain drugs during pregnancy certainly doesn't help and is probably more likely to damage an already vulnerable fetus even more—though it does not seem to uniquely cause autism if other kinds of preexisting risks are not also present.

Other Risks to Fetal Development. There are many things a woman hopes to avoid during pregnancy. Many things that do appear to increase the risk for autism also increase the risk of other developmental problems: One of the risks more specific to autism seem to be viruses that cross the placenta into the baby's developing nervous system. The most well-known example of this is the rubella virus, which in one study done in New York in the 1960s appeared to increase the risk of autism sixtyfold. In the 1960s, before a vaccine for rubella was available in the United States, a large number of autistic, deaf, blind, deaf-autistic, deaf-blind, blind-autistic children were born as many pregnant women were exposed to the rubella virus for the first time, without having developed an immunity to it from earlier exposure. There was a similar spike in the rate of autism documented in southwestern London years later among an immigrant population with no previous exposure to rubella.

Other pregnancy risks that are risks to any pregnant woman seem to increase risk no more and no less for mothers of children who subsequently develop autism: These include receiving abdominal X-rays—especially in very early pregnancy, and abdominal bleeding—such as through rupture of the placenta. Often these events present very difficult personal and moral dilemmas and, at the time, it can be hard to know what to do. One mother whose son, Craig, I followed for some time, was born quite retarded and autistic. He was born to her late, after she thought she could no longer have children. Before being X-rayed for some gastrointestinal distress, Craig's mother had signed a waiver declaring she wasn't pregnant. As it turned out, she was in her second month of pregnancy. The hospital, upon seeing the pregnancy on the X-ray, advised an abortion, which the mother declined on religious grounds, perhaps a clear decision at the time. However, when the boy's condition revealed itself, the mother and father sued the hospital for causing Craig's autism with the X-ray. It seems pretty clear that the X-ray alone was unlikely to have caused Craig's autism: His mother *was* older. The family history suggested some probable mental retardation or other developmental problems in an uncle living in another country. The important thing is that, from our present understanding of these things, we have no way of knowing what the main risk factor for Craig was, or if there even was a main risk factor—not the opinion the parents' attorney had hoped to hear. The moral of the story is that for any given child there is not likely to be a one hundred percent sure-fire way to know what caused a particular case of autism.

A very bad early pregnancy with much early bleeding, a ruptured amniotic sac, or cervical incompetency, or multiple miscarriages in other pregnancies or believed miscarriages that turned out not to be miscarriages—these are all stories of mothers with children who turn out to have disabilities. Similarly, stories of long, long labors at home followed by long rides to the hospital and C-sections, deliveries of hypoxic births (blue babies) followed by difficult resuscitations, or babies who didn't feed, lost weight, didn't sleep, had seizures—these are all stories of mothers whose children turn out to have disabilities. The really tough thing to remember as you go over and over a story like this in your mind is that these can also be dramas with happy endings—and are for many children and their families. It would be great if we had a crystal ball and could tell what lay ahead after every scary episode. But we don't.

Whatever the effects of prenatal and birth events may be, or whatever their effects in combination with genetic events are, it is likely that changes in the brain that can result in autism are already present by the time of delivery. Most recently, one study has found protein differences in the heel-stick blood of newborns who turn out to be autistic or mentally retarded compared to babies who turn out to develop typically or to have cerebral palsy. This suggests to us that whatever is different about the brain is already at least somewhat different by the time prenatal brain development is complete. (We do not yet know how early in pregnancy these differences might be detectable.) Since such a high percentage of children with autism also have some mental retardation (up to 70 percent), it is no surprise that the two groups might test the same. It does give us a clue, however, that whatever causes the autism is not likely something that only starts to happen after the birth.

ANOTHER CHILD WITH AUTISM?

What should you do if you find yourself in a situation in which certain risk factors seem to indicate why your child or a child whose family you are helping is autistic or otherwise disabled? For a couple that has already had one child with autism, thinking of each of these risk factors as potential vulnerabilities or triggers of autism can be valuable. Unfortunately, there are no rock-solid probabilities to give. What you have here is some information to help inform the difficult decision of whether to have another child or not.

Why Does This Particular Child Have Autism? Some people will have just read the preceding section with the desire to understand, if possible, the factors that may have contributed to their child's autism. The important message for them is that they may never know for sure. It can be incredibly frustrating to have such a major life event remain unexplained or only partly explained. I can tell you that every couple of years for the last 20 years I have seen someone try to fill this "need-to-know" void—with a diet, with a drug, with a vitamin, with a therapy that inexplicably and vastly improves how the child sees the world. Especially early on in the process of trying to answer "Why me?" "Why did *I* end up with a child with autism?" there is a strong and absolutely understandable vulnerability and receptivity to these theories that purport to tell you why and then tell you what to do about it. Unfortunately, it isn't that simple: There isn't an "allergic" autism for which there is a diet. There is not a vitamin-deficiency autism for which there are easy-to-take, nice safe vitamins. Whether a child's autism comes from heredity, from an early gene mutation, from a difficult pregnancy, or a traumatic birth, or some combination thereof—once the child has autism, the work to be done is based on who the child is and what he knows and doesn't know, what tools he has for learning, and what tools he needs to develop.

Risk Recurrence If You Have a Child with Autism. If you are the parent of a child with autism, you can look at the odds for the birth of a child with autism that were discussed earlier in this chapter and then add or subtract from that number depending on how "loaded" or at risk you feel your family tree is for autistic disorders and notably autistic "personalities" (or what was called broader phenotypes or "oak trees"). You can consider whether there are possibly triggering factors that may have interacted with genetic vulnerabilities that might exist in your family tree and that precipitated the problems of the child currently diagnosed with autism. Remember that there is no way to know for sure what your risk recurrence is. (In my experience, most families overestimate their risk, worrying that every dislikable, antisocial, or alcoholic relative might have a touch of autism.)

Looking at the bigger picture, my personal feeling is that parents should be encouraged to think of the protection that can accrue to a family and to a marriage by also raising a typically developing child if the autistic child is an only child. This is not easy to do. Thinking about having another child, one who doesn't have autism, can raise feelings of guilt about potential emotional abandonment of the child with autism. This does not seem to be how it goes however. There are other reasons we will discuss in later chapters about how having typical siblings in a home may be therapeutically beneficial to a child with autism. Having a child with autism makes a remarkable difference to parents. Over time, as the child is better understood, he is in fact less disabled in the eyes of these loving caregivers who understand him best. This parental scaffolding is probably the single most important protective factor any child with a disability can accrue. It takes much energy for the parents to support this scaffold. Most often, the presence of a typically developing child as well as a child with autism in the home puts things into perspective and strengthens the supports that parents can provide.

Parents should be encouraged to have open and objective dialogue with one another about what it would mean to add to a family with a child with autism, discussing the upside and the downside. Parents might compare this type of difficult conversation to drawing up a will. Parents of young children are scarcely at a stage of life at which they wish to discuss the banal practicalities of whether their 50 percent interest in the family home should be left to their spouse or to their child. Nevertheless, few would argue that if something happened to their spouse, they would hope their spouse's last wishes were in writing. It can be just as hard as discussing what you would want for your family if you died as it is to stop pointing fingers at who may have the "bad" genes and really assess if there is any evidence for a particular family to be below average, average, or at greater-than-average risk of having another child with autism.

Eagle Eyes on the Lookout for More Autism. Another group of readers will consist of those who already have an infant or are pregnant again since the diagnosis of the child with autism. After one child is diagnosed with autism, it is no surprise that subsequent siblings are watched with eagle eyes from day one. For me, a great day at work is one in which I have an anxious mom bring in her new baby who she fears has autism, too, and be able to dispel her fears and show her with one hundred percent certainty that her baby is perfect.

On average, the mother of a child with autism who does not feel her new baby or baby-to-be is genetically at risk and is having or has just had a good pregnancy and delivery—after a particular difficult pregnancy or a particularly difficult delivery with the child with autism, can probably breathe a pretty deep sigh of relief. If the list of possible risk factors changes notably between children (and remember, this includes a new spouse), there is likely a basis for less worry. Also, it is important to remember that as many as one out of four siblings of children with autism have some language or speech difficulty. That first trip for a hearing test is not necessarily déjà vu. Most siblings who would fall into the up to 25 percent with early-onset language problems experience only transitory delays that require no or only brief therapy.

THE IMPORTANCE OF EARLY INTENSIVE INTERVENTION

It almost seems to go without saying that children with autism need early and intensive interventions. It has been so frequently stated that, for many who work with young children with developmental disabilities, it is almost a mantra. Like a mantra, it is something that can be repeated so often and so fervently that we may cease to reexamine the basis for the universal acceptance of this statement. At this point in our understanding of neurodevelopmental disorders, it is quite important that we *do* reexamine this statement, as fairly recent developments in neuroscience have amplified and changed what we know about the importance of early intervention.

The main concepts behind intensive early-intervention programs for children with autism are *plasticity* and *transfer of function.* Both of these concepts suggest that a brain that is atypical in its development can be reorganized by intervention so that development can then proceed more typically.

In the case of plasticity, the idea is that the developing brain does not yet have "seated" or fixed locations associated with specific functions the way an adult brain does. For example, we know from studies of stroke patients and brain-injured soldiers that "insults" (injuries) to very specific regions of the brain can result in the loss of very specific abilities, such as loss of the ability to recall names or recognize faces. The work of writers such as neurologist Oliver Sacks documents many fascinating and sometimes peculiar neurological injuries that result in odd patterns of behavior. Oliver Sacks, in fact, wrote an account of a high-functioning woman, Temple Grandin, entitled *Anthropologist on Mars.* However, Dr. Sacks does not suggest that Temple Grandin has an insult to a very particular part of the brain, nor does anyone else. In autism, the brain is wired differently; differences are microscopic, not the relatively crater-like lesions associated with explicit brain damage.

THE DEVELOPING BRAIN AS A MAP WITHOUT ROADS

We know that autism, like many neurodevelopmental conditions, is not a straightforward insult to a very particular part of the brain. Instead, the young brain is plastic and malleable, and experience, as well as the natural course of development, can and does reshape it. Even in a typically developing brain, experience wires recognition and understanding.

It is possible to think of the brain of a young child with autism as a tract of land without roads: There will be some obvious places for roads to go: These will be the natural flat smooth valley bottoms with no vegetation and a hard, packed surface. For some children, this means that the effects of intervention will be quickly and fairly easily achieved with just a little bit of special attention.

Certain tracts of the brain are intended to carry certain kinds of information, just as certain topography can support a freeway.

However, there will be some other places where roads can be built, but only with the use of a little more construction machinery: Some trees might need to be knocked down and a hard surface of packed gravel added. These correspond to changes in the brain that require more persistent work, take longer, and require more expertise.

Finally, there are other places in which you would only build a road if there were no other way of getting from point A to point B. These are your tunnels, bridges, and steep mountainside grades. In fact, in these difficult construction situations, you may not be building on solid earth at all, but in the air or underground, creating an artificial, manufactured way of achieving your goal. In some cases, interventions are designed like this, such as when a child is taught to communicate using pictures or a mechanical device. In these cases you are achieving your goal, but not getting there in the most "natural" way. There is still a lot we don't know about the brain, but in some cases information may be stored or processed in the brain in areas usually intended for something quite different. For example, deaf children who sign may use the opposite side of the brain in which language and grammar are stored to instead store the direction and speed of signing, which for a deaf individual essentially represents grammar.

WHAT KINDS OF THINGS RESHAPE THE BRAIN?

It is reasonable to assume that since the plastic brain is reshaped by experience, it can be reshaped by experiences we would consider both good and bad for the child, and by things that happen both before and after the child is diagnosed. Early intervention takes advantage of plasticity by giving the child's brain increased exposure to good experiences (that is, enrichment). Enrichment consists of those things we have reason to believe will best promote reshaping to enable more typical functioning. Enrichment experiences can be defined as experiences that allow the child to reorganize how things are processed in the brain. This reorganization is sometimes referred to as a transfer of function, especially when reorganization involves building a new "road" or taking a different "route."

The concept of transfer of function is related to the concept of plasticity: "Transfer of function" stems from the idea that certain areas of the brain are destined to be enabled to carry out certain functions. If we assume that a particular brain region is, for some reason, particularly at a disadvantage, early intervention should be targeted to provide sufficient stimulation to help to transfer the functions usually handled in the disadvantaged region to a more enabled part of the brain.

This is where teaching strategies that utilize special modalities of information delivery come into play. For example, a child who does not extract meaning from auditory information (words) adequately might be helped by having other information-delivery systems in use at the same time. Since many children with autism do seem to have auditory-processing problems, many teaching approaches incorporate the use of pictures or objects along with auditory information to enable transfer of function from visual to auditory information processing. The rationale for doing this is that a child may be better able to store information partly based on visual recognition in a different region of the brain from that in which purely auditory information might be processed or stored. The auditory information gets tagged onto the visual information, and then the child has a new "pathway" for retrieving the meaning of the auditory information in the future; he can associate it with a visual "carrier" that contains the auditory information. It is important to understand this kind of process in order to be able to judge what type of teaching strategy may be best for a particular child: In the example just given, you would want to make sure that the child with the auditory-processing problem was not just given visual information to process because, while that might help him recognize what was going on, it would not help him "tag" and store the auditory information along with the visual and later be able to retrieve its meaning. In the field of early intervention, there is much talk about this sort of "multisensory" learning.

THE "WINDOW OF OPPORTUNITY"

The concept of early brain development suggests that early intervention occurs during the "window of opportunity" in which the brain is young and malleable. I have found in my clinical work, however, that parents may, out of understandable anxiety about their child's condition, interpret this "window of opportunity" too narrowly. We all continue to learn throughout life. Also, we now know that the learning curve for acquiring different kinds of skills is not quite as once thought, with a rapid acceleration until five to eight years of age and a tremendous leveling thereafter. The window of opportunity is never fully closed. It is never bolted shut, nor is it triple-paned. The picture is a bit more complicated.

Rat Tales. More recent studies have told us some very interesting things about the brain. To go to a very simple model, we can look at the work of neuroscientists who study a great many rats. In one series of experiments, there were up to four groups of rats: The first group lived in a rather large cage that resembled a messy toy box that was rearranged from time to time. This was meant to represent the natural environment in which a presumably savvy, feral rat might live. A second group of rats regularly attended a rat-like Outward Bound, which for humans means climbing trees, swinging from ropes, and challenging oneself with a number of scary physical challenges. For this second group of rats it meant climbing tiny rope ladders, crossing tiny rope suspension bridges suspended over long drops, and so on. A third group of rats was taken from their cages daily and exposed to a forced gallop on a mechanically driven wire wheel (think of using a treadmill at the gym and not being able to control the speed or length of workout). The fourth group, referred to by the researchers as their "cage potatoes," were confined to a smallish cage, in which there was not much to do but reach over to suck on the nutrition tube. These rat studies have been done a number of ways—younger rats, older rats, rats treated a longer time, a shorter time, etc. What effects did these different learning environments have on their brain development? With humans, you can only observe and guess—not know for sure. With rats, one finds out for sure by "harvesting" the brain. Not surprisingly, the "cage potatoes" had brains wired with the fewest connections. The feral rats living in the messy toy box had the most connections. "Outward Bound" graduates were generally rated a cut below them. The rats that went to the rat gym were generally a cut below the "Outward Bound" rats.

So what do we take from all of this and apply to our understanding of how children's brain development may be influenced by different sorts of experience? It seems fairly clear that a varied, complex environment that was not too repetitious and predictable—the messy toy box that was changed from time to time—provided the most enrichment. Structured experience that was challenging and required active problem solving—the Outward Bound experience—was also beneficial, since, even though it became more repetitious and predictable over time, it offered a sense of mastery too. Activity alone (the wire wheel) that was both repetitious and predictable and did not require active problem solving (though it did involve sustaining alertness—a groggy rat was likely to get tossed to the floor of the cage), was not as enriching for brain development as conditions in which the rat had to take a more proactive decision-making role in what he'd do. The rats that lay around and were made to do nothing made nothing of themselves (that is, of their brains).

It is a big leap from rat experiments to early interventions for children with autism, but we can certainly form some hypotheses: The first would be that an early intervention experience that provides novelty and diverse forms of stimulation (that is, the opposite of predictable and repetitious) and that requires active responding might be most beneficial. Second, interventions in which children have experiences actively and continuously presented to them might be seen as slightly less beneficial than more self-initiated exploration. These general principles make sense and are common sense. However, teaching children with autism based on these principles presents some special concerns: First, many children with autism prefer repetition to novelty much of the time. Second, many children with autism prefer predictability rather than new situations much of the time.

So where do we go from here in learning from the rat model? The rats are not neurodevelopmentally disadvantaged rats with a condition (like autism) that inhibits the tendency to seek out varied, self-initiated learning experiences or to derive pleasure from such experiences. So, with autistic children, we may have to rely on adult-initiated teaching (like the forced "Outward Bound" experience)—even though self-initiated learning experiences may be more enriching for the brain. However, we should keep in mind the likely importance of more active self-initiated learning as a preferred modality of learning, one that can be used when there is a tendency for exploration rather than for the repetitiveness and preference for predictability that often characterizes autism. Therefore, teaching strategies that allow the child to be increasingly self-initiating are (if we stick to rat-brain theory) going to be important for brain development, and reorganizing the brain from having an atypical structure to having a capacity for more typical functioning. Therefore, we likely should aim to move the child from responding to forced stimulation to responding to self-initiated problem solving. Teaching strategies that move from highly repetitious trials (that enrich via increasing the overall amount of responses required) to strategies that, for example, give the child an opportunity for self-initiative, like choosing how or which activity to pursue next, need to be considered as adding another dimension of important stimulation for the brain-rewiring process.

Needless to say, we can also hypothesize from the rat tales that it is important to keep children from being couch potatoes (human cage potatoes) and limit time spent without exposure to novelty at all, such as engaging in some repetitive activity for long periods—be it something as simple as rocking or flapping, or something seemingly more complex, like lining up Leggos over and over again or watching and rewinding the same 30 seconds of a Thomas the Tank Engine video.

CHAPTER CONCLUSIONS

In this chapter, we looked at the possible origins of autism. We reviewed various areas of study such as genetics, epidemiology, and prenatal and birth factors. While we know some things about how these factors bring about autism, there is still more we do not know. Autism often runs in families, but often seems to have multiple causes. What we do know from basic research is that intensive and early interventions are likely quite important for children with autism. We know this from studies of how the brain develops and from studies of how the brain can be shaped by experience. In the next chapter, we will begin to examine the origins of the patterns of behavior that characterize autism.

CHAPTER TWO

When Atypical Development and Typical Development Cross Paths

Where and when do things start to go wrong developmentally for the child with autism? When is it that the "signal" which is sent out to the child—is received differently from the way it is received by other children? When is it that the child first looks at something, hears something, touches something, but the information that he gets is somehow different from what other children understand from that same experience?

Studies of how newborns scan a mother's face show relatively random inspection of its features, with the baby's eyes wandering to the shape of the mother's face as well as its interior features. However by four months, it is normal for infants to have locked on to the eyes and mouth as the centers of the "action" on Mom's face. Are autistic babies doing this, too? Or, is this why we hear "I knew there was something wrong almost as soon as he was born—he never looked at me!" Maybe, for some babies, the brain wiring that helps them realize that the eyes and mouth are the face's main sources of signals isn't working from the very beginning. However, we also know that some babies with autism absolutely did make fantastic eye contact at first—but then this ability diminished or disappeared. If we could know with perfect accuracy what happened and when for each baby who was subsequently diagnosed as autistic, we might be able to start to separate out different causes for the autism.

The same observations can be made about how a baby processes sound: At first, we expect babies to coo and gurgle in a way that is pretty much the same for all babies the world over. Amazingly though, by the time the baby is six to nine months old, the sounds babies produce have a lot to do with the sounds in the baby's language environment—the "ba-ba-ba," "de-de-de" we recognize in English. But, we know that some parents of children later diagnosed as autistic felt their baby never gurgled cooed or made much sound at all—from the very beginning. This is one reason many parents first suspect deafness. Other parents suspect ear infections—because the early cooing and babbling falls off—and is never replaced with the "ba-ba-ba" type sounds of the world around them. Just like the problem posed by early facial attunement, the development of sound production leaves us wondering If we could know with perfect accuracy what happened to sound production and when for each baby who subsequently was found to be autistic—we might be able to start to separate out different causes for the autism.

Do You Need to Read This Chapter? This chapter is a bit more theoretical and abstract than the others. It is designed primarily to inform the educator or other treating professional who is seeking to draw together seemingly disparate observations of how learning proceeds in children with autism. It is also designed to help an educator or other therapist understand how to design tailored interventions. Some parents may wish to gain this same kind of perspective. In that case this chapter may be informative for you as well. However, if you're at the point where you just want the bottom line on what should be done for your child, or whether your child's program or proposed treatments fully meet his needs, please feel free to skip this material at this point; you can always come back to it later. This material may be a useful framework for someone who has seen many different kinds of children with autism—but many seem less essential to the interests of someone with one autistic child in mind.

Patterns of Atypical Development in Autism Defined. The development of a pattern of behavior arising from primary deficits in processing information and from the ways the child develops or doesn't develop ways around those deficits can be thought of as comprising an *atypical ontogeny*. This means that the sequence of development is different, but predictable once we know that the child has autism. An atypical ontogeny is when an atypical developmental sequence of interrelated behaviors occur which are more or less successful accommodations to learning differences defined by a child's underlying neuropathology.

THE CONCEPT OF PRIMARY, SECONDARY, AND TERTIARY LEARNING DEFICITS

An Introduction. Analyzing the earliest symptoms of autism can be regarded as the first step in deconstructing what is wrong with the way a child with autism is taking in information. By tracing back from the earliest reported problem (like not babbling English-language sounds), it is possible to paint a picture of which senses might be processing information in an atypical fashion. These early processing problems can be referred to as a type of *primary deficit.* In a minute, we'll survey a potential list of these. For now, the important point is to realize that these primary deficits are not what make for the child's diagnosis. (For example, an absence of babbling English-language sounds is not one of the diagnostic criteria for autism.) Instead, the diagnosis is typically based on observations about the things that do or do not happen as a result of the primary deficits. For example, a lack of babbling (when there's no hearing loss) raises a clinician's suspicion of autism. (However, babies who go on to have other problems besides autism also may not babble. This can include babies who are eventually described as having receptive language disorders, for example.)

It is the lack of babbling, *not* the actual failure somewhere in the process of selectively perceiving, attending to, and processing sounds of the surrounding language environment, that gets enumerated as a clinical observation in support of an early suspicion of autism. The failure somewhere in the perceiving, attending, or processing stage is what is being called the primary deficit. The failure to develop babbling of speech sounds can be regarded as a *secondary deficit* (that is, derived from the primary deficit). Similarly, if the baby responded to an inability to selectively perceive or attend to sounds by continuing to make odd little sounds that were neither infant coos and gurgles nor expected babbling for children in his language environment, we could think of that as another kind of clinical observation in support of the diagnosis of autism, and also as a kind of secondary deficit. So, there might be two babies that had something making them unable to perceive or attend to language sounds in the expected fashion. In one case the baby might not babble at all, and in another case, the baby might babble, but with the odd little sounds that parents often describe as "speaking his own language," "speaking Martian," etc. Basically the same primary deficit might produce two somewhat different secondary deficits—being silent or speaking Martian, and either of these secondary deficits would be raise our suspicion of autism.

THE MATRIX OF ABILITY AND DISABILITY

Every Child's Profile of Deficits Is Different. But why would one baby adapt one way and one another way if they had the same underlying problem (failure to perceive or attend to language)? One part of the answer might lie in whether things were going wrong at the perception or attention stage. At the perception stage, this might mean that the baby was hearing, but was somehow perceiving a very "noisy" signal—like a radio with a lot of static. If the problem was at the attention stage, this might mean that the baby didn't focus on the sound for long because the sound seemed unimportant, like hearing a car pass outside. In autism (unlike in a "pure" language disorder) it may be that there is often "another reason": This might depend on what other primary processing abilities were operating as expected and whether there were other kinds of primary deficits. For example, in young autistic children, there also may be primary deficits related to social events not being very important, and so those things are not given attention either. If the sound being heard is a social sound (like a human voice) it may be disregarded just the way the sound of a passing car may be disregarded by someone else—because it is perceived as no more important. In this way, primary disabilities start to cascade with the failure to perceive or attend to sound, possibly compounded by a failure to attend preferentially to human-produced sounds. On the other hand, a child with a purer receptive language disorder wouldn't also lack the primary deficit of low importance for things social. That child might therefore prefer sounds coming from people—even if not understood—and in the process of orienting to a speaker might pick up non-speech cues (like body language) that would help him figure out what was going on.

Origins of the Matrix of Ability and Disability. Cascading primary deficits and interacting primary strengths and weaknesses can be thought of as a *matrix of* *ability and disability*—with whatever abilities that are strong and intact stepping in to compensate for processing abilities that are not able to function as expected. One baby with profound auditory processing problems might not perceive speech sounds and non-speech sounds as different in the way that is expected and might not respond to sound at all, becoming quite silent at the age that babbling is expected. Another baby, less affected, might be able to make this distinction, but not well enough to filter out specific sounds he was hearing all the time, so he begins making odd little sounds instead. As you might imagine, we might want to think about intervention for these different patterns of vocal production differently—something we'll come back to later in detail.

Patterns of primary deficits and subsequently different secondary deficits (depending on the matrix of ability and disability) might have implications for other later developments that might contribute to the child's picture of clinical concerns, too: For example, if the child babbling odd little sounds actually thought he was repeating the same thing each time to signal a response to what he thought he was hearing, he might get very frustrated and irritable that the world around him was not contingently responsive to his signals. This child might become easily aggravated, have tantrums readily, become more aloof (having given up trying to communicate), or instead (or in addition) become quite independent as an adaptation to frustration at not being able to communicate. Independence might not seem like part of a larger problem; not all adaptive responses to an underlying disability will be seen as symptoms. But a child with a hair-trigger temper might seem to be a problem. This problem, basically a failure to find a way through his matrix of ability and disability to accommodate to his primary deficit (failure to perceive or attend to language), might be construed as a *tertiary* level disability (in other words, a reactive symptom). Like primary signs of a disability, tertiary signs will not be diagnostic either. Something like a tantrum can obviously be caused by any number of things—a general communicative failure (as in the preceding example), or by factors not related to underlying primary disability (like failure in an effort to sway the opinion of others, or being tired and irritable). Again, as you might imagine, we might want to think about intervention for these different kinds of tantrums (as tertiary signs) differently— something we'll also come back to later in detail.

Building Treatment Plans: Considering What's Primary, Secondary, and Tertiary. The next step in viewing this basic way of thinking about the child's learning process as having primary, secondary, and tertiary factors is to clarify how these concepts can be used to think about developing individual treatment plans: In other words, if we are going to plan how to help this child, how can we use this model to figure out what we should do and where we should start? If the child throws tantrums easily, is it necessarily appropriate to give him medicine to make him less likely to show hair-trigger frustration? Change his diet to see if he becomes more mellow? I would argue not. Instead, what needs to be done first is to deconstruct the nature of the problem—the hair-trigger temper or the hyper-independence—and figure out *why* the child acts this way. Has the child learned to get angry quickly because that makes everyone around him take notice and do nothing but try to soothe him until his need is met? If so, a tantrum can be viewed as an adaptive strategy for a communicative failure. If we looked back at this situation and saw that this tantrumming child is making unintelligible sounds when others might use words, we might recast the tantrumming as the child's just not expressing himself in a way we'd like him to be able to communicate. Maybe teaching this child to lead the adult's hand to things he wants would ease frustration. This is a familiar adaptation that many children with autism come to on their own. In the context of our discussion here, hand leading can be thought of as a secondary sign (and a diagnostically contributory symptom) to an underlying primary problem related to failure to communicate by other more typical means. If the child has started hand leading on his own, it can also be regarded as a successful *self-accommodation* to the underlying primary disability. It can be considered successful because it assists the child in compensating for lack of communicative means, and also prevents tertiary signs of the primary disability, like tantrums.

If the child is silent, maybe not realizing the communicative value of sound at all, he might be a child who also lacks a preference for social stimuli and orients little toward speech sounds in particular, or toward people in general. Hand leading may not be a natural self-accommodation for this child. Starting to teach communication through a non-social stimulus, maybe by clarifying meaning with strong visuals, would help this child understand better. This suggestion still falls into the category of helping the child make a better accommodation to his primary deficit—his difficulty with processing sound. Better still would be a strategy that could help sound make sense, like slowing down sound, repeating sound, making sound melodic, or making sounds atonal. As we'll talk about later, there are interventions that have incorporated strategies such as these. The only point here is that, depending on a given child's matrix of ability and disability, the compensatory strategy that will work best is likely to vary. Deconstructing the child's secondary and tertiary signs can lead to a better understanding of what that child's matrix of ability and disabilities contains and how stronger abilities come into play when weaker ones fail, and may thereby indicate which strategies are likely to be effective.

Using this model, the foregoing examples of treatment strategies are obviously not meant specifically to apply to any one autistic child or to autistic children in general, but rather to exemplify a way of thinking about how children learn when they are faced with "wiring" limitations. As we discussed in the last chapter, there is good evidence that "rewiring" can occur. However, what is fundamentally different in the approach to doing that and what is presented here, is the idea that there is enormous—though systematic and understandable—variation among children with autism (due to the matrix of ability and disability), and that, therefore, it will be beneficial to individualize "rewiring" (treatment) when we have a specific idea about which circuits currently work and which don't work well. Everything we have said before about the possibility of changing the wiring pertains, but what specifically needs to be changed, and how to effect rehabilitation—or, more accurately, *habilitation* (building new circuitry)—can be examined by thinking in terms of primary, secondary, and tertiary signs of the child's underlying neurodevelopmental problem. To use a metaphor from the last chapter, we need to discover where to build roads and what equipment to use.

Primary, Secondary, and Tertiary Deficits Equal Innate, Virtual, and Indirect Symptoms. A slightly different vocabulary for thinking about the concepts related to atypical development in autism would be to think first of primary deficits as "innate" deficits: things the child is born with or acquires because of some atypical maturational pattern that might be influenced by genetics, environmental insult, or a combination of the two. Next, the secondary deficits can be characterized as "virtual" deficits, in the same way we think of the term "virtual reality." The deficits exist because something underlying them has created them, and they form the reality of the child's view of the world. Sometimes the virtual world of the child is one that works fairly well with various self-accommodations to the underlying primary problems, such as when the child has figured out that doing for himself is likely to be more efficient than trying to communicate his needs to others. Finally, the tertiary deficits can be seen as epiphenomena—not symptoms arising from innate deficits like the secondary (virtual) deficits are, but rather resulting from a failure to develop a self-accommodation that meets the child's objectives.

PATTERNS OF ATYPICAL DEVELOPMENT IN AUTISM

One way to think about what happens from the time the baby's genetic makeup is determined at conception until the signs and symptoms of autism become clearly recognizable is by using this model of atypical development in autism. An atypical but predictable pattern for development results from a given autistic child's atypical neurology. The model is useful as a way of thinking about the interrelation among primary aspects of perception known or believed to influence development in a way that forms autism. As shown in the above diagram, the developing fetus starts off with an already established set of genes, the genotype. However, everything that happens thereafter—in utero, during the birth, and possibly for some period of time after the birth—modifies the genotype into something called the phenotype. The phenotype is the exact way in which the genes are expressed in this particular child. Less than optimal events at critical times in the pregnancy and delivery (sub-optimality) are thought to sometimes trigger sub-optimal brain development by changing the environment in which the brain can grow and develop—as was discussed in chapter 1. After birth, the brain the child is born with is already shaped by both genotype and phenotype. The initial "wiring," and the things that are different about it, constitute the child's innate, primary deficits. All the things that happen subsequently will modify these primary deficits. Depending on the rest of the child's wiring, the "matrix of abilities and disabilities" is formed, which defines how the child's brain can decide to try to compensate for the things that are weak by relying on the things that are stronger. This can be thought of as the basis for the child's "virtual," or secondary level of disability, not the actual areas of the brain and their immediate functions that are different, but how these differences get expressed in a particular child. Each child will be more (or less) successful at compensating in different spheres of functioning. Some self-accommodations the child will come up with will be better adapted to the world around him than others. A child who is not able to self-accommodate well is going to develop maladaptive symptoms (partly failed accommodations) like screaming, tantrumming, and being self-injurious or aggressive to others out of frustration and a failure to have developed more successful means to get needs met. These partly failed accommodations are the indirect symptom or epiphenomena of the child's underlying disability. They represent a tertiary level of difficulty.

Diversification of Behavior and the Emergence of Symptoms. As children grow, they can do more things, such as walk, reach, and intentionally search for objects and use them in planful ways. So, as their behavioral repertoire becomes more diversified, the pattern of secondary and tertiary signs and symptoms become more reflective of the matrix of ability and disability, and thereby more obviously autistic. The matrix of ability and disability might be partly predicted by the child's genotype—by which "autism" genes that child has inherited—but it is not identical to the genotype, because of factors that influence phenotypic expression and opportunities a given child has had to make self-accommodations.

In the next part of this chapter, we will use this theory and formulation of how atypical development in autism gets started to move from a developmentally based description of how symptoms of autism emerge to the major thesis of this book—that autism can be most usefully characterized as an assortment of autistic learning disabilities and as autistic learning styles arising from a child's matrix of abilities and disabilities.

PRIMARY INNATE DEFICITS
AND AUTISTIC LEARNING DISABILITIES

The Building Blocks of Autistic Learning Disabilities. What are some examples of primary deficits? There are several candidates that might hypothetically have a pervasive effect on processing all sorts of incoming "signals." Some have been suggested over the years as possible core deficits in autism. It is important to think of these difficulties, if they do exist in a particular child, as not unique to autism, and not necessarily diagnostic of autistic spectrum disorders. These are difficulties that also may be contributing factors in any number of neurodevelopmental syndromes, such as attention deficit disorder (ADD), obsessive-compulsive disorder (OCD), or mental retardation. This is certainly not to say that all of these disorders are essentially the same as autism. Rather, autistic spectrum disorders arise from the matrix of ability and disability in which a pattern of strengths and weaknesses coexist and mutually influence one another.

For example, a tendency to perseverate (think, say, or do the same things over and over) coupled with poor auditory processing speed might result in repetitive echoed speech, which is often, though not always, a symptom of autism.) The first tasks should always be to look at the problem symptom, like echoed speech, and deconstruct it—break it down to its parts. In the case of echoed speech, primary components might include difficulties in processing auditory input fast enough, and the tendency to be repetitive. In this example, the "matrix of disability" is where these two separate difficulties of processing speed and perseveration work upon each other and then combine with relatively OK auditory memory to make for echolalia, a secondary, or virtual, deficit, and a possible symptom of autism. But, in the absence of social deficits, echolalia may not indicate autism.

Primary deficits can be thought of metaphorically as rheostats, gateways to what is in the brain: These primary functions (like processing speed) can be thought of as having certain settings for optimal functioning. But, often, a number of these primary functions are not set at advantageous settings for the child with autism. The settings can be changed. It may be that in some cases settings on these rheostats change just as a result of development and typical experience. Most of the time the child will need help to change the settings. However, we have to identify what needs to be changed before we can make a plan to change it.

We will discuss seven areas in which these initial psychophysiological phenomena that we are going to call primary deficits may have thresholds that are innately different for children with autism. It is not intended as an exhaustive list but as a fairly comprehensive one. This model of organizing information-processing difficulties is being offered as an organizing framework for understanding the things that set children with autistic spectrum disorders apart from others, not as a systematic review or representation of any particular areas of research.

ATTENTION/ HABITUATION/ NOVELTY RESPONSE

Attention Shifting. The first interesting possible area of primary or innate deficits is that one involving thresholds related to attention. What gains a child's attention and what holds it, and for how long, arguably has a lot to do with what gets learned. The ability to learn from and process incoming information has to do with shifting away from one kind of stimulus when there is no new information associated with it, and deciding what to attend to next. We are accustomed to thinking of children with autism as resisting change and doing poorly at transition times—problems at least partly involving the shift of attention. When most of us see something quite new, we attend for a while and then, at some point, decide that no new information is coming in and shift focus. For example, when a fire engine comes down the street with sirens blaring, we are likely to look at it. If it stopped in front of us for several minutes but no one came out of it, no one went into it, it didn't move, and you stopped puzzling reasons that that might be so, you'd be ready to shift your attention and continue walking down the street—even if the sirens continued to blare.

We know that children with autism often seem to have problems attending and shifting attention. In my clinic, which is just next to our hospital's emergency ambulance bay, ambulances frequently roll up, sirens blaring, just like in the previous illustration: Parents of little children at the clinic being evaluated for autism will lead their child to the window, pointing enthusiastically after the ambulance, only for us all to see how apparently oblivious the child is to what's going on. Why is that? Maybe the child doesn't follow a point. But he hears. He sees. In an instance like that, there seems to be something fundamentally wrong with the child's basic brain systems, with his attention "rheostat" that should indicate something to which almost everyone else can't help attending.

On the other hand, something seemingly smaller may catch the attention of this same child, but he then proceeds to attend too long. For example, the wind often blows hard through the leaves of the poplar trees outside my clinic window, and the same child might stand by the window and stare at the trees for several minutes. Why does he continue to stare at the windblown trees? Not a lot new is happening, but the child's attention-regulation "rheostat" doesn't seem to say "Enough already!" or "OK, this is boring now." Attention may be too hard to get, too hard to shift, or both.

Lack of Curiosity and Preference for the Familiar. To some extent, many children with autism seem to have an innate preference for sameness and familiarity that is exactly the opposite of most children's preference for novelty. Another way to put this would be to say that these children who prefer sameness and eschew novelty are children who lack curiosity. In a new place, it is not uncommon for autistic children to hone in on the familiar in the same way their siblings might hone in on what is new. Children with autism often arrive at one of my clinic playrooms, look around at shelves of new toys, and make a predictable (to parents) beeline for the one thing that is exactly the same as a favorite toy that the child also loves to play with at home. Twenty minutes later the other toys may still be unnoticed and untouched.

Lack of curiosity (or aversion to novelty) can be seen as a big problem for little children: If a child with autism comes into my clinic playroom, beelines for one toy, and is still playing with it 20 minutes later, he has had one learning experience. (Arguably, he has had even less than one learning experience if he selected an already familiar toy.) In this same 20 minutes, a typically developing sibling may have had 20 learning experiences if that child has successively picked up 20 new toys, and checked out how each works. So, in just 20 minutes, the child with autism is 19 learning experiences behind his sibling. Think of the cumulative impact of his lack of curiosity in just the first two or three years of life!

We consider it innate, a "given," that young children will be interested in many new things. Of course, we also expect there to be innate difference in temperament—such as how readily children will explore a new place, whether they prefer to explore on their own or need to bring a parent along, and how easily overwhelmed they may be by new things. The child with autism often seems extreme in this respect, physically running away from a new object that is introduced too assertively, or even assaulting a new object or throwing it away as if it were a substantial threat. Sometimes it is difficult to draw the line between a child who is "slow to warm" and one who has such an aversion to novelty that it stifles curiosity and learning and becomes maladaptive. When drawing distinctions such as these, it becomes particularly important to realize how something like aversion to novelty is a primary deficit, and not a symptom of autism. Embedded in a characteristic matrix of disabilities, an aversion to novelty might be one part of autism, but on its own, it may represent something much more benign, like temperament, or something that can dampen learning overall, like mental retardation.

Later we will talk in detail about all the implications for learning that an aversion to novelty or a lack of curiosity might confer on a child. For now, it suffices to say that it is important to be aware of this aversion for each child with an autistic spectrum disorder—because figuring ways to get the child to be less averse to new things, and therefore more curious, is likely to have a positive effect on his ability to learn new things.

REINFORCER SALIENCY:
THE ABILITY TO FIND REWARDS THAT WORK

Another innate difference that sometimes characterizes children with autism and that may also characterize children with some other kinds of neurodevelopmental disorders is the absence of rewards that can meaningfully motivate the child (reinforcer saliency). Anyone who has used any aspect of an applied behavior analysis/discrete trial training type program for a child with autism knows that initial successes often hinge on whether the tutor or therapist can find something the child will "work for." For some children, the list of rewards or "reinforcers" is long, including foods, toys, sensory stimuli, and sometimes even social praise. For other children with autism, the basic tendency to organize behavior to achieve a desired goal does not seem to exist. This difficulty needs to be distinguished from the child who simply does not yet have cause-and-effect reasoning, but does have things he wants. For some children, no one food seems preferable to another. If something that child drinks—say, apple juice in a sippy cup—is withheld pending a desired performance, the child may simply lose interest in trying to obtain apple juice and in the future be suspicious of drinks offered in that sippy cup.

Fortunately, most children with autism do find at least some things rewarding: Often the most reliable things on the lists are favorite foods, followed by sensory rewards (like tickling, bouncing, or swinging). Some children have toys that can be held out as rewards; for just a few (who have not yet been explicitly "taught" to want social praise), an adult's smiling face, clapping, or an encouraging tone of voice may be perceived as a reward.

Finding meaningful rewards is likely a factor that pervades all aspects of a child's openness to learning. We can think of reward saliency in the context of the child's matrix of abilities and disabilities, such as by considering whether the child will work for any kind of social praise or whether that area is disabled too. Similarly, some autistic children who are drawn to novelty will work to solve a problem that makes something work and causes a new and interesting sight. Those who are also uncurious and averse to novelty will not be so motivated.

It logically follows that anyone working with a particular child with autism wants to have a mental or actual list, a *reward hierarchy*, of the things that motivate this child—and how important each item on the list is for him (that is, how hard he will work for it). The most rewarding things can be reserved for teaching the most difficult, newest, initially least interesting, and otherwise intrinsically unmotivating things. For example, a child who has severe problems with a perseverative behavior (like a five-year-old boy I saw recently who tried to "chin" everyone who came into physical contact with him) might require a very highly valued reward whenever he tolerated some (relatively acceptable contact) *without* chinning.

Children Lacking Response to Most Rewards. The most difficult situations are presented by those children on the far end of the reward saliency continuum, those who are very passive and don't really seem to care in any way what they get and what they don't get. Remediating this primary difficulty and simply building a reward response as an initial step in implementing any other treatment may be an important part of any planning for such a child, irrespective of what learning target is being addressed. One four-year-old would only work for the opportunity to flourish grosgrain ribbons. He had many. For him, it was the only place to start—until he learned more things, had more experiences worth repeating, and so had expanded his reward hierarchy.

AROUSAL REGULATION

A somewhat related innate deficit that some children with autism may have occurs in the domain of arousal regulation. In the 1960s, when autism was first coming to be understood as a brain-wiring problem, there were theories that tied autism to defects in the particular areas of the brain believed to be responsible for "fight or flight." These parts of the brain—such as the amygdala and limbic system—still play a part in speculation about the shape autism actually takes in the brain. From an evolutionary perspective, there is clearly value in knowing when to fight or flee. If you can't respond to these basic social exigencies, you do indeed have a disabling learning deficit. However, children who are developmentally unable to tell safe from hazardous are protected by their parents. So if the amygdala is involved in autism, as data suggest, and the amygdala governs the intensity of reaction to things, how do problems in arousal regulation fit into understanding the learning experience of children with autism?

Sensory Under- and Over-Responding. Indicators of arousal-regulation difficulties are present when the child with autism "turns off" or overly "turns on" to some sensory "channel." Some children with autism seem to be easily over-stimulated by sensory stimuli that others would regard only casually—or that would elicit only a passing alerting response. Over-stimulation might take the form of covering ears to certain sounds, avoiding certain textures on the fingertips or body, or hopping and flapping when something spins or makes a certain loud noise. Parents often feel uncomfortable when they see children do these things because over-arousal behaviors are seen as deviant. Adults generally do not like to watch children with autism engage in signs of over-arousal, and behavioral methods can certainly be used successfully to control such behaviors.

But what can we learn from the occurrence of these behaviors? For one thing, they suggest to us which sensory channels have an attenuated or otherwise deranged "bandwidth." This in turn can narrow the learning experience: If a child won't touch certain things because of the way they feel, he may not be exposed to things other children his age do touch and from which they consequently learn. A child who covers his ears to certain sounds is showing his inability to attend to, and also an inability to learn anything from those sounds. So, as we begin to look for features of treatments, we need to consider which sensory "channels" may need "amplification" and which may need "muting."

Self-Accommodations to Over-Arousal. Arousal-regulation difficulties that are associated with autism include both hyper- and hypo-sensitivities on all the sensory channels. Auditorily hypersensitive children may cover their ears at noises that don't disturb others particularly, like a garbage disposal, a vacuum, a blender, or other low-pitched growls. Typically, it is a particular kind of noise (frequency or hertz) rather than loudness (decibels) alone that causes an over-stimulated response. For some children it is certain combinations of the frequency and decibels, such as very loud noises with deep reverberations—motorcycles, thunder, or planes taking off—that are over-stimulating and aversive. Sometimes, the autistic child's "rheostat" seems so miscalibrated that he can even respond quite unfavorably to sensory stimuli that others don't even consciously perceive, like the flicker or hum of all those wall-to-wall fluorescent lights on the ceilings at K-Mart stores.

The Hard-to-Arouse Hyposensitive Child. On the other hand, the child may have arousal-regulation problems that are manifested by under-responding: The most classic example is seen in the experiment many parents perform of clapping pot lids behind the toddler who doesn't even startle, even though a hearing test a week later shows her auditory nerves work just fine. While some children may be hypo-sensitive to sound, others may be hypo-sensitive to kinesthetic sensory input, such as seeming impervious to pain.

We sometimes think of behaviors such as rocking from foot to foot, toe-walking, and flapping hands or arms as "self-stimulatory" behaviors. This term reflects the hypothesis that these behaviors occur to induce stimulation, which can sometimes seem the case when observing a bored, disengaged, or avoiding child with autism who seems to be making his own focus for his attention. Arguably, this does occur in states of hypo-arousal. However, much of the time these same behaviors are seen when the child has been exposed to overexciting things, like a spinning musical top. In those situations—quite possibly more common—the flapping or rocking seems to be a way of "short-circuiting," and discharging excessive arousal.

Behavioral Manifestations of Hyper- and Hyposensitivities. Over- or under-responding to sensory inputs from each of the sensory modalities is found in children with autism: Hyper- and hyposensitivities are also prominent in the vestibular (or movement) sensory domain. Some children seem to crave motion stimulation such as bouncing and swinging, which does not seem to tire them after a while, as it does other children. In fact, some research has pointed to vestibular under-arousability by showing that some children with autism don't get dizzy like the rest of us. Other children with autism are incredibly averse (over-aroused) by vestibular stimulation. Sometimes the arousal-regulation difficulty is one in which reactivity fluctuates so that something once responded to as aversive becomes highly sought. A paradoxical observation—something I've heard from parents more than once about their child's arousal-regulation peculiarities—is that something that was once very aversive and overarousing later becomes something the child craves. One little boy, Rory, was terrified at his first encounter with a merry-go-round. His mother, thinking it was a worthy challenge to help him overcome this fear, managed to gradually desensitize him. Within a short time, Rory was asking incessantly about the possible presence of merry-go-rounds when taken to a new place; he loved to ride them and was highly distressed when merry-go-round riding would end for the day. When last I saw them, Rory's parents were spelling out "merry-go-round" lest it trigger a new round of requests. The same thing happens with elevators and escalators.

Having odd olfactory responses and smelling and eating a narrow food selection is not as likely maladaptive a sensory hypo-response as ignoring some other kinds of sensory information, but such behaviors serve to further underscore the various ways in which over- or under-responses to sensory stimuli occur in autism: Children averse to certain tastes are fairly common, and in general it is not at all abnormal for many young children to avoid strong tastes altogether. There are, however, some children with autism with the opposite taste response: One mother told how she had to hide onions, as her seven-year-old son would eat them all raw.

Sensory over-responding is also sometimes present in response to certain types of visual stimuli; some children with autism seem to crave the opportunity to view serial vertical lines—telephones poles along a freeway, chain-link fences on the perimeter of a playground, or lines drawn by the child for his own amusement on a chalkboard or piece of paper and then viewed from the periphery of vision.

We recognize each of these behaviors to be abnormal, but they also represent underlying difficulties with wiring and that may distort the information attained by the child from his surroundings. (This distortion is what is sometimes referred to as "stimulus over-selectivity.") To the extent that these perceptions are distorted and then experienced as more rewarding or aversive than they might be for other children, they may have an impact on the types of situations and experiences the child seeks out or avoids, and what aspects of those experiences he focuses on. Whether or not the child has hyper- or hypo-sensitive responses to things is generally included in a clinical history to decide whether or not a child might have autism. However, it is less usual to go the next step and use that information to construct a picture of how these hyper- and hyposensitivities might shape how the child sees his world.

PERSEVERATION

Many children with autistic spectrum disorders engage in behaviors that they repeat so often that one wonders what they mean to the child, or whether, after so many repetitions, they can mean anything at all. Depending on what is being described as the matrix of the child's disabilities, perseverativeness may take a variety of forms. There can be simple repetitious vocalizing, like uttering "Gee-due, gee-due," over and over, without anyone's being certain of the exact meaning or context for saying "Gee-due." Older children with more advanced language skills may repeat a question like "Go to Burger King after band practice?" even when the child knows the answer. Other children perseverate with physical actions, like the "chinning" described earlier, or with repetitive hand-flicking or wrist-turning movements. Still other children engage in repetitious play ranging from simple activities like repeatedly pulling the handle on a "Speak N Say" to complex repetitive play like staging the landing of United Flight 2030 at LAX to go see Grandma in Santa Monica, over and over again. At first, perseverative behavior may seem interesting because the child seems so intensely involved in the activity, or because the activity itself seems quite interesting. (The very first time I saw Adam's Flight 2030 routine I wondered how his parents could think he was autistic. After Flight 2030 had been reenacted verbatim for the fifth time in five minutes, I understood much better why Adam's parents had come.) The point is that the underlying nature of the problem is the same—a tirelessness with non-novel activity. Perseverativeness can be considered a primary innate trait that overlaps with a failure to habituate and the accompanying failure to prefer novelty that was discussed earlier. In the void created by an absent drive to change activity, or innovate, perseverativeness has fertile ground in which to grow.

Silk Purse from a Sow's Ear: The Up Side of Perseveration. Most perseverative behaviors, however, differs from a broken record. Often, the longer the child perseverates, the more intense, rapid, or frequent the repetitions become. Most parents can see the "point of no return" coming—that point at which the perseverative behavior has taken on a life of its own, where interfering with it will certainly provoke a tantrum or some other very negative response—like the child hurting himself or another person. What does this pattern of increasing excitement while engaged in a perseverative behavior suggest? To the extent that perseverativeness is self-perpetuating and excitatory, it is a kind of motivation to do more—albeit more of the same activity.

To this end, when perseverativeness is an observed trait in a child, it can be regarded as a possible strength as well as the obvious and more often described weakness. When we examine perseveration in the context of a child's matrix of abilities and disabilities, it is possible to see perseverative behavior as both strength and weakness: On the plus side, if the child prefers repetition, repetitious tasks may produce more focused and sustained attention than tasks requiring flexibility and dynamic problem solving. Stacking a ten-block tower with ten blocks of the same size may be more enjoyable than being asked to figure out any way to make the ten blocks look like a car. On the minus side, perseverative behavior can be regarded as mental "down time," a time when no new stimulation is being received.

From the point of view of intervention, perseverative tendencies can be leveraged to influence motivation in a child who may otherwise have low motivation, or what was earlier described as low reinforcer saliency (i.e., not having many things he cares much about). On a number of occasions, I've been brought videos of a lackluster child working with a therapist. The child demonstrates complete disinterest in what is being taught and in what is being held out as a reward for a successful performance. Then I notice that there is much discussion on the video about not letting the child "stim," have his "stimmy" toy, or have a certain item because he "stims" too much. Interestingly, those who utter such statements are tacitly acknowledging exactly what that child does find reinforcing, namely, the "stimmy" thing. The child might be uninterested in his therapy because all the things he's interested in have been taken out of therapy! How can a balance be achieved so that this very goal-directed motivation (clearly seen when the "stimmy" toy is present) can be utilized to achieve new learning?

From the viewpoint of some behavioralists, the more the child "stims," the more he will want to "stim," and that is bad simply because such behaviors appear abnormal and serve as mental down time. OK, fine. However, what is often *not* recognized is that the "stimmy" action may be an in-road to establishing more self-sustaining behavior in an otherwise passive child who is apparently unmotivated to do anything. By thinking of the perseverativeness as innate, *and* as a possible strength, and not just a weakness, it becomes possible to design specifically tailored interventions. As we'll discuss in chapter 8, "stimmy" objects can be successfully used as motivators (positive reinforcers) for other things that it may be desirable to teach the child. Some curriculum models that will be discussed also capitalize on this innate quality of many children with autism by designing highly repetitious or predictable programs, giving the child a "dose" of the repetition he seems to crave, letting the perseverativeness of the routine be its own reward for the tasks that constitute the routine. The point is that as one more specifically targets a child's innate difficulties (say, perseverativeness and low reinforcer saliency), ideas about how the child can be taught can emerge from referring back to an understanding of the primary problems underlying autism.

PERCEPTUAL INCONSTANCY/DISTAL-PROXIMAL PREFERENCE

Perceptual Inconstancy. In the 1970s, autism research was just getting started. One early idea to emerge was that of "perceptual inconstancy," the notion that children with autism might not be experiencing sensory input—visual, auditory, tactile, or vestibular (movement)—in the same ways as others, or that perhaps these perceptions were "inconstant," or varying. If this were true, think about how disorganizing it could be: Imagine that every time you entered a room in your house and turned on the lights, the illumination seemed different—100 watts one day, 400 the next. It would be one thing if you had a rheostat on your light switch to control the illumination, but what if you didn't? Maybe you would repetitively switch the lights on and off trying to figure out what the lighting would look like the next time the lights went on. I am not saying that this is why so many children with autism are drawn to switching lights on and off, but rather that you would probably try to come up with strategies for organizing your observations about what was going on around you. One general strategy might be to avoid things that gave you perturbing input. (For example, a few years ago, I experienced an eye condition that, for several months, caused my perceptions of illumination and color to differ in each eye. I got in the habit of waking up with only my "good" eye open for a while before facing the more uncomfortable task of dealing with the odd input from the other eye.) "Virtual" disturbances of this sort may explain why some sensory stimuli that were once considered very aversive, like Rory's merry-go-rounds, can become an obsessive focus for repeated experience.

Proximal versus Distal Sensory Inputs. Related to this idea that children with autistic spectrum disorders may have difficulty perceiving perceptual input in a constant fashion is the idea that children with autism may tend to be more oriented to "proximal" rather than to "distal" sense receptors. Proximal sense receptors are those dealing with sensory input that is very immediate to the body—things that are touched, put in the mouth and tasted, or smelled, and the way the body is moved. Distal receptors include vision and hearing, which pulls in input that occurs outside of the child's own body. Autistic children more often seem less aware of distal inputs, and more aware of proximal inputs, as if they live in a world of their own that consists of an encapsulating bubble that is sometimes drawn very close around them. Some of this poor distal-proximal attunement balance may simply be a very delayed aspect of maturation, since infants are much more proximal, becoming more distally attuned as they mature. For other children with autism, it may be that some sensory channels have more "noise" than "signal" and the preference is to tune into "channels" with less static.

For some children with autism, thinking in terms of which of the senses seem turned up the highest and which seem turned down the lowest, and which get clear reception and which don't gives us some clues as to what sensory information is actually being received and processed—and what kind of weight it is given as the child tries to make sense of it. Thinking in terms of a particular child's difficulty in balancing sensory receptors may help us "turn up" rheostats that are "turned down" too low, and "turn down" the ones that are "turned up" too high. Temple Grandin, a person with autism who has written incredibly cogently about what it is like inside her experience of autism, long ago invented a "squeeze machine": Arguably, the squeeze machine "turns up" her vestibular input, creating a better homeostasis and a mood state that feels good to her.

PROCESSING SPEED

Perceiving Sound. An important innate feature of information processing is processing speed. How quickly information is perceived, made sense of, and responded to has much to do with how we can handle those inputs. The processing-speed difficulty that has probably received the most attention in trying to understand children with autism is auditory processing speed. In this case, the concern is with three things: First, how quickly is auditory information perceived and attended to or not. ("It's a sound! Is it directed to me?"). Second, the sound needs to be registered in some way that involves meaning ("Is it speech? What am I being told or asked to do?" or "Does this sound call for a response?" or "What is that sound? An angry dog?") Third, the sound needs to be transformed into an expressive product. This may be a mirror of what went in, or a more complicated response. If there is too much of a slowdown during perception or early extraction of meaning, the very temporary traces of memory that hold exact words and sounds long enough to make sense of them can be expected to disappear. Once they are gone, it may be impossible to reconstruct what has been said. It becomes impossible to get to the level of longer-term memory. For example, try to recall if your husband or wife told you when she'd be home from work today. You might well remember *what* she said, but it is unlikely you remember all the exact words she said. This is because you heard her, extracted the meaning, and then automatically decided whether to store that information for a short or long time. If you never understood in the first place—because she spoke too quickly, you didn't realize she wasn't speaking to you, or she spoke too quietly—the rest of the processing would never have happened.

Extracting Meaning. It is known that children with autism have processing-speed problems when it comes to sound perception: The earliest bits seem to go OK, which is how we can tell the child is not deaf. One idea is that slowed processing speed results in distortion so that the last sound of what is said masks earlier sounds before the brain has had an opportunity to extract any meaning: For example, if someone spoke to you in Spanish, and you spoke only rudimentary Spanish, you might still be trying to translate the first word while the rest of the sentence had been spoken and disappeared. Sometimes children with autism, seemingly aware that they will not be able to process a whole sentence, will just repeat the last few words. This is a kind of echolalia and may serve the function of letting the listener know that the child is at least partly "in" the conversation, or that the child is acknowledging the topic: Q: "Michael, do you want juice?" A: "Want juice?" meaning I hear you, I'm with you on this.

Just as there are methods for addressing other innate information-processing difficulties, there are approaches for addressing auditory-processing delays (which will be addressed in chapters 6 and 7). However, as is the case with other innate disabilities, the treatment must be planned with the matrix of disability in mind—using stronger, less affected (or unaffected) capacities to help compensate for processing-speed difficulties.

Processing Speed Delays in Other Sensory Domains. Auditory-processing difficulties are probably the easiest to conceptualize. It is also easiest to see how delays in auditory processing can have a profound impact on language development and, as a result, on much of learning.

There is no reason to believe, however, that these processing-speed difficulties don't exist in other domains: There has been some work, for example, on recognition of faces and emotional expressions in children with autism. Both these areas are weaknesses for many children in the autistic spectrum, possibly because of the difficulty of extracting what are relevant features for attention. (One can speculate that one source of the popularity of Thomas the Tank Engine among children with autism is that he only has a few clear, unambiguous, unvarying facial expressions. When Thomas is mad, you know he's mad!)

AFFILIATIVE ORIENTATION

An area of innate social response that might be described as a dimension of primary disability universally seen in all children with autism is an apparent lack of affiliative drive. The basic desire to be with, do with, and be like others seems diminished. This difficulty can be described as innate because under normal circumstances children are not taught to want to be with others rather than to be alone. They are not taught to find other children interesting; they just do. Of course the quality and contingency of care that a child receives has a lot to do with how sociable and warm a particular child is, and there are more innate, temperamental qualities to affiliativeness as well. We know from studies done in the 1960s that families of children with autism are no less warm than other families. That is not the reason the autistic child appears to lack a strong desire to be with others.

Affiliation and Evolution. Lack of affiliativeness can be seen as an innate disability from the perspective of evolutionary psychology as well. Evolutionary psychology, the study of the adaptive or survival value of innate behaviors or preferences, would suggest that an infant who is not affiliative risks loss of care. Initially, parents are driven to care for infants because of the infant's helplessness. Over time, anything the child does that is seen as organized, adaptive, or social strengthens the parents' love and desire to take care of the child even more. However, our social values today are not what they were at the time that man evolved on the African savannah. It is possible to imagine that, at that time, it was absolutely necessary for a child to put out love-engendering signals if his parent were going to put in the effort to help him survive. A sick or otherwise atypical child who did not engender affection probably did not survive because he failed to elicit the extra care he needed. Today, the fabric of society helps bind all of us.

Affiliation and Learning. In practical terms, a basic lack of affiliative drive means that the child is not particularly drawn to things just because those things involve human activity and interests. Many of the learning opportunities from which infants and toddlers naturally benefit involve wanting to watch others and then be like them. Many children with autism imitate other people poorly. The pervasive effects of not readily being motivated to imitate others are felt in learning all sorts of skills. Learning through imitation of either adults or peers is often a major area of learning disability for the child with autism. Addressing this difficulty will be covered in chapters 4 and 8 as we discuss social learning and play. In the context of this chapter, affiliative drive can be thought of as another primary area of disability in autism that can be addressed by considering the child's matrix of abilities and disabilities and devising ways to use strengths to compensate for weaknesses, as we see in treatments in which primary rewards of food or sensory stimulation are paired with affiliative responses (smiles, a positive tone of voice) so that affiliative responding is learned.

THEORY OF MIND

"Theory of Mind" Defined. A final type of innate process that has received much attention in the experimental research on autism is a concept called "theory of mind." What this refers to is the in-born response that humans have to understand that others maintain states of consciousness parallel to their own.

Earliest manifestations of problems in this area of functioning can be observed when an infant fails to follow a parent's gaze or fails to perceive markers like facial expression that "speak" for themselves. While the failure to develop pointing is often regarded as the earliest indicator of difficulties in developing theory of mind, it may be that, even earlier, infants with this difficulty fail to respond to habitual parental facial expressions that precede rewarding (or punishing) social contingencies. This might include things like an infant's failing to smile in response to a parent who raises her eyebrows and smiles before picking the infant up for a cuddle, kiss, or feeding.

Problems in deriving information using this form of perception have been referred to as an absence of a theory of mind, or by the catchier, and quite accurate term "mindblindness." While most theory of mind research has been fairly cold, cognitive, and clinical (Does a child who was out of the room know that another has hidden something from her?), the idea of essentially "mind-reading" by examining the actions of another is clearly a prerequisite mental ability in learning to be sympathetic or empathic, evoke guilt, and experience shame, to name a few things we come to expect of toddlers.

It has often been argued that lack of a theory of mind is the core deficit in autistic spectrum disorders, though some who have made this argument have eventually shot themselves in the foot by showing not everyone with an autistic spectrum disorder displays a lack of theory of mind in all situations. (Actually, such findings more likely indicate the range of phenotypic penetrance of this trait—that is, the degree of severity.) From the perspective taken here, autism and related disorders are seen as falling across a spectrum and so are the basic deficits that combine to form different kinds of autistic spectrum disorders. Nevertheless, an absent theory of mind (in its purest, cognitive sense) in combination with a lack of affiliative orientation can be seen as core to many (though certainly not all) of the signs and symptoms of autism that form as different primary innate disabilities interact within the matrix of ability and disability and form the secondary, "virtual" symptoms of autism.

SECONDARY "VIRTUAL" DISABILITIES AND AUTISTIC LEARNING DISABILITIES

Secondary Disability and Signs of Autism

As we have discussed the idea of primary innate deficits of different kinds, I have hoped to convey the idea that there are basic aspects of seeing the world that are likely quite different for the child with autism. These differences can be regarded as in-born differences, some things that have developed differently with regard to the capacities of the child's brain. This book is not the place to read about what parts of the brain are likely affected and why, but good overviews of such work are given in the Further Readings section for this chapter. These are important questions for learning more about the basic underlying cause of autism. But from the point of view of treatment, it is necessary to start with what is observable and figure a way to reorganize behavior to better adapt it to learning and socializing. "Better" can be construed to have meaning on two levels: Behaviors can be trained and shaped to be as normal as possible, and treatment can be thought of as actually having the potential to change the brain itself, as discussed in chapter 1.

The Concept of Acquired Deficits and Virtual Disability. Now, to build on the concept of primary or innate deficits, we can begin to explore more secondary or acquired deficits. These are difficulties acquired as a result of the child's trying his best to figure out what is going on, but using somewhat faulty apparatus (defined by his primary deficits). There are a number of ways to think and talk about these secondary or acquired deficits: They are acquired when a primary ability or capacity for taking in information should be operating but isn't working well. The defective understanding that results can therefore be thought of as an *acquired* deficit rather than one that is innate or intrinsic to the child's wiring.

Another way of thinking about these acquired deficits is that they are "virtual" disabilities. The term "virtual" refers here to the important distinction that the acquired deficit exists because the more basic innate abilities fail to function properly. We assume that the innate deficits have a physiological basis in the brain's neuroanatomy or neuro-chemistry, even though we may not presently be able to point to the exact location. By contrast, secondary deficits, what can be thought of as acquired or virtual disabilities, are not intended to be construed as having a locus in the brain, but are the result of poor integration of the circuitry—not enough wires, wires in the wrong place, poorly insulated wires, wires with poor conductivity—so the information gets distorted in ways that form one or more characteristic signs of autism.

So, for example, we talked earlier about innate primary deficits in (auditory) processing and perseverativeness. Let's say that both of these primary deficits occur in a child. But let's also say that this child has intact auditory memory. The result may be repetitive echolalic speech. Essentially, repetitive echolalia can be seen as emerging from the matrix of abilities and disabilities: the disability being a failure to auditorily process sounds rapidly enough to extract meaning, coupled with a tendency to repeat things; the ability being the child's using relatively good auditory memory to store what he hears. The concept of a matrix of ability and disability simply becomes a way of thinking about interactions among innate problems and the acquired or virtual disabilities that can result.

Obviously, there is no physical "matrix of abilities and disabilities" in the brain. Therefore, it is also not likely that there is a specific place in the brain in which a "virtual" symptom of autism, like echolalia, is produced. This type of reasoning may be helpful not only for thinking about where symptoms come from, but also for thinking about any genes that in the future may be associated with autism—meaning that there is unlikely to be an echolalia "gene," but there are possibly genes with functions more closely tied to the more innate deficits (like speed of auditory processing) discussed earlier.

Self-Accommodations. Some secondary or "virtual" disabilities can also be regarded as self-accommodations to the innate defects: When a person's leg is injured and he can't walk properly, he may limp instead; but the leg is still used for locomotion. When a child can't understand what is being said, he may echo and get a response that is related to the specific intent of what was meant; so to some extent, he is still communicating. Limping is a self-accommodation to not being able to walk properly, and echolalia is a self-accommodation to not being able to talk properly. Nobody teaches us to limp. Nobody teaches a child to echo. Over time, limping may distort the musculature needed to restore proper gait. Over time, echolalia may distort the ability to communicate, especially if it is so successful that there is no incentive for a revised effort. (One way that echolalia can be "too" successful for the child is if the listener does not require further communicative effort, like having the child repeat what has been said a bit more correctly.)

As we go over each area of autism symptoms in subsequent chapters, we will discuss how each of the areas of innate disability can enter into the matrix of abilities and disabilities—unique to each child—and emerge with various self-accommodations. Understanding the origins of these self-accommodations, which themselves are the symptoms of autism (and also sometimes other neurodevelopmental disorders), is the first step in understanding an individual child's treatment needs. As symptoms of autism are understood as self-accommodations to innate disabilities, targets for treatment become clearer. This is because it can be very helpful to deconstruct each symptom into its primary, innate elements to know what really needs to be treated, to get closer to treating the underlying brain difference that it may be possible to remodel, and to be better able to analyze other symptoms that may later arise from the same matrix of abilities and disabilities.

TERTIARY EPIPHENOMENA:
FAILURE TO SELF-ACCOMMODATE TO PRIMARY DEFICITS

Pathognomonic (Defining) Diagnostic Symptoms and Specificity (Uniqueness) of Symptoms. Children with autistic spectrum disorders begin with some primary difficulties that can be traced to how they initially perceive and process incoming information from the world around them. This is what has been referred to here as "innate" deficits. These deficits combine in a way that is unique in each child: Stronger, intact abilities step in to compensate for weaker abilities (the concept of a matrix of abilities and disabilities). Characteristic patterns of compensation like this, in which stronger innate abilities rather automatically help compensate for shortcomings can be viewed as "self-accommodations," as in the example of echolalia. Characteristic patterns of self-accommodation, like echolalia, come to be seen as pathognomonic or defining features, as echolalia can be for autism. However, the whole syndrome of autistic spectrum disorders is defined by no one pattern of self-accommodation, no one symptom. Other children with other neurodevelopmental disorders might develop echolalia too, and for the same reasons. However, if another child does not also have other innate deficits that can be associated with autism, such as a lack of social affiliativeness, a lack of capacity for theory of mind, etc., that child's full matrix of abilities and disabilities may not produce a complement of self-accommodations that specifically constitutes an autistic spectrum disorder. Instead, that child might just have echolalia, but have intact social relatedness and intact capacity for theory of mind, and so have some sort of language disorder. On the other hand, the child might have echolalia, but also have a global set of social, linguistic, and motor innate impairments, and be best characterized as primarily having mental retardation. Each individual self-accommodation that is pathognomonic of autism, though not necessarily unique to autism, can be thought of as an autistic learning style or an autistic learning disability. To the extent that the self-accommodation is successful, we will want to focus on that pattern of compensation as an *autistic learning style*. To the extent that the self-accommodation is unsuccessful (and can be improved by intervention), we will want to focus on that pattern of compensation as an *autistic learning disability*.

This is to say that every child with autism (just like every child without autism) learns in a certain way that results from his strengths coming to the fore and, one hopes, helping him overcome his weaknesses. Special education is all about identifying children's strengths and helping children best use their strengths to overcome their weaknesses. When children do not automatically form adequate self-accommodations, the purpose of a special education is to design better accommodations, so the child can use innate strengths to overcome innate weaknesses.

Pathognomonic (Defining) Diagnostic Symptoms versus Indirect Symptoms. There are times, however, when strengths and weaknesses do not fall together in a way that makes for a natural self-accommodation. The child's natural attempts to compensate for his difficulties short-circuit—and there are *failed* self-accommodations. We discussed earlier the child who has auditory-processing difficulties and learns to echo (use good auditory memory) to hold on to what he has heard long enough to actually process it or to just repeat it to indicate that he is on the topic with you. What about the preverbal child? He can't take advantage of auditory memory in the same way (recreating the auditory input to get another chance to process it). The preverbal child, even if he does have receptive language capacity, cannot repeat to let you know he's on the topic.

So what happens? Say the verbal child is repeating "Danny want juice?" and this gets him juice. But, if Danny is preverbal, he may want juice, but have no way to indicate it. This child is subject to a whole set of behavioral difficulties—indirectly arising *epiphenomena* that are not really signs of autism, but frequently occur when there are failed self-accommodations (like no echolalia).

These indirect symptoms may include screaming, physical tantrums (like throwing oneself on the floor or dropping suddenly to one's knees), aggression toward others (hitting mom), aggression toward objects (throwing or breaking whatever is nearby), running away from the source of frustration, or even self-injurious behavior (like hitting oneself in the head, head-banging, hand-biting, scratching, or pinching). Therefore, we can think of maladaptive behaviors such as these as a tertiary level of symptoms. These are not unique signs of autism, but phenomena that are well recognized as characteristic of autism, particularly in young, or poorly socialized, or poorly taught children with autism.

Recognizing Failed Self-Accommodations for What They Are. The hardest thing for parents is that these indirect symptoms are often at their worst and most uncontrolled right before the child starts any intervention. Usually, a parent's primary complaint may be that the child doesn't talk, but also recognizing that the way he tantrums and resists makes it seem that it will be impossible to teach the child. Typically, before any treatment, not only has the child failed at successfully accommodating to some key innate disability, his parents have not yet had the opportunity to learn to help their child either. The child has failed to self-accommodate, and the parents do not yet know how to offer successful strategies to improve his capacity to self-accommodate.

Intervention in the form of special-educational strategies is, of course, a key way to help the child accommodate to his innate difficulties more successfully, thereby reducing frustration and converting failed self-accommodations into successful accommodations. This is a really important first step for most children. For parents, learning to do something to reduce the severity and frequency of outbursts and aggressive, frustrated, and injurious behaviors is the first sign of hope.

Tertiary Symptoms of Autism and Functional Behavior Analysis. If a child shows tantrums, aggression, self-injury—any of these possible tertiary signs of autism— he is showing us that he may not have adequate means to understand what is going on, control what is going on, and/or communicate about what is going on.

Parents and teachers just know the child is one unhappy little cookie. Children who are hitting themselves, biting others, or screaming do not seem happy. In addition, it is unpleasant for those around the child to tolerate these behaviors. So, epiphenomena are associated with three difficulties: the child is unhappy, the parent or teacher is unhappy, and the child is failing to get his needs met without he and/or the adult feeling unhappy because of the undesirable behavior the child uses to get his way.

So how should such a behavior be handled? How do we deconstruct a situation in which the child's bad behavior can be described not only as a "negative" or "undesirable," but as a tertiary symptom of his autism, as a failed self-accommodation? How do we fix the underlying problem? Usually, when the tertiary symptom or epiphenomena (the tantrum, the hitting) is studied carefully, it is possible to identify why the child is doing what he is doing.

Those working from a behavioral perspective would call analyzing the cause of the problem behavior—a *functional analysis*. For those who already know what a functional analysis is, read on, as an alternative strategy for using the results of a functional analysis will be explained. If this is a new concept, a functional analysis is sometimes described as the "ABCs" of understanding an undesirable behavior.

The "ABCs" Revisited. The "A" stands for understanding the *antecedents* of an undesirable behavior. Most behaviorists would say that it is likely that something has not gone the way the child has wanted it to. Perhaps the child wanted to watch "Blues Clues" and his older sister turned on "Barbie Goes Shopping." The child then head-butted his sister (or the TV). Let's say head butting is a frequent problem, and that the head butting is addressed to whomever or whatever the child sees as having thwarted his desires. The "B" is for *behavior*, in this case, head butting. So, head butting is what we wish the child wouldn't do; the behavior we would like to change. "C" is for *consequences*. Let's say that the older sister runs sobbing from the room saying "Tyler's head butting me again!" Meanwhile, Tyler changes the channel until he sees "Blues Clues." Worked pretty well from his perspective.

From Tyler's autistic point of view (which is not clouded by empathy for his sobbing sister, nor is his self-esteem diminished by her screams of "I hate you!"), head butting is an efficient means to an end. It is likewise for the child who has experimented with shrieking until he discovers the most efficient decibel level and pitch to get caregivers to drop whatever they are doing to run around and figure out what he wants

A conventional behaviorist's solution to this dilemma might be to change the consequences the child receives for the undesirable behavior so that the effectiveness of the undesirable behavior (say, shrieking) is thwarted. In this case, as soon as the shrieking begins, the parent might be advised to move the child into his bedroom where he will presumably be away from whatever triggered the shrieking, and where the shrieking will, one hopes, become a less successful appeal to those accustomed to running around trying to figure out what he wants and getting it for him. If the child disliked removal to his room, this technique might indeed be effective in reducing shrieking. However, if the child preferred removal to his room and whatever he could be doing in there instead, we might expect only to have temporarily distracted him from his screaming. In that case, screaming will resume as soon as he remembers what he wanted, and has someone in whose proximity he can shriek. But let's focus on the best-case scenario, in which isolation was undesirable and reduced shrieking. Was isolation really an effective intervention?

It could be argued that the intervention was not successful in terms of teaching the child anything positive and adaptive. The child may have learned not to shriek, but we have no real reason to believe that this child will not start head butting next. This is because the deterrents put in place to end the shrieking did nothing to address why the child shrieked in the first place. In our example, we have assumed that an undesired behavior is due to unhappiness over the controlling older sister's inexplicable choice of "Barbie Goes Shopping" over "Blues Clues." The real problem is that except for head butting or shrieking, a child may have come up with no effective, acceptable way of indicating his TV preference. The child is experiencing a communication failure. The child needs a positive adaptation he can use, not just a behavioral deterrent.

The head butting (or shrieking) can be considered epiphenomena of an autistic symptom, which in this case is a failure to understand language. Maybe just prior to his sister's changing the channel, Tyler's mother told him that three half-hour segments of "Blues Clues" were enough for today, and it was now his sweet long-suffering older sister's turn to watch what she wants. But maybe Tyler didn't understand a word his mother said except the "TV" part. Maybe hearing "TV" made him hopeful that he would see more "Blues Clues" (since he lives in a very solipsistic little autistic world). So, he was really bitter when he saw Barbie.

A functional analysis of this situation shows that the *antecedent* was the arrival of Barbie on the TV screen, the *behavior* (response) was head butting, and the *consequence* was a sister who exited the room so that Tyler could regain control of the remote. What conventional functional analysis of the behavior might miss is that the whole situation was caused by a communication failure. Yes, you can stop head butting by giving a time-out to a child who doesn't like a time-out, but nothing has been accomplished prophylactically. The child is likely to simply try to find another way to get his way. It may turn out that his new strategy is also an undesired behavior, like the shrieking we mentioned earlier.

An Additional Step in Functional Analysis. The functional analysis does not address a press to communicate, or how the child might communicate given that the shrieking or head butting can be seen as a failed self-accommodation. This is to say that the child has not come up with a more successful self-accommodation than head butting or shrieking. Using our model of viewing the child with autism as comprised of innate deficits and successful and unsuccessful accommodations to these innate deficits, the first step would be to classify the head butting as an unsuccessful accommodation. (In fact, Tyler accomplished a result that most fairly could cause us to view his accommodation as partly successful.) But, while the head butting may have been successful in getting him immediate access to the TV, it was not adaptive. It was not a response that built skills in getting along with others. It did not improve acceptable communication skills. (And, we can assume, it did not get him his desired television viewing for long.)

What would be most helpful in this situation would be to deconstruct the problem by seeing Tyler's head butting as a maladaptive communicative act that needed to become more adaptive. If, for example, Tyler had a picture of a "Blues Clues" character to indicate what he wanted, and if Tyler's mother had an "All done" system or a "Your turn/"My turn" system that he understood, the situation might have turned out differently. Such strategies would have given Tyler a more successful accommodation to his primary problems in processing or expressing language. Of course, it would be ideal for Tyler to be able to say "Mommy, I want 'Blues Clues' please." This would be a great long-term goal. However, all children make steps in learning a new skill, and the steps that the child with autism makes need to be defined by that child's matrix of ability and disability. For many children with autism, the visual modality is relatively strong, and so giving the child an accommodation that uses picture-based communication can be a successful way of showing him how a relative strength (visual knowing) can overcome a relative weakness (lack of understanding of a spoken word).

One can better use functional behavioral analysis by looking at the inappropriate behavior as a failure to understand or communicate a need. The behavior that follows is therefore undesirable. By figuring out what constitutes the components of the failure (i.e., lack of verbal understanding or lack of nonverbal or verbal expressive communicative means) and how the child might use a mental "strength" to compensate, it is possible to greatly reduce the inappropriate behavior not through negative reinforcement (or punishment), but by helping the child increase his capacity to solve problems effectively.

ATYPICAL DEVELOPMENT AND DEVELOPMENTAL STAGES

Learning follows a developmental sequence. In this chapter, we have talked about the concept of "atypical ontogeny," the atypical developmental course of children who have innate problems in receiving, processing, and sending information. In the case of autism, frequently occurring innate disabilities co-occur in typical patterns that form a unique ontogenetic (developmental) profile that professionals have come to refer to as autistic spectrum disorders. While there are individual differences in each child's learning profile, there is always a matrix of ability and disability, a place where innate strengths find a way to help the child self-accommodate for his innate weaknesses. In the next chapter, we will enumerate these as a collection of *autistic learning disabilities.*

In addition, we have discussed what happens when the child's disability is such that successful self-accommodations do not arise. In this case the child may fail to get his needs met at all and be abjectly withdrawn, or passive, or he may develop maladaptive ways of getting his needs met by intimidating others with behaviors that they find frightening or irritating. All children with disabilities, however, need to be helped to find the most productive way to deal with the limits imposed by their innate disabilities. This involves enhancing relatively stronger skills so that better accommodations can be achieved. It involves supporting the child through the expected developmental stages so that, just as for a typically developing child, the child with autism can build upon the simpler stages of knowledge as more complex concepts can be added to further represent what is going on.

Remediating Atypical Development Developmentally. Typically developing children start by viewing their world in a very sensory and very "motor" way. They know what something is by feeling it, handling it, looking at it from different perspectives—sometimes even mouthing it. This gives way to the child's needing to have a classification system for all these sensory images, and that's where language comes in. If the child with autism is still processing information about his world on a sensory and motor level and is not using language (because it makes no sense, or is not retained), he needs to learn language in a way that plays to his particular strengths, that is, with consideration to his matrix of abilities and disabilities. If the child is very visual, sensory and motor input should be very visually attractive to increase its salience. The young, autistic, language-learning child still needs those sensory and motor inputs for language learning, but because the auditory "channel" is turned down, turned off, or distorted, we need to rely heavily on very salient visual stimuli, along with sensory and motor stimuli, to devise a language-teaching situation that helps the child with autism compensate for lack of auditory signal.

We instead see some remedial-education methods that use two-dimensional flash cards, which the child is shown but cannot touch, turn over, and explore in multiple dimensions (size, weight, texture, and so on). While using good visual stimuli is a good way to help the child compensate, we do not, at the same time, want to move away from simultaneously activating the developmentally typical processes used in a typically-developing child's acquisition of understanding, namely, the sensory and motor inputs. All of those inputs build a database that the semiotic (language meaning) system uses later. If we move away from the developmental aspect of the learning model when teaching children with autism, such as by trying to teach language with flashcards, we teach a behavioral response to the flashcards, not real language. This is why we hear of children "mastering" certain vocabulary via flashcards, but not yet being "ready" to generalize what they are learning. Generalizing is part of mastery and is integral to words having meaning. It is a lazy solution to use flashcards with children with autism because it may make a better self-accommodation by helping the child rely on stronger visual skills, but it does not contribute to the developmental foundation that is also needed. Without that developmental foundation, it will be difficult for skills to become "generalized," in other words, self-generative.

To reinforce this point, let's go back to the example of Tyler wanting to watch "Blues Clues." Let's say someone decides that because Tyler has good echoic capacity and some imitation skill he can be taught to verbally request "Blues Clues" by learning to vocalize one sound at a time. If Tyler is taught to get "Blue Clues" on TV by vocalizing "B," and later "BL," and later, "B-L-U," he is being taught a skill that allows him to compensate by using relatively stronger rote imitation skills, or rote auditory memory skills. However, this teaching may have nothing to do with the developmentally very early achievement of certain communicative acts like gaze, pointing, and vocalizing, which in a typical baby, are the context in which the meaning intended by "B" or "BL" or "B-L-U" rests. Without those earlier aspects of communicative meaning in the linguistic sense (not just the "I-make-this-sound-and-I-get-this-thing" cause-and-effect sense), there is little impetus to try to "generalize" what the spoken words really mean and how they can be used in other communication contexts.

The challenge in helping children to learn is several-fold: We must first identify innate disabilities, as these show us the errors being made in apprehension of stimuli that need to be processed for recognition of important social, linguistic, and cognitive information. Second, we must identify self-accommodations formed through the child's matrix of abilities and disabilities in which stronger and more intact functions are automatically deployed to make sense out of information that is missed or misapprehended because of innate deficits. Third, we must recognize how barriers to learning, such as tantrums, aggression, and even inattention, can be viewed as failed self-accommodations. Fourth, we must devise teaching that minimizes barriers to learning by showing the child more efficient compensations. Finally, we must teach developmentally, so that foundational skills are not omitted and so that what the child learns is meaningful, generalizable, and adds to understanding, rather than being limited to being functional only in the specific situations in which the skill is first taught.

CHAPTER CONCLUSIONS

Autism is not a simple problem. As discussed in chapter 1, there are multiple factors that might influence why a particular child has it. What we do know is that there are not yet any straightforward ways to undo what is wrong with how a brain is put together—no medicine that changes biochemistry or brain structure in some mysterious way and results in autism's just disappearing.

Some researchers labor to find a neurogenetic or biochemical pathway to a cure. There are certainly things to be learned from the efforts of such investigators. I, however, am not such an investigator. The approach being taken here is more pragmatic: My starting point is not the neurobiology or biochemistry, but the capacities it initially defines. Once a child shows signs of autism, those signs must be read very carefully to understand exactly what is wrong. That is the first step in remediating any problems the child has or will have.

It is easy to believe that a treatment that fits one child labeled "autistic" will also help the next child. The label of "autism" (not to mention all the other autistic spectrum labels) is really just a heading for a series of difficulties that often occur together. In many incredible ways, autistic children can seem astounding similar—in their love of Thomas the Tank Engine above all else, their endless fascination with any kind of spinning top, and so on. Those observations are clues that lay on the surface. In this chapter we have just begun to explore what primary problems in learning, knowing, and understanding create such phenomena. In the next chapter, we will focus more closely on how the innate, primary problems interact with an autistic child's more intact abilities to form characteristic autistic learning disabilities.

Autistic Learning Disabilities Defined: How Strengths Compensate for Weaknesses and Form Autism

WHY DO WE NEED THE CONCEPT OF AUTISTIC LEARNING DISABILITIES?

An analysis of autistic learning disabilities is meant to assist in the move from observations made during diagnostic or psycho-educational assessment to specific teaching strategies. The concept of autistic learning disabilities provides a method for systematically examining how different symptoms of the autistic spectrum disorders have a direct impact on how the child with autism learns. The concept of autistic learning disabilities is based on understanding how receiving and processing information can be different for a child with autism compared to a typically developing child. It is a developmentally based method for looking at learning in the autistic spectrum disorders.

In the preceding chapter, we discussed the origins of the kinds of learning difficulties that are experienced by children with autistic spectrum disorders. Some of these difficulties were defined as innate difficulties or deficits. This means that these are conditions that the child with autism probably had from birth, or around the time of birth. These factors, such as how much drive for novelty a child has, how quickly the child can process auditory information, how perseverative the child tends to be, are basically traits which affect the ways that a developing autistic child's apparatus can come to apprehend the world around him, make sense of what is taken in by the senses, and do things like produce an immediate response, or store information meaningfully for later use.

What makes the autistic spectrum disorders a distinctive syndrome is that these innate disabilities tend to be certain ones. Conversely, the innate abilities or mental aptitudes of children with autism also tend to be of a certain sort. These characteristic strengths often include auditory memory, good "procedural" memory (that is, being able to picture how to do things), visual-spatial understanding, and visual-motor coordination. Therefore, the developing child with autism, just like any child, has a characteristic set of strengths and weaknesses; just like any child, we support the autistic child's growth by emphasizing talents and helping the child with autism come up with strategies to overcome weaknesses.

A wonderful thing about child development that all parents experience is learning what their child's strengths are: With typically developing children, one child may be particularly precocious in terms of motor skills, pleasing his former-high-school-quarterback father with the fact that he can catch a Nerf ball really well by the time he is 11 months old. A mother who considered a career in the symphony may be particularly thrilled to observe what seems to be perfect pitch in her three-year-old daughter. Parents of children with autistic spectrum disorders feel no differently about their child's strengths. A father who is bedeviled by maps may be especially impressed by his seven-year-old with autism who can draw three-dimensional maps of the route to Aunt Fannie's house (although he may refuse to say hello to Aunt Fannie when they arrive). Another child with autism may endlessly annoy parents by being able to detect and reject minute amounts of crushed Remeron in whatever food it's put in—but there is also an element of pride in the child's incredibly sensitive palate.

Whether a child is typically developing or has an autistic spectrum disorder, that child will have strengths and weaknesses in how they perceive things and learn. When those strengths and weaknesses form characteristic patterns that we associate with the autistic spectrum disorders, they can be referred to collectively as *autistic learning disabilities.*

How Unique to Autistic Spectrum Disorders are Autistic Learning Disabilities? Most of this chapter is devoted to describing the range of autistic learning disabilities—characteristic ways in which learning may likely be different for the child with an autistic spectrum disorder. The term "autistic learning disability" is intended to refer to specific impairments in learning that are strongly—though not necessarily a hundred percent associated with autistic spectrum disorders. (In fact, all signs of autism are seen at least occasionally, and some, frequently, in children with other neurodevelopmental disorders.) In this chapter, autistic learning disabilities will be enumerated to demonstrate the many ways in which the child with an autistic spectrum disorder may be apprehending and responding to things around him differently from others. Not all children with autistic spectrum disorders have every one of the autistic learning disabilities you will read about. Some children who have one or more of these autistic learning disabilities may not necessarily meet full diagnostic criteria for autism or even for another pervasive developmental disorder. The presence of autistic learning disabilities raises the index of suspicion that the child might have an autistic spectrum disorder but is not a method of diagnosis by itself. Some siblings of children with autism may show a few of these autistic learning disabilities—but socially and communicatively not be disadvantaged the way a child with autism may be. The term autistic learning disabilities is not meant to be a reified construct to be studied as a distinctive entity. Rather, the intention is to use the concept of autistic learning disabilities as a heuristic device for understanding how teaching may need to be modified when a child has certain characteristically autistic ways of processing information.

This Chapter as an Introduction to "Part II-Autistic Learning Disabilities Described." The purpose of chapter 3 is to define what autistic learning disabilities are and how they set the autistic learner apart, creating a need for different teaching strategies that are specific to how a particular pupil with autism can best learn new things. In order to fully understand the point of view taken in Part II of this book, you will really need to look at this chapter (even if you skipped the earlier chapters of Part I, which were a more detailed analysis of thinking about the origins of autistic learning disabilities).

When we begin Part II, we will focus on each of three areas of autistic learning disability. These areas broadly follow the triad of social impairments in autism—in social interaction, communication, and activities and interests. In chapter 4, we will cover both description and treatment of what is meant by social autistic learning disabilities. Communication, the focus of so much treatment in autism, and also the source of great differences among children within the autistic spectrum, will be covered in three chapters: Chapter 5 will define communicative autistic learning disabilities. Chapter 6 will deal with treatments of these communicative autistic learning disabilities in preverbal or nonverbal children. Chapter 7 will deal with treatments of communicative autistic learning disabilities in verbal children who are within the autistic spectrum. Chapter 8 deals with identifying and treating the third area of the autistic triad of social impairments—the child's interests, and relating to the word of objects. Chapter 9 moves outside core symptoms of autism to a specific focus on how the full spectrum of autistic learning disabilities has an impact on the development of adaptive skills and how these can be treated when autism-specific learning styles are taken into account.

THE DEVELOPMENTAL VIEW OF DSM-IV CRITERIA
FOR AUTISTIC DISORDER

Why Do We Need Diagnoses?

How the DSM-IV Criteria for Autism Work. When autism is diagnosed in the United States, the clinician is probably using a diagnostic standard called the DSM-IV, the *Diagnostic and Statistical Manual of the American Psychiatric Association (Fourth Edition)* that was published in 1994. Use of a diagnostic standard is designed to ensure that there will be agreement among doctors in different places as to what is being called autism, or where the line is being drawn between autism and PDD. There are, however, differences in how the DSM-IV criteria for autism are actually used, because doctors with different degrees of specialization in autism tend to judge the qualities and range of severity for each symptom differently. There are many adjectives used in the DSM-IV criteria to describe symptoms of autism, like "diminished," "abnormal," "impaired," or "atypical." These words are interpreted to indicate different thresholds of severity by different professionals. It would be ideal if doctors had some sort of videotaped glossary of each symptom of autism that showed several examples of children doing things that were intended to be interpreted as meeting the criteria for various symptoms of autism, so that everyone could be similarly calibrated about when "lack of awareness of others" really was "marked," or "ability to make peer friendships" was really "impaired." This, unfortunately, isn't the case. It's one reason why the same presenting symptoms can be differently interpreted at different diagnostic centers.

Some clinicians feel it is helpful in certain situations to use the term "autism" rather than "PDD" or "PDD,NOS" because the dividing line between these may mean access or no access to certain autism-specific services the clinician feels should be helpful to a particular child. This further muddies decision making about which specific behaviors are "marked," "pervasive," or "lacking."

The 12 diagnostic criteria for DSM-IV Autistic Disorder are grouped into three areas—social development, communication, and activities and interests. Within each area are four specific criteria, each representing a different area of symptoms. Generally, the first criteria in each of the three areas are the ones that can be detected at the earliest ages, and the latter ones in each area are the ones that become apparent later on in development.

Understanding What Autism Is and What Mental Retardation Is. Each of the DSM-IV criteria should be evaluated according to the child's level of mental development so that developmental disability or mental retardation is not confused with autistic symptoms. Mental retardation can be thought of as an additional, overlaying problem. When children are young, which is when much diagnostic assessment is taking place, almost all children with autistic spectrum disorders show some evidence of below age-expected development in either language skills, non-language skills, or both.

Because of this overlap between autism and mental retardation, some of the most clinically useful research on diagnosing autism suggests that each diagnostic criteria be rated according to the child's *nonverbal* level of mental development. This is a very helpful way to think about the symptoms of autism because *verbal* ability is part of many signs of autism. By judging signs of autism in accordance with a child's nonverbal ability, there is a further check that other types of language delay are not confused with autistic symptoms. This is because children with non-autistic language delays tend to have better nonverbal communication skills than children with autism given their overall nonverbal developmental level. Nonverbal functioning includes non-language abilities, which for young children can be assessed by how well they can put together puzzles, sort things, and copy actions they've seen. This can be contrasted with verbal intelligence, which involves language use and understanding and is always affected in certain ways in autistic children. Therefore, a measure of mental development for the purposes of assessing autistic symptoms not due to overall mental retardation alone is best estimated through the child's functioning in areas not directly affected by the presence of the symptoms of autism—like nonverbal intelligence.

Using nonverbal (nonlanguage) intelligence as a way of estimating an autistic child's general level of mental development is not a perfect indicator, but it does provide a basis for separating many of the effects of mental retardation from the autism itself. Nevertheless, the majority of autistic children have some degree of mental retardation as well, so it is important to find a way to measure it separately from the symptoms of autism. By using the child's nonverbal IQ (nonverbal mental age) as a baseline, we are essentially asking "How does this child's behavior in each autistic symptom area compare to what a child should typically be able to do at this mental age?" Once there is a general fix on the child's nonverbal mental age (which a professional obtains via a combination of testing the child's intelligence, observing the child, and interviewing the parents), it is possible to assess the child for the presence of autistic symptoms—given his overall developmental level or possibly present level of mental retardation.

Knowing If a Child with Autism Also Has Mental Retardation. Many parents ask "How can you tell if my autistic child also has mental retardation?" What is mental retardation anyway?   As we talked about in chapter 1, population studies of children and adults with autism have consistently shown that 70 percent of those with autism have some degree of mental retardation as well. This means that full scale IQ is below 70 (where 100 is average). Full-scale IQ is a weighted average of language and non-language abilities with language becoming more weighted as the child matures. IQ is simply a score on a test that gives us some idea of how a child will develop over time. It tells us something about how fast or how slow new things will be learned. Since children with autism tend to have very "splintered" IQ scores, an overall average number cannot be viewed quite as meaningfully and in quite the same way as when an average represents less variation. ("Splintered" means that some areas of intelligence—like language or non-language skills—are significantly different from others.) However, a very broadly estimated developmental level (for which an IQ score is just one measure) is needed to estimate whether a child's symptoms and developmental milestones (or lack thereof) are due to autism or to overall degree of developmental impairment.

It is particularly hard to know if the youngest children with autism have any mental retardation, because they tend to be very uncooperative on formal tests of intelligence. Examiners then have to rely on reports and observations of how sophisticated the child's spontaneous problem solving, play, and language skills can be in order to make some estimate. Over time, as instructional control is established and there has been an opportunity to teach the child, the child's capacity can be better estimated. This means that many clinicians may defer adding a diagnosis of some degree of mental retardation in very young children or not mention it at all. One can certainly appreciate not wanting to be wrong about saying a child has mental retardation when the child is in fact just very badly behaved. However, it is important to have some clinical sense of how delayed development may be so that the diagnoses of mental retardation and autism are not confounded.

Developmentally Based Diagnostic Assessment. A straightforward way to respond to the need to examine the symptoms of autism according to the child's level of development is to start with a diagnostic checklist that associates expected milestones in normal development with each of the symptoms of autism. (As is done in Table 3.1). In this way, the developmental age of the child is considered as each symptom is evaluated. The clinician essentially asks "If this 36-month-old child is at the 12-month level, should we be expecting him to ___ yet?" with the blank being whichever symptom is being assessed. In the table below, there is a developmental schedule of milestones related to the symptoms of autistic disorder that can serve as a guide for developing this sort of understanding of the diagnosis.

Boundaries of Autistic Disorder and PDD,NOS. To be diagnosed as having Autistic Disorder using the DSM-IV criteria, a person must be considered to have positive symptoms on six of the 12 criteria. At least two of the criteria met must reflect difficulties in social development; at least one criterion must be met

TABLE 3-1

DEVELOPMENTALLY ORIENTED
DSM-IV CRITERIA FOR AUTISTIC DISORDER

"... at least 2 signs from A, 1 each from B & C; ... at least 6 overall."

A. QUALITATIVE IMPAIRMENTS
IN RECIPROCAL SOCIAL INTERACTION:

1. **Marked impairment in the use of multiple nonverbal behaviors such as eye-to-eye gaze, facial expression, body posture, and gestures to regulate social interaction.**

    Developmental Examples:
    A social smile in response to listening to caregiver (MA: 1-4 m.)
    Vocalizes in response to a social smile and talking (MA: 1-6 m.)
    Anticipatory reach to be picked up (MA: 6-10 m.)
    Responds to an inhibition on command (MA: 7-17 m.)

2. **Failure to develop peer relationships appropriate to developmental level.**

    Developmental Examples:
    Looks on with notable curiosity about peers (MA: 6-9 m.)
    Parallel play (MA: 20-24 m.)
    Associative group play (MA: 36-42 m.)
    Cooperative play (MA: 42-48 m.)

3. **Lack of spontaneous seeking to share enjoyment, interests, or achievement with other people (e.g., by lack of showing, bringing, or pointing out objects of interest).**

    Developmental Example:
    Social reference: shares pleasure/information (MA:8-14m.)

4. **Lack of socioemotional reciprocity.**

    Developmental Examples:
    Anticipatory excitement at initiation of care (MA:1-4 m.)
    Discrimination between familiar and unfamiliar adults (MA: 3-8 m.)
    Repeats a performance that is laughed at (MA: 8-17 m.)
    Emotional reaction when caregiver is sad/hurt (MA: 24-30 m.)

B. QUALITATIVE IMPAIRMENTS IN COMMUNICATION:

1. **A delay in, or total lack of, the development of spoken language (not accompanied by an attempt to compensate through alternative modes of communication such as gesture or mime).**

    Developmental Examples:
    Listens selectively to familiar words (MA: 5-14 m.)
    Pointing/using gestures to get wants met (MA: 11-19 m.)
    Labels several familiar objects/pictures (MA: 17-30 m.)

2. **Marked impairment in the ability to initiate or sustain a conversation with others despite adequate speech.**

    Developmental Examples:
    Simple nonverbal interactions, e.g., pat-a-cake (MA: 5-12 m.)

Jabbers expressively, imitates words (verbal MA: 9-18 m.)
Uses words to make needs known (MA: verbal 14-27 m.)
Relates stories (verbal MA: 48-54 m.)

3. **Stereotyped and repetitive use of language or idiosyncratic language.**

    Developmental Examples:
    Repeated babbling of C-V combinations (≤ verbal MA:18-24 m.)
    Echos 2 or more of last 2 words heard (≤ verbal MA: 24-30 m.)
    Refers to self by pronoun (verbal MA: 24-32 m.)

4. **Lack of varied spontaneous make-believe play or social-imitative play appropriate to developmental level.**

    Developmental Examples:
    Carries and hugs a teddy bear or doll (MA: 14-18 m.)
    Concrete, repetitive play (MA: 24-32 m.)
    Understands simple fairy tale (MA 36-42 m.)

C. RESTRICTED, REPETITIVE, AND STEREOTYPED PATTERNS OF BEHAVIOR, INTERESTS, OR ACTIVITY:

1. **Encompassing preoccupation w/ 1 or more stereotyped & restricted patterns of interest, abnormal either in intensity of focus.**

    Abnormal at any MA; Developmental Counter-Example:
    Persistently imagines being a fantasy character (e.g., fireman, ballerina—MA: 36-42 m.)

2. **An apparently compulsive adherence to specific nonfunctional routines or rituals.**

    Abnormal at any MA; Developmental Counter-Examples:
    Insists on having transitional object along (MA: 18-24 m.)
    Knows what comes next in bedtime routine (MA: 36-42 m.)

3. **Stereotyped and repetitive motor mannerisms (e.g., hand or finger flapping, or twisting, or complex whole-body movements).**

    Developmental Examples:
    Hand flapping/ tensing when excited (not >MA: 6-9 m.)
    Rocking on all fours (just prior to crawling)

4. **Persistent preoccupation with parts of objects.**

    Developmental Examples:
    Most objects go into mouth (not >MA: 12-16 m.)
    Interest in strongly sensory stimuli (e.g., Pat-the-Bunny)
    (MA: 12-16 m.)

1. (**Bold-face** type from: *The Diagnostic and Statistical Manual of the American Psychiatric Association.* 4d ed. Washington, D.C.: American Psychiatric Association, 1994)
2. From: Siegel, B. "Toward DSM-IV: Taking a developmental approach to autistic disorder." In Pervasive *Developmental Disorders: Psychiatric Clinics of North America.* Vol. 14. No. 1. Edited by J. H. Beitchman and M. Konstantareas. 1991, March, Phila.: W. B. Saunders. Pages 53-68

in the communication domain of development; and at least one criterion must be met in the domain of atypical activities and interests.

If the child has a less severe form of the behavior described in a criterion, which may contribute to a diagnosis of PDD,NOS. If no criteria are met in the domain of atypical activities and interests (Section "C") but the child does show a variety of signs in the domains of social and communicative development, the diagnosis of PDD,NOS is also used. Sometimes PDD,NOS is used when the child is so young that many of the developmental criteria are seen as still too difficult to assess, so less than six criteria overall are currently felt to be clearly met. Therefore, some doctors may say the child is "too young to tell." This is problematic, because clinicians who are very experienced with young autistic children can tell fairly accurately from the early profile of symptoms that *are* met which ones will become positive as development progresses. The younger a child is, the less specifically autistic signs will likely be. However, a clinician who knows the research in this area and is experienced with young autistic children can most often tell if a child is autistic by the child's second birthday and sometimes sooner.

One of the problems in using the diagnosis of PDD,NOS is that the lower limit is not clearly specified. It is clear that to receive a diagnosis of PDD,NOS, a child should have difficulties in some of the areas listed in the social (Category "A") and the communicative (Category "B") domains. Some clinicians might give a diagnosis of PDD,NOS to a child who meets as few as two criteria for PDD,NOS (that is, one from "A" and one from "B"). Although this is not strictly incorrect, it matters a great deal which criteria the child meets, as some of the problems that PDD children have are also common in children with related problems like developmental language disorders. That's one reason that a diagnosis of PDD,NOS needs to be made by someone experienced with autistic spectrum disorders. For instance, "a failure to develop peer relationships appropriate to developmental level" may be due to autism—as when a child actively avoids or ignores peers, or may be due to being hyperactive and intrusive—as when peers don't want to play with the child because he is too bossy. Other children lack peer relationships because they don't talk, and peers walk away when they are not answered. Other children are shy or anxious and cling to parents or the teacher, and they too may not be the most fun playmates. An experienced clinician limits a positive rating on this criterion to the child who lacks interest in peers, seems not to know how to join a group in a way peers find socially appropriate, or actively avoids those who approach him.

All of the criteria need to be assessed in terms of whether the *quantitative, qualitative,* and *developmental* characteristics of symptoms meet criteria. If not, just about every neurodevelopmentally disabled child, every delayed child, every mentally retarded child can be seen as meeting some criterion for autism.

SHOULD AUTISM BE SEEN AS ONE OR AS MANY DISORDERS?

The Lumpers versus the Splitters. A popular pastime among academic mental health professionals is to debate whether we have too few or two many categories to characterize disorders like autism. Much effort has been expended (some of my own included) in trying to determine whether we wouldn't be better off to call all children with signs of autism "autistic," or whether we wouldn't be better off describing some children as autistic, some as having PDD, some as having atypical autism, some as having atypical PDD, and some as having Asperger's syndrome, and so on. What is this debate really about? A way to get more research grants? What do we hope classification research will lend to our understanding of autistic spectrum disorders?

There are two camps of autism classifiers, referred to here, for lack of a more pompous-sounding scientific term, as the "lumpers" and the "splitters." The "lumpers," as the name implies, see the autistic spectrum as just that—a continuum of severity, number, and frequency of related symptoms that tend to co-occur. "Lumpers" feel that all of these children have similar treatment needs, and services should not be withheld from one over another because one child happens to meet five of twelve criteria and gets labeled "PDD," while another is judged to have six, is labeled autistic, and can then receive many more services.

The "splitters" on the other hand, focus on the fact that not all children with symptoms in the autistic spectrum have the same difficulties, that there may be different "autisms" arising from different origins (different genes, different neuroanatomical features, different neurochemistry), and that these different groups may have different kinds of abilities, disabilities, and outcomes. "Splitters" might also argue that the connotations of a full syndrome of autism, or "classical" autism, may be too pejorative a label for many children afflicted with just some of the disabilities associated with the "broader spectrum" or "broader phenotype" (as discussed in chapter 1).

If you ask me, I think both groups have a point. I would describe myself, and this book, as having come full circle on this issue. Let me explain, and then call me what you will: What is important about attaching a "label" is that it's a heads-up that this child will likely have some things he can and cannot do well. As was said earlier, of the 12 symptoms of autism in the DSM-IV, children only need show positive signs in six of the areas of concern (as well as meet some other requirements as to which signs they show and when each started) to qualify for a diagnosis of autism. This assessment results in a number of combinations of symptoms that a child might have and still rightly be classified as "autistic." Further, if the child has only a few concerns, she might be labeled as PDD,NOS or as having Asperger's syndrome. (An earlier volume—*The World of the Autistic Child*—details how these criteria work.)

Not only might the number and combination of symptoms vary, but the severity and frequency of the symptoms might vary as well. In addition, cutting across the range of autistic spectrum diagnoses is mental retardation. Seventy percent of those with autism have some degree of mental retardation in evidence by adulthood, and of the remaining thirty percent, two-thirds have verbal IQs in the borderline or mildly mentally retarded range. This fact means that not only are those with autistic spectrum diagnoses different according to which symptoms are present, but they also differ by an overall factor that speaks to the likely rate of learning and how complex the mental abilities they will develop will likely be. All these factors affect treatment response and, ultimately, prognosis.

Using the Autistic Learning Disability Concept to Address Lumping and Splitting. My preference is to "lump" together all children with some positive symptoms of autism—those with autistic disorder, PDD,NOS, etc., and to describe them as all having some "autistic learning disabilities." The next step is to ascertain which autistic learning disabilities a particular child has and design learning experiences for that child based on his learning disability profile. In essence, each symptom needs to be assessed separately to determine whether the child has difficulties in that dimension, how impairing that symptom is to him, and what he already does, if anything, to compensate for that problem. This approach of regarding each symptom separately, as something in need of separate treatment consideration, might be viewed as the ultimate form of "splitting."

This is certainly *not* suggesting that every child with any sign of autism, no matter how mild, should be called autistic instead of that child's current diagnosis (if any). This is not to suggest that there should be many more programs for autistic children so that all children with any of these signs can have access to them.

We have known for a long time that many signs of autism are present in children who primarily are handicapped by mental retardation, a language disorder, or anxious, obsessive traits. As awareness of autism increases and diagnostic tools improve, more children accumulate more "labels" as finely tuned ways of examining learning weakness are developed and used. It does seem possible that one reason more children are now labeled as having autism is that some children are so labeled even when there are just one or two, developmentally transitory signs (such as signs that are present only when the child is still a toddler and preverbal).

Some of the signs of autism, like delayed language development with echolalia, are not unique to autism per se and need to be carefully examined to see if echolalia in this particular case comes with other signs of autism or not. For example, an echolalic child with good, compensatory nonverbal communication strategies such as directing gaze and pointing can be taught further compensations very differently from an echolalic autistic child with no pointing and no joint gaze (looking to see if what he's looking at is also being looked at by the person with whom he's trying to communicate).

If the child does echo, and even if he isn't autistic in any other way, it may still be helpful to deconstruct the origin of the echoing by examining it from the perspective of what kind of innate processing defect and compensatory strengths it might reflect.

Echolalia (we will talk about different kinds later) can be considered an autistic learning disability because it often characterizes autism. The autistic learning disability model is a way of inventorying all the kinds of learning problems we think of as possibly problematic for a child with an autistic spectrum diagnosis and considering what it may mean for learning and remediation.

TABLE 3-2

DOMAINS OF AUTISTIC LEARNING DISABILITIES
AND CATEGORIES OF DSM-IV AUTISTIC DISORDER

Qualitative Impairments
in Social Interaction Social Autistic Learning Disabilities

Qualitative Impairments
in Communication Communicative Autistic Learning
Disabilities

Restricted, Repetitive, and
Stereotyped Patterns of Behavior, Nonsocial Autistic Learning Disabilities
Interests, or Activities

AN INTRODUCTION TO THE THREE DOMAINS
OF AUTISTIC LEARNING DISABILITIES

Symptoms of autism can be broadly grouped into three domains. This is also true for the three broad domains of autistic learning disabilities. Each domain of autistic learning disability (ALD) corresponds to a category of DSM symptoms for autistic disorder. As in the DSM, a few different types of symptoms, manifested by certain patterns of behavior, can be described within each of the three domains. While the specific symptoms of the DSM-IV criteria for autism have been studied in great detail, the criteria for ALDs is something new, meant not to be used instead of the DSM, but rather to help move clinicians from enumerating symptoms to enumerating areas in which the autistic child's learning deficits exist. Table 3-2 (above) shows how the three domains of ALDs and the three categories of DSM symptoms for autism correspond.

Each area of the three areas of autistic learning disabilities can be briefly defined in terms of what aspects of perception and information processing they encompass, what the learning implications of such problems in perception and information processing are, and what qualities of the child's experience and learning are influenced by having a particular autistic learning disability.

SOCIAL AUTISTIC LEARNING DISABILITIES
AND DSM "IMPAIRMENTS IN SOCIAL INTERACTION"

The core symptoms relate to *social development.* Autism is literally defined by the presence of primary social impairments. A child without difficulties in the domain of social understanding is not autistic. Children with social impairments that result from emotional abuse or neglect, or who may be socially immature because language development is impaired and communication is difficult are also considered not to have the kind of primary social impairments associated with a diagnosis of autism. Social autistic learning disabilities correspond to Category A in the DSM-IV criteria for the diagnosis of autistic disorder "Qualitative impairments in reciprocal social interaction." Table 3-3 shows how we can move from what DSM describes as social impairments to what can be described as social autistic learning disabilities.

The first DSM-IV set of diagnostic criteria for autism, "impairments in reciprocal social interaction," maps onto three main areas of social autistic learning disabilities. DSM symptoms marking deficits in reciprocal social interaction are the most universal and specific of the three areas of autistic impairment. Similarly, social ALDs can be thought of as uniquely autistic.

Lack of Awareness of Others. The first social ALD area is lack of awareness of others. The child who is unaware of others and what they are or are not doing fails to apprehend a great deal of experience that feeds into the child's development of how and why people interact in the ways they do. The child is "in his own little world," and often seems unaware of things that don't already have meaning and associated positive consequences for him.

Lack of Social and Emotional Reciprocity. The second area of social ALD is lack of social and emotional reciprocity: When a child is uninterested in doing things to please (or even displease) a parent or teacher, the child lacks the fuel that drives the social "engine" that powers much early learning. Sharing experiences, getting noticed, and being praised are intrinsic to learning and often missing or greatly diminished for the child with an autistic spectrum disorder.

TABLE 3-3

CHARACTERISTICS OF SOCIAL AUTISTIC LEARNING DISABILITIES

LACK OF AWARENESS OF OTHERS

Definition:
　　Physical size of the child's domain of awareness of what is going on around him seems less than for others his age.

Learning Implications:
　　Child fails to apprehend many things going on around him that others might notice.

Qualities:
- Foremost motivation is to please self, rather than another
- Instrumental learning style—more readily learns things that result in self-satisfaction

LACK OF SOCIAL AND EMOTIONAL RECIPROCITY

Definition:
　　Child does not clearly demonstrate sympathy, empathy, or altruism in a way that guides pattern of interactions with others.

Learning Implications:
　　Child is uninterested in learning new things to earn attention or approval of caregivers or other adults.

Qualities:
- Lack of desire to please others
- Low response to social praise and/or physical affection
- Lacks concern about the effect of his behavior on others

LACK OF SOCIAL IMITATION

Definition:
　　Child does not seem to be motivated to copy actions or attitudes of others.

Learning Implications:
　　Child does not learn readily through incidental or purposeful models.

Qualities:
- Low level of interest in peers
- No interest in rule-oriented or imitative (parallel) play
- Does not change in response to peer pressure/norms/interests

Lack of Social Imitation. The third area of social ALD is lack of social imitation: Typically, children learn new things by "automatically" copying other children and adults because most things that others do are somewhat or very interesting, merely because someone else is engaged in that activity. When this conduit of receiving new information is blocked, a main source of possible input is closed.

COMMUNICATIVE AUTISTIC LEARNING DISABILITIES AND DSM "IMPAIRMENTS IN COMMUNICATION"

The second area of impairment associated with autism comprises problems in using language communicatively (communicative ALDs). This can range from not understanding or using spoken language at all to having an above-average vocabulary but having little to say that is truly reciprocally conversational. Some of the specific difficulties that comprise the criteria for the type of communication impairment associated with autism are not unique to autism. However, these difficulties are ones that are very common in autism. This second area of impairment, communicative autistic learning disabilities, corresponds to Category B in the DSM-IV criteria for autistic disorder, "Qualitative impairments in communication." (see Table 3-4.)

The "qualitative impairments in communication" map onto four main areas of communicative autistic learning disabilities. The first two communicative ALDs involve receiving and sending communicative signals through nonverbal means. The second two communicative ALDs involve receiving and sending communicative signals through auditory channels.

Deficits in Understanding Body Language and Facial Expression. The first communicative ALD involves understanding body language and facial expression: Before speech ever emerges, body posture, gesture, and facial expression serve as a first language. After spoken language develops, body language and the face serve as additional "signals" that can reaffirm, contradict, or qualify the importance and urgency of what is being said. When a nonverbal "signal" is not received, decoding verbal communication is naturally a lot more difficult. For

TABLE 3-4

CHARACTERISTICS OF COMMUNICATIVE AUTISTIC LEARNING DISABILITIES

UNDERSTANDING BODY LANGUAGE AND FACIAL EXPRESSION

Definition:
> Child appears to have poor comprehension of gestures or facial expressions.

Learning Implications:
> Child misses paralinguistic "signal" that should qualify or even take the place of words. The child who does not look or show an expressive facial reaction to words may be seen as noncomprehending or even defiant.

Qualities:
> - Likely to ignore pointing/other hand gestures designed to influence behavior.
> - Likely to ignore positive facial expressions (smiles or nods of encouragement) designed to influence behavior.
> - Likely to ignore negative facial expressions (frowning, shaking head "no," or stern expressions) designed to influence behavior.

EXPRESSIVE BODY LANGUAGE AND FACIAL EXPRESSIVENESS

Definition:
> Child does not use a full or subtle range of facial expressiveness or body language to convey emotions communicatively.

Learning Implications:
> It may be difficult to ascertain if the child has comprehended a verbal or nonverbal "signal," especially in the absence of a linguistic response.

Qualities:
> - Lack of a physical response (approaching, sitting down when asked) may be taken as inattention (e.g., the child's having an attention deficit disorder).
> - Lack of physical response taken as noncompliance/defiance.
> - Child's reaction to events hard to "read."

UNDERSTANDING SPOKEN LANGUAGE

Definition:
> Child may initially comprehend mostly words with visual analogs because of strong visually based information-processing skills; may have processing-speed delays that selectively result in "masking" of what is said subsequent to the processing "bottleneck." Understanding is likely at least partly limited by topic, context, and person speaking—i.e., salience/attention to what is being said.

TABLE 3-4 (CONTINUED)

Learning Implications:

Many autistic children need language teaching with mnemonic use of two-dimensional and three-dimensional materials, and visually based actions to acquire language content. Content and context of teaching must also take into account interface with social autistic learning disability factors.

Qualities:

- Child may demonstrate comprehension of key words, and then use context cues to "fit" likely fuller meaning.
- Apparent "selective hearing"/"selective listening"; child responds reliably to some things (like a TV jingle), but not to others (her name).
- Words or phrases once heard may not reappear increasingly or ever again.

USING SPOKEN LANGUAGE

Definition:

Language is more often instrumental in content (designed to get a need for the self, or a self-interest, met) than expressive (sharing information/interests, chitchat). Autistic language may be marked by immediate echolalia or delayed echolalia, be telegraphic, or be marked by other idiosyncratic phrasing or use.

Learning Implications:

Earlier, language tends to be used to get needs met when it is either the only way or the most efficient way to do so. Later, development of spontaneous use and expressive functions are closely tied to talk about higher-interest areas.

Qualities:

- Immediate echolalia may have a range of functions such as to mark a turn in the conversation, indicate assent, or request clarification/further information.
- Delayed echolalia may be self-directed play, rehearsal of meaning, or larger segments as unparsed single units of meaning.
- Prosody (tone of voice) may be sing-songy or flat, but without cadence tied to word meaning.

many children with autism, the ability to make sense of the spoken word is often impaired as well.

Deficits in Expressive Body Language and Facial Expressiveness. The second area of communicative ALD considers expressive body language and facial expressiveness. If a child hasn't received, or has only partly received a verbal or nonverbal communicative signal, it will be difficult for the child to "send" any contingent or otherwise meaningful response. From the perspective of teaching the child with autism, disability in this area means needing to know what is received and what meaning is being attributed to nonverbal signals. Until the child with autism can be helped to attend to and process nonverbal communicative signals, this major compensatory strategy typically used by non-autistic children with language-processing disabilities is closed as well.

Deficits In Understanding Spoken Language. The third area of communicative ALD, understanding spoken language, is often the most impairing educationally. For many children with autism, the specific reason that they don't speak or that language is significantly delayed often requires assessing what other ALDs are present in order to gauge the likely efficacy of different treatment approaches. Remedial strategies for communication deficits must take into account the likelihood that there are communicative ALDs in understanding and using nonverbal communicative signals (a weakness), as well as the likelihood that there is a more intact capacity in visual memory and visual spatial abilities (strengths). These kinds of difficulties, as well as those presented by the ALDs in understanding and using nonverbal communication, will be discussed in chapter 6.

Deficits in Use of Spoken Language. The fourth area of communicative ALD is the use of spoken language. Again, there are characteristic impairments and characteristic strategies for remediation, such as focusing on the child's strongest areas of interest to motivate the communicative use of language. These will be discussed in detail in chapter 7.

NON-SOCIAL AUTISTIC LEARNING DISABILITIES
AND DSM "PATTERNS OF ACTIVITIES AND INTERESTS"

The third area of impairment associated with autism has to do with the atypical behaviors that are observed when one watches the child with autism interact with the objects in the world around him. This includes how the child with autism plays (or doesn't play) with toys, and whether the child focuses on just one part of an object (like a part that spins), or plays in a repetitive, and at times, almost frenzied fashion, performing the same action over and over. This third area of impairment largely corresponds to Category C of the DSM-IV criteria for autistic disorder, "Restricted, repetitive, and stereotyped patterns of behavior, interests, or activity."

Atypical "patterns of behavior, interests, or activities" map onto three main areas of non-social ALDs. The first two involve different disturbances in processing basic sensory inputs in a way that results in characteristic autistic symptoms that also represent barriers to learning. The third involves disturbances in how children with autism do or don't play with toys and other common objects, and how this in turn reflects on the child's capacity to internalize the meanings of objects and actions in the world around him. A fuller description of nonsocial ALDs as well as treatments for them are in chapter 8.

Abnormal Thresholds in Sensory Processing. The first area that has strong implications for a child's ability to learn is the characteristic ways in which children with autistic spectrum disorders can over- or under-attend to certain kinds of sensory information—tactile (touch), olfactory (smell and taste), vestibular (movement), visual, and auditory. Fundamental to meaningful information processing is knowing how relevant or irrelevant different continuous sensory inputs are perceived to be. When certain inputs are over-responded to), other inputs might be missed—like when a child stares at a row of chain links and fails to observe other activity on the playground, or stares at a glittery object, missing what is being said by the person holding it. When certain sensory inputs are not considered relevant, information is missed, and the perception of his surroundings that the child then creates is altered. This faulty picture, developed from disorganized perceptual experience, can go on

TABLE 3-5

CHARACTERISTICS OF
NON-SOCIAL AUTISTIC LEARNING DISABILITIES

LACK OF IMAGINATION IN PLAY

Definition:

    Children with autism tend to show little fantasy, limited representation of social situations, and limited language use as part of play. _

Learning Implications:

    Play should be a medium for practicing real and imagined social rules, including corresponding practice of associated language meaning, with language driving play and play driving language.

Qualities:

- No reenactment/rehearsal of socializing behaviors through play.
- No action as symbols to associate to verbal expression.

STEREOTYPED AND REPETITIVE INTERESTS

Definition:

    Children with autism tend to eschew novel objects and actions and prefer familiar actions with new or old objects, which in the absence of imagination in play, leads to a limited, stereotyped, and repetitive play repertoire.

Learning Implications:

    Aversion to novelty goes hand in hand with low curiosity, which should be a "lever" usually available to motivate learning. There therefore tends to be limited learning through exploration. Time spent in repetitive activity can be seen as mental "downtime" because no new information is being processed.

Qualities:

- May selectively focus on one sensory aspect of one kind of object ("flickability" of stringy materials).
- Unusually slow satiation with objects may initially appear to be very good concentration—before the persisting pattern of use of the object is seen as repetitive.
- May prefer routines and rituals because novelty is minimized and such a pattern may complement communicative autistic learning disabilities (i.e., visually versus language-based understanding of action).

to be quite a shaky foundation, making it difficult for the child to make full sense of events that follow.

Stereotyped and Repetitive Interests. The second area of non-social ALD can insidiously corrode the autistic child's ability to learn. Time spent at repetitive or stereotyped routinized play or other activity is essentially mental down time. The more time so spent, the less time for mastering new information. In addition, the great sense of satisfaction or even excitement that many children with autistic spectrum disorders experience when engaged in repetitive activities speaks to its self-reinforcing qualities.

Lack of Imagination in Play. The third area that has strong implication for the child's ability to learn is the lack of imagination in play that is virtually always notable. Play should drive language, and language should drive play, and so when either is absent, the other suffers. Remediating one provides the foundation for improvements in the other to occur in an ongoing and dynamic fashion.

HOW ARE AUTISTIC LEARNING DISABILITIES SHAPED?

In Part II of this book, we will begin an analysis of each area of autistic learning disability by developing an understanding of where that autistic learning disability arises. It is really helpful to understand what kinds of basic processing problems (primary, innate deficits) contribute to each area of ALD or each symptom of autism. With this understanding, it becomes possible to begin to think in terms of an individual child's autism. The child's DSM symptoms and ALDs can come to be seen as road maps showing where failures in apprehending and processing information occur. By thinking in terms of how these basic processing problems form the learning problems that we associate with autism, we can begin to explain the causes of learning failures. The ALDs, like the DSM symptoms of autism, are mostly not innate disabilities (as that term was used in the last chapter), but rather partly successful or failed self-accommodations to the child's innate disabilities. We can begin to see how some signs of autism are actually the child's automatic (and impressive) attempt to "rewire" around some of his own problematic circuitry, such as when instrumental communication like hand-leading is used because the child cannot resort to either verbal or referential nonverbal communication.

Designing treatment based on the perspective given in these last two chapters sometimes involves identifying activities such as self-accommodations already in place and helping the child to get them to work even more efficiently. Sometimes treatment involves starting from the point of failed self-accommodations and showing the child a way to operate more efficiently and thereby reduce his frustration and isolation.

I think of treatment for autism by visualizing water flowing down hill in a rocky stream, finally reaching a lake below. When there is a boulder in the stream, the water flows around it. Flow between tightly packed rocks may be slower, but all the water still flows down hill. Children's mental development can work the same way: When there is an obstruction to their information-processing (the boulder), the information flows around it—and gets to the lake (the child's understanding of the world) via a more circuitous path than if there were no boulders in the stream. Boulders may slow the flow, and really big boulders may dam parts of the stream and divert some water altogether. (Some children don't learn to communicate orally; some never have truly reciprocal peer relationships.) The trick to making sure that as much water gets to the lake as possible is motivation—teaching the child things he feels there is a reason to understand. The water in the lake represents the things that the child with autism has come to understand, because he was motivated to master and retain that knowledge. As long as the instruction continues to be meaningful and motivating to the child, the water will continue to flow. Water finds a way to flow or seep to its destination if it can. Our job is to engineer it.

CHAPTER CONCLUSIONS

In the next six chapters we will examine how the child's self-accommodations— or lack thereof—create a list of treatment issues for us to use to help children with autistic spectrum disorders. I will continually try to emphasize from where each autistic symptom comes, expanding upon the autistic learning disabilities model that has just been outlined. This is intended to allow the reader to think creatively about any symptom in any individual child with autism, to understand what innate disabilities and partial accommodations make up this child's way of expressing this symptom, and then, to learn how to go about remediating the specific problems that underlay the child's symptom and ability to learn.

PART II

Autistic Learning Disabilities and Autistic Learning Styles

What Makes the World
of the Autistic Child Different?

In the first of the three parts of this book, we took a look at what happens to the perceptions and information that are the basic inputs into the brain of the child with autism. Rather than looking at these issues from a neurophysiological point of view, we looked at signs and symptoms—a grouping or cluster of symptoms that reveal an underlying problem. A blind child has a different set of data to work with because he doesn't see. A deaf child has a different set of data to work with because he doesn't hear. We have some idea about how the worlds of the deaf or blind are reshaped by the phenomena of not hearing or not seeing. But how does autism give children a different data set? What's missing from their data set? What might they intensely focus upon in a way that deafness predisposes a deaf child to learn sign language so readily? How do we rewire around the weaknesses and utilize relative strengths as best we can? How do we come to understand this profile of weaknesses and strengths—autistic learning disabilities and autistic learning styles? How can information about how the profile is different for each child be used to individualize treatment plans?

In Part II, we will discuss a range of autistic learning disabilities that alter how a child with an autistic spectrum disorder sees the world. We will progress from this discussion into figuring out what we can do to help children compensate for each of these disabilities—once an individual child's particular ALDs and autistic learning strengths are identified. Then, in Part III of this book, we will examine how each of several well-known methods for treating autism rates when it comes to addressing a specific area of autistic learning disability. Understanding and using this approach allows parents to pick and choose among program features that may benefit their child. It also allows teachers and other therapists to design and tailor programs based on an individual child's needs.

CHAPTER FOUR

Social Autistic Learning Disabilities

What Are Social Autistic Learning Disabilities? In this chapter, we will discuss how disabilities in forming a social understanding of the world are central to defining autism. These difficulties in social understanding affect the way the child sees the world, the ways he can learn. We will describe some teaching approaches specifically aimed at helping the child affected by different aspects of these social autistic learning disabilities. Each major aspect of social ALDs will be fully described in this chapter. Each major area of social ALD can be traced to underlying and innate primary deficits that the child with autism experiences. These deficits, along with relatively stronger areas of perception and function, come together to form the characteristic signs and symptoms we consider to be the social hallmarks of autism. By understanding how these patterns form to create the social hallmarks of autism, we can start to understand how the learning process is systematically and predictably altered for the child with autism. Once we understand how learning is altered, it is much easier to figure out how to teach.

Steps in Understanding Social ALDs. Treatment design follows from deconstructing social ALDs back into primary, innate deficits to be remediated. In this way, it is possible to tailor an intervention approach specifically for the learning problems that exist in a particular child. (This might sound a little abstract right now, but all it means is that, for example, teaching something like peer play skills needs to be done differently for a child who understands language fairly well versus a child with little receptive language.)

THREE KEY DIMENSIONS OF
SOCIAL AUTISTIC LEARNING DISABILITY

Each social autistic learning disability is closely related to and overlaps the others. As a group, they emphasize three broad dimensions of social behavior in autism that stand as significant barriers to learning in the same ways that other children of the same age do. These three areas of social autistic learning disability were introduced in the last chapter (see Table 3-3). Social differences that affect how children with autistic spectrum disorders can learn can include a lack of awareness of others, a lack of response to social reward, and a lack of social imitation. These key dimensions of social ALDs can best be explained in a chronological order that reveals how parents usually begin to note that children with autistic spectrum disorders are viewing the world differently. These differences can be highlighted by describing various situations and reasons that the learning differences of the child with autism become increasingly apparent as the child interacts more with his world and is increasingly expected to respond to it. Difference are especially apparent when the child begins to have experiences with other children—siblings, relatives, day-care mates, or children of the same age who attend enrichment programs or preschool with the child.

RESPONSE TO PRAISE:
THE FUEL FOR THE SOCIAL ENGINE

How Does Lack of Response to Social Reward Affect Learning? Perhaps the most important way in which the learning ability of children with autism differs from others is in their poor response to social praise and encouragement. For parents, as well as teachers, it is a given that a child wants praise and attention and generally wants to please key adults. Of course, no child wants to please all the time, and the reason we call the "Terrible Twos" the "Terrible Twos" is that they mark the stage at which the toddler begins to derive pleasure from being defiant.

What goes on with an autistic child is quite different. If he appears defiant, it is because he is more interested in pleasing *himself* than in displeasing *you*.

This un-self-consciousness is undoubtedly part of the "mystique" of autism. The child runs on a different kind of power supply than everyone around him. Classrooms, and by extension, all teaching, even informal activities like a parent reading to his child are predicated on the assumption that the child is interested in you and therefore interested in pleasing you. If a parent reads to a child, the parent can usually assume that the child will be interested when the parent makes the story sound really interesting.. This gives the parent the "go ahead" to use story time as a place to teach new ideas. The typically developing child's interests and attention can be counted upon to follow the parent's.

What preschool is all about is the child's ability to transfer that desire to please mommy or daddy onto the teacher so that the teacher is viewed as she who must be obeyed and pleased. If the teacher did not have this tool at her command, her classroom life would be difficult. Now, picture this from the point of view of the child with autism: The teacher is no more important a focus than any randomly selected pupil. If the teacher lacks this magical salience (and the authority) that parents should have, why should a child sit in circle because the teacher said so? Why not look around the room and decide where else to go that might be more self-satisfying?

When I go to visit a preschool in which a pupil is pointed out to me as questionably autistic, I like to watch what happens at circle time. On many occasions, I can pick out the child who I am going to be asked to observe simply by the fact that he has a large or vigorous-looking instructional aide seated behind him in the circle. Her purpose will be to obstruct his attempts to escape. When circle starts to get very language-intensive, the young subject of my observation will make his break. Let's say he runs to the bunny cage in the back of the room. He tries to poke his finger at the bunnies through the wired mesh. He comes close to being bitten by the biggest bunny who thinks the little finger is food. (This is because he doesn't check back to see if an adult thinks what he's doing might be dangerous. We'll get to that problem later.) Often, in a typical preschool, this type of behavior is viewed as immature or poorly socialized, and the parent is frequently told that the child is not "ready" for preschool—try again next year. What can be missed here is that this child is not running away *from* the teacher. He is running *to* the bunnies. (He also does not look back to see if he will get in trouble for trying to "feed" the bunny his finger.) The hyperactive or poorly socialized child will look back at the teacher or aide as he escapes, often giggling with satisfaction. (He *is* running away from the teacher.) The child with autism never looks back. The running away is directed at satisfying his own interests—not at thwarting the teacher. However, many teachers more accustomed to the poorly socialized child, rather than the one with autism will see the child with autism, as defiant and, in any case, potentially disruptive to other pupils in the class.

Nevertheless, after getting the boot from a few more preschools, the more socially disconnected nature of the "defiance" shown by the child with autism is usually pinpointed. Sometimes, the child with autism may first be thought to have a hearing problem, or an emotional problem—*if* the teacher does conclude that the behavior is not directed at defying her. However, the core difficulty is a lack of desire to do certain things just to elicit a positive response from those in caregiving roles. This is the part that is core to autistic spectrum disorders. Of course, children vary in this respect in terms of severity and pervasiveness of this type of trait. Some children with autistic spectrum disorders who may be more emotionally tied in to parents may take notice of their parents' reactions—but no one else's, or may "tune in" only when the social cues from an adult are literally "in their face." For other children with autism, the desire to please is partly regulated by how "noisy" the social environment is—how many kids there are, how many are doing different things, how much talking there is, and the presence of other stimulation that he is not able to fully process. In a "noisier" environment, some children with milder autistic spectrum disorders turn off or shut down to social contingencies, but don't do so nearly as much in one-to-one encounters. This is a clue to why one-to-one home-based teaching can be so helpful for some children.

INSTRUMENTAL LEARNING STYLE

What Motivates a Child with Autism? If a child with autism is not motivated to do things to please others, what does motivate him? Children with autism are motivated to please themselves. In the last section we talked about how the child who didn't want to participate in circle ran *to* the bunnies, not *away* from the teacher. He was motivated to see bunnies, not for the teacher to think he was a well-behaved boy, a good listener, etc. It is easy to see how this organization of behavior is not compatible with being a ready and willing pupil.

All of us have some things we prefer to do that are more pleasing than other things. The difference for children with autistic spectrum disorders is that they will consistently choose to do the thing that is most pleasing to themselves, even if it displeases someone else. One of the things that I think gives children with autism an air of inscrutability and makes getting through to children with autism rewarding is this sense of detachment and living in their own world according to their own rules. Most children with autism certainly "march to the beat of their own drummers." There is a benign obliviousness, rather than a defiant rejection of what others want or expect. Some of this seeming detachment is a result of the absent theory of mind we discussed earlier: The child with autism can't "read" your mind, and so it makes it more difficult for you to read his. Some of the lack of desire to please key "others" is based in a lack of an affiliative orientation, a natural desire to be part of a group of similar individuals, be it a family, a sibling group, or a class. Just as we depend on the child to want to please people, we also assume that the child wants to fit in with his peer group. This is most often *not* the case for the autistic spectrum child. He is happy doing his own thing and appears to have little use for adopting the ways of the group. This was the quality that neurologist Oliver Sacks was writing about when he described Temple Grandin, a very intelligent woman with autism as an "anthropologist on Mars." Some children with autism will observe others but have no intrinsic drive to be part of the scene. In the words of a teenager with Asperger's syndrome, who was asked what two five-year-old boys might do with a couple of plastic triceratops, he replied, "Bang them together in some sort of Jurassic Park-type activity." Asked if he thought that would be fun, he replied, "Not very."

In any case, the job of intervention is to diminish or end the state of autistic detachment and replace it with a functional affiliativeness. An interesting biography of an adult with autism, Jessy, written by the woman's mother, Clara Claiborne Parks, is entitled "Exiting Nirvana": The title neatly illustrates the dilemma of working with children with autism—they may be quite happy in their detached little world. It is we who decide for them that it would be better if they struggled to understand how to join our world.

Motivation and Group-Based Instruction. What an instrumental learning style means in a learning context is that the child cannot be expected to strive to please others in the same way as other children. He will not be motivated to learn things just because those around him are being told, "Oh! You're so smart!" "What a great job!" "Clever boy!" These compliments as well as a sense of pride in one's own accomplishments, which allows the feelings of being praiseworthy to be sustained, are usually absent unless they are explicitly taught. They can be taught. Initially, however, this presents a significant problem for teaching a child with autism, or molding his behavior at home into more mature forms.

Lack of Response to Praise and Group Instruction. Teachers work under the assumption that a child will respond to praise, as has already been described. One important element of this is that verbal praise is something that can be used to direct the behavior of several children simultaneously, and need not be directed to a particular child. If all preschoolers were as "deaf" to praise as many very young children with autism are, every preschool class would behave like a herd of cats—adorable, warm, and fuzzy, but following their own lead.

Fortunately, while autistic children may not start off wanting to please the teacher, they do start off with *a* desire to please—themselves. By structuring activities so that the child derives some pleasure, satisfaction, or material gain from the teaching situation—that is, something he wants—he can be persuaded to take part in activities with instructional value. Children with autism can be thought of as running on different fuel: If most children are powered by gasoline, children with autism can be said to be powered by diesel. If you put gas in a diesel-powered vehicle, it's not going to go anywhere. A major area for developing instructional approaches for children with autism is to reorganize their motivational priorities so they can be helped to learn more readily and eventually to respond to the same kinds of motivators as other children. When this starts to happen, the child with autism may be able to begin to benefit from learning opportunities inherent in a wider range of circumstances.

It is one thing to note that the child with autism doesn't respond to social praise. It is another thing to restructure the learning environment so that the child is consistently motivated by something other than social approval. Then, it is another thing still, to address how social approval can come to be motivating. Picture a group of little preschoolers wearing signs that say "Will work for praise." Imagine one child whose sign says "Will not work for praise." Working for social praise is such a given that when we think about early education environments for young children, we don't always realize that if you turn off that channel, you have a very different experience. If the child cares little or not at all about the teacher's appraisal of him, he has much less reason to pay attention to figure out what he should be doing. If the child doesn't care if he earns the teacher's approval, why would he want to show evidence that he's learned something new? What this means is that many children with autistic spectrum disorders, at least at first, are going to learn very little in a group-based educational setting that is predicated on the idea that if the teacher says or does something, it is going to be interesting to understand whatever "it" is, just because it was the teacher's idea to teach the children about this topic. So, for example, why learn your colors? Because the teacher wants to know if you know what color shirt she's wearing? If you're interested in having her praise you, you might put on your "thinking cap" and try to give the right answer. If you see no reason to care, there's no reason to attend, no reason to think about it, and no reason to answer.

ESTABLISHING INSTRUCTIONAL CONTROL

Alternatives to Group-Based Teaching. When I talk about this inability to learn in a group-based setting with parents, I often hear "But, if he can't go to school, how is he going to learn anything? How is he going to learn to get along with other kids?" These are completely logical questions. It is not that the child can't ever go to school or ever benefit from normal school experiences, but that the child must first learn *how* to benefit from group-based instruction. This is an extra step in the educational process that usually does not have to be taken when the child is developing as expected.

Paired Association Learning. A common way of addressing this type of deficit is to teach a positive response to social praise by pairing it with nonsocial reinforcers—things the child currently *does* want. The most obvious and "classical" of these reinforcers is food that the child likes given in exchange for something we consider a learning experience. This is certainly not the only way to teach a child to respond to social praise, but it is the most basic and simple way. Once the child has had the opportunity to benefit from these teaching strategies aimed at making social praise and adult attention more worthy, the child becomes more ready to benefit from a wider range of educational environments—and from all kinds of experiences in which response to social attention is the coin of the realm.

IMITATION AS THE GATEWAY TO EARLY LEARNING

Why Is Imitation Important? Imitation is a very crucial conduit through which the one- to four-year-old child normally takes in a tremendous amount of information. Throughout that period of development when language has not yet been established as an internalized means of narrating and planning behavior and problem solving, imitative schema (maps) guide typically developing children through practice and mastery of new skills. Originally, psychologists referred to key aspects of this process as "assimilation," meaning that the child would first see something new, and then take parts of what she saw into herself and reenact what had been observed as self-initiated activity. Later, the child could be described as taking the newly acquired information and being able to use it to "accommodate" variations on the theme: A toddler seeing a new type of sand toy in the sand pit at the playground might be expected to first watch as a slightly older child added sand, turned a crank, and extruded small blobs of sand. If this looked incredibly interesting to the toddler, she might be expected to run up to the toy and either join in, or, if she was a more shy child, wait for the older child to leave the toy alone, and then pounce on a chance to imitate what she had just seen. That imitation of the first child's use of the sand-cranking machine would be "assimilation" of a new play schema. Later, the toddler might decide to pour water or small stones through the machine instead. She might decide to turn the machine upside down and see what happened if the sand went in the other end. The results of all these little "experiments" would allow the toddler to construct a database of information about this type of sand toy; first, by assimilating what she had seen the other child do, and second, by conducting her own experiments to "accommodate" the results of new information produced by her experiments with the sand-cranking machine to her understanding of how things like this might work.

Imitation as an Experimental Method. When a child with autism lacks the ability or drive to imitate things in the world around him, he fails to engage in critical self-initiated experiments that should allow him to construct a world of meanings for the objects and activities he sees. Imitation is a complex ability, and it is also a complex disability. Difficulties with imitation can be thought of as a convergence of at least two main areas of innate disability that may affect children with autism. As we discussed earlier, much of what we recognize as formal symptoms of autistic spectrum disorders can be seen as the result of multiple and converging innate disabilities that coexist in a way that makes for a characteristic pattern of disability as well as possible adaptations. This coming together of innate deficits was referred to earlier as the "matrix of abilities and disabilities" through which the child's difficulties as well as strengths form self-accommodations to what he cannot process in the usual ways. We will now examine possible components of a failure to imitate, with the goal of developing a better understanding of which underlying innate deficits may need to be addressed for a particular child when lack of imitation is identified as a learning deficit.

Imitation and the Desire to Be like Others. The first component of an innate disability that contributes to problems in imitation is the lack of an affiliative orientation. A big part of imitating is wanting to be like, and do like others. Typically, we do not *teach* our children to imitate; it is just something they begin to do spontaneously. When a child lacks the expected amount of drive to be like others, to be where others are, or to do what others are doing, the drive that underlies learning through imitation is gone or diminished. A child who is shy may seem to lack a desire to join with others, but this can be distinguished from autism because, in the child with autism, the lack of desire to join in is pervasive and present across many situations, but in the shy child it is usually most notable with groups of peers, in busy situations, or around relative strangers.

Imitation and a Theory of Another's Mind. The second innate ability that underlies imitation is the capacity for a theory of mind. When a child copies the actions of another, he implicitly reflects the understanding that there is something salient, something to be understood, a positive experience to be gained by doing what another is doing. Imitation is a way of "assimilating" what is in the mind of another through experiencing the experience of another. This explains the attraction to imitating peers: Peers have minds of similar complexity and organization, so the child can most readily "see" what it is that the peer is doing. (This may also explain why some parents and teachers note that autistic children will imitate a bad behavior more readily than a good behavior: Bad behaviors tend to be mentally simpler behaviors to execute. A bad behavior, like biting or hitting, is often a means to an end, which does not require theory of mind, just simple cause and effect, to understand.)

Imitation and Novelty Seeking. A third innate ability that drives imitation is response to novelty. As we discussed, children with autism often have the opposite response to novelty from other children. They tend to run from novelty rather than seek it. The typical toddler is most likely to want to imitate something rather novel and salient, something that really catches his attention. Therefore, Barney is more interesting to copy than Peter Jennings. The child with autism, however, does not attend to novel things as readily, and so, in avoiding novelty, misses the salience that novelty brings—the Barney traits (purple-ness, bulbous-ness, gawkiness) that might otherwise seem captivating. This is not to say that children with autism don't like Barney—many do. However, it is more likely that Barney's familiarity and the repetitiveness of what he does, not his novelty, makes him attractive.

In many ways, the absence of imitation, or a low or limited level of imitation, is probably one of the biggest learning handicaps of a developing child with autism. There is so much he should be taking in via observation of others. Lack of observation of others has a pervasive effect on the amount of information the child takes in. This failure to "assimilate" new information, in turn, profoundly affects the child's ability to "accommodate," or to develop further information by relating new experiences to existing schema.

How Children Learn Imitation. Let's go through an example that demonstrates learning through imitation in a typically developing child that may provide a model for the way children with autism also can be taught to imitate: The 14-month-old gets a present. It is a stuffed cow. The father waves it around, saying, "Cow! Cow! Moo! Moo!" He tickles the baby with it. The baby is interested, thinks this is very cool, grabs for the cow, waves it, and says, "Ca-Ca! M-o-o-o-!" several times. He gets a lot of parental attention for having done so well at this little lesson. Later, the 14-month-old's five-year-old sister is playing with her farmyard set, and the 14-month-old toddles through her neatly arranged corral, grabs a plastic cow, and shows Dad, saying, "Ca-Ca! M-o-o-o!" A behaviorist would say that the 14-month-old has "generalized" what a cow is. We could also say that the 14-month-old "assimilated" his dad's cow use, and then accommodated his newly acquired cow schema to include plastic cows as well as stuffed cows.

Imitation and the Behavioral Concept of "Generalization." Understanding how and why a 14-month-old imitates is critical because we often hear behaviorally oriented teachers commenting on how something the autistic child has learned hasn't "generalized" yet. What is meant is that the child has learned to respond to one example of a learning target, but has not shown the predilection to use that information elsewhere. For example, a child might learn to "touch cow" using a six-inch, hard rubber cow, but will not yet "touch cow" if a larger, soft-flocked cow is used. Why not? How is the process of learning different for the child with autism? He has not learned through imitation. Usually, the procedure is to "motor prompt" the child with autism, taking his hand and putting it on the cow (rather than the pig) when he is asked to "touch cow." The prompt is used less and less until the child can discriminate between a cow and a pig on his own. When he does this correctly, he gets half a pretzel stick or some other treat he likes.

There are several key differences in the learning process so far for the 14-month-old and for the child with autism. First, the autistic child's actions are motivated by cause and effect, not a desire to imitate (that is, to do like, or be like someone else). He has figured out what to do to get the pretzel stick. (He did not use theory of mind—"I will have fun if I do this with this cow, too!" but rather simple cause and effect.) He did not begin the activity spontaneously, but his behavior was systematically "shaped" to "touch cow" starting from the level at which he was physically shown to do it. (He did not seek novelty.) The child with autism likely engaged in this activity with no social reference to the teacher before or after identifying the cow. (There was no affiliative orientation motivating a desire to do as the teacher had done.) There was no "generalization" because critical components of the learning experience—the novelty seeking as part of the learning experience, and motivation to engage in this activity because someone else interesting did it first—were lacking.

What does this mean? Is motor prompting not a good way to teach children with autism? No, it doesn't mean it's not a good way of teaching. It can help the child attend to something he might otherwise avoid attending to. Giving a food reward sustains and organizes attention around a goal (the food), which is important for the child when social attention alone is not that relevant. It does work to teach specific examples, and sometimes in the process, the child becomes interested enough in the materials or in the way the teacher is teaching to retain this information in a qualitatively different way that promotes assimilation and accommodation. In this case, teaching must include materials that are intrinsically interesting to the child to increase the probability that the materials themselves will stimulate the desire to learn more, just as they do in a typically developing child.

This slightly different understanding of imitation should help one understand how to construct teaching situations. If the child *is* interested in some qualities of the teaching materials, there is a chance that the child *will* become increasingly interested in the teaching interaction. By providing opportunities for imitative learning for children with autism in a way that stimulates the same innate functions that govern more typical patterns of learning through imitation, there is a better chance that acquired information will be retained, used, and added to, as it is with a typically developing child. The point is that an aspect of typical development, like imitation, can be deconstructed into its innate components—affiliative drive, theory of mind, and novelty seeking (things we talked about in chapter 2)—to describe how, why, and when imitation promotes learning. In the case of autism, the first step in remediation of the failure to imitate is to deconstruct it into these same innate components—affiliative drive, theory of mind, and novelty seeking. Weakness in any of those areas, or often in all three, will limit imitative learning. Any of these possible innate weaknesses must be addressed to improve capacity for imitative learning. By bolstering the underlying deficits (such as by using intrinsically interesting materials so the novelty of the materials benefits rather than inhibits learning) we model typical development of imitative learning and thereby give momentum to the generative, motivating qualities of learning through imitation. Said more simply, the child with autism may start to imitate after he has been stepped through imitation of an activity, and it has turned out to be fun.

So, imitation can be increased by manipulating the novelty of the teaching materials: A child with autism may be happy to imitate "waving" using a twirling battery-operated pom-pom with flashing lights, but may remain uninterested in waving a baton. Similarly, imitation can be increased by tweaking the "affiliative-drive" component of imitation, such as when a peer provides a model of an activity that is developmentally at the child with autism's own level, and so is more readily experienced as interesting. In the next section, then, we'll discuss how peers fit into learning.

SALIENCE OF PEERS

Why Are Other Kids So Interesting (Or Not)? Another important dimension that sets the learning style of children with autistic spectrum disorders apart from peers is that they do not seem to find peers salient in the same way that other children do. Put very simply, peer pressure means little. From as early as 18-24 months of age, peer pressure should mean something. (For example, I remember visiting a day-care center for typical toddlers at which it was the practice to bring a potty-trained two-and-a-half-year-old into the room with the 18- to 24-month-olds and encourage the 18- to 24-month-olds to "watch" while the two-and-a-half-year-old used a potty chair successfully, while basking in the lavish praise of the teacher.)

There is peer pressure, and there is peer pressure: No one wants to raise a child who becomes a six-year-old slave to fashion, or a seven-year-old who thinks he won't be able to face his friends if you don't buy him the latest Harry Potter video the weekend of its release. However, being responsive to peers can be seen on a whole different level in the case of children with autism. We can do this by looking at the study of ethology, the social and adaptive function of how groups of animals behave together. We can see that higher mammals all have organized ways in which they relate to peers. Interestingly, just as in humans, much of it can be described as play. What are juvenile animals playing at? Life. Play for young animals, as well as for young children, is practice for the roles and relationships they will have as adults. Children tune in to peers as a way of learning and practicing skills of group membership. Belonging to a group is intrinsically important, and an ethologist would argue that this behavior has evolved in humans from the behavior patterns of animals for which affiliation with a group equaled safety. This casts an importance on teaching affiliative behavior that we usually don't even think about when children with autism refuse to play with others. Play is not just so the child can occupy his time, and not look different. Play readies children for social relations as adults.

When I speak with parents of children who are brought for an autism assessment, the child's disinterest in peers is often initially regarded as individualism, as his seeing peers as uninteresting, or else is simply regarded as something the child is not good at because he has had very limited exposure to peers. Certainly, there are individual differences in how sociable children are, just as there are for adults. Certainly, many children with autism have distinctive and well-defined odd or narrow interests that may not be shared by age mates. Certainly, skill and successful interactions with peers increase as a result of experience.

Nevertheless, for many parents, lack of salience of peers is the first really convincing sign of autism: A parent might tell me of going to Gymboree class and watching her 22-month-old rush away from the peer group as soon as she lets the child off her lap so she can help raise the unfolded parachute that all the other toddlers rush under screaming with delight. With many "enrichment" classes for children as young as eight months, parents may notice that their infant is the only one not taking much notice of other infants as the teacher chirps on about Mozart, Bach, and Beethoven. (It is not unexpected, however, for all the babies to ignore the teacher in this sort of "lesson.") The early differences in eschewing peers that parents notice can be important *specific* indicators of autism since many other early signs of autism, especially early language delays alone are seen in infants and toddlers with everything from ear infections or bilingual homes to those with language disorders or mental retardation not associated with autism.

Development of Interest in Peers. The preference to be with peers compared to adults starts late in the first year of life and is quite marked by the preschool years in typically developing children. Distressed children of any age do tend to retreat to their parents. Anxious children cling to their parents more than those who are not anxious. A calm and alert three-year-old in a familiar room with his mother and a familiar peer, however, will most likely prefer to do something with the peer rather than his mother for much of the time.

We have already discussed the importance of imitation for learning—with an emphasis on its applications in acquiring concepts or language. However, social skills are partly learned imitatively too—and are driven by this desire for peer affiliation and acceptance: Recently, I visited an Early Start class for children with autism. On my way there, I passed a Head Start class for typical preschoolers. They were assembling outside their classroom, and their teacher was asking them to "line up." One child (a born leader, we can guess) had taken this very literally (as preschoolers will do), and was balancing on a four-inch-wide painted line running along the sidewalk paralleling the outside of the classroom. Within 30 seconds, *everyone* was balancing on this line, watching one another and evaluating their own and one another's success—having a great time. The desire to "do like" and "be like" others was in full force.

Why Peer Pressure Is Important to Teachers. The foregoing story of preschoolers lining up is a mundane example, but teachers of preschool-aged children regularly capitalize on this tendency. Very often, instructional activity has been organized so that children with a lower level of mastery of the activity can benefit from seeing others perform the activity. Think about circle time in a special-education preschool class that might have a child with autism in it. The teacher asks, "What's the weather today?" She helps out by handing the first child a cloud with Velcro on the back. The child comes to the front and sticks the cloud on a board next to a picture of the school. The next child is asked, "Is it cloudy, or is it sunny?" This child is offered a choice of a cloud and a sun, and picks the cloud without help, as does the third child. By the time it's the fourth child's turn, there has been plenty of opportunity to observe the correct response and do what the other children have all done. If that fourth child is a child with Down's syndrome—he will likely be chomping at the bit for his turn and probably will pick the cloud (as imitation is generally little affected by Down's). He will likely pick the cloud even if he understands little or no language, because he will simply want to imitate the other children. However, if the fourth child is a child with autism, the modeling of the desired response by the first three children has probably meant little. It is very likely that the first three turns have not left him chomping at the bit for *his* turn. He probably won't pick the cloud—or spontaneously do anything with his cloud, just because it has been handed to him. If the most interesting thing he can think to do with the cloud is to flick it, he will flick it.

A child with autism who has marked difficulties with imitation is not going to benefit from circle time or any type of group activity predicated on the idea that his performance will be amplified and motivated by peers having performed the same or similar task. Much of early childhood group-based instruction assumes that a new child will want to become more like others in the group and be motivated to engage in the focal activity because everyone else already finds it fun and interesting. One manifestation of how peer pressure is used as a teaching strategy is that preschools tend to have rolling admissions—with kids entering the program throughout the year—as they turn three, four, etc., rather than all starting together at the same time. This way, the teacher is aided by children familiar with the routine who provide needed models for newer pupils.

Low Interest in Peers and Implications for Learning. There are two obvious and important conclusions we can draw from our observations about the difficulties children with autistic spectrum disorders have because peers lack salience for them: First, group-based instruction that naturally relies on the whole group's wanting to participate and attend together is likely going to lack the intrinsic motivational value it has for typically developing children compared to children with autism. Without this source of motivation to attend and participate, the child is likely to learn less, much less, than a child for whom the situation is intrinsically motivating. Second, the child must be helped to see peers as interesting. Once this is accomplished, the child can begin to benefit from instruction delivered in ways more typical for others at the same point in development. Sometimes we hear terms like "incidental learning" or "social learning," which refers to the fact that children learn many things they are not explicitly taught and that have not been broken down for them into smaller components. It seems likely that this type of learning is fairly minimal while peer salience is low, and these methods, which will be examined in more detail later, require some prerequisite building of interest in what it is that peers do.

DESIGNING TREATMENTS FOR
SOCIAL AUTISTIC LEARNING DISABILITIES

The preceding sections have discussed the ways in which the child with autism learns differently because of his inability to construct an understanding of how people interrelate, why they interrelate, and the way they get new information from doing it. Now, we will discuss a number of ideas for helping children with autism overcome these barriers of social incomprehension.

MOTIVATION

The Art of Giving Reinforcement

The first task in starting to work with a child with autism is to decide how you are going to motivate that child. There is plenty written about the science of giving reinforcement. There are many different kinds of "reinforcement schedules." We can talk about these. However, I would argue (and some might disagree) that teaching anything using reinforcement procedures of any sort is more of an art than a science when it is well done. This means that a parent or teacher can certainly be as good at this as any behavioral specialist when just a few basic principles are kept in mind.

Anyone who has ever taken a basic psychology course, had a dog, watched a public TV program on training horses, or visited Sea World is familiar with the idea that giving a rat, a dog, a horse, or a whale a piece of food can be a persuasive means of getting that animal to do what you want. Basically, it is not all that important to the animal why you want him to do the foolish thing you want him to do; it is only important that after he does it, he will get a desired food reward. This will work for children with autism too, and for the same reasons.

It is not a bad idea to use food rewards to motivate a child with autism to do a task. It is just not a very sophisticated way—and not one that is likely to instill an intrinsic love of the task. It may not increase the likelihood of the child's being motivated to do that task again without a promise of the beloved food reward. So how do you motivate a child with autism to want to do things that are good for him to learn without putting him on a high calorie diet?

Pairing Nonsocial and Social Rewards. The first principle, which has been discussed a bit already, is that the child with autism needs help to learn to value the same kinds of social rewards that the rest of us value. Whether at home or at school, both parents and teachers rely on the child's responding to social praise, positive evaluations of performance, and acknowledgment of empathetic, sympathetic, and altruistic acts as good behaviors worth repeating in the future. When these types of social praise are paired with forms of reward the child currently cares about, eventually, the social praise alone will take on reward value. A main approach to teaching children with autistic spectrum disorders to overcome their failure to respond to social praise is to pair praise with tangible rewards, things the child does value. It is important to remember this goal. When a child is given a treat and a "Good Job!" for successful task completion, it is not just success on the task that is the goal: In later life, it will be far more important that the individual be motivated by social praise than that he be able to complete a ten-block shape sorter. This means that social praise accompanying tangible rewards for successful performances should resemble the kind of social praise to which you'd like the child to respond in the future when the tangible reward is no longer used.

The aspect of the instruction that involves putting tangible rewards and social praise together is critical. The balance between keeping the child motivated, helping the child become more self-motivated, and helping the child work for social praise alone is what moves the child toward a greater degree of independence in the future. That balance is maintained by several factors: the reinforcement schedule used, the reinforcers used, and the integration of reinforcers into teaching so that reward becomes intrinsic to the learning experiences the child has.

Reinforcement Schedules. The term "reinforcement schedules" refers to how often the child receives a reward for keeping with an activity and for completing it successfully. There are basically three types of reinforcement schedules: fixed, ratio, and variable. A fixed schedule means the reward comes at a completely predictable time—which could be every ten seconds, every ten minutes, or every time a piece goes in the form board. In this system, the child gets the expected reward if he is doing what he is supposed to be doing when it is time for the reward. With younger children, shorter intervals between rewards are used to increase the chance that they will continue to succeed, and to retain interest in the activity by associating it with lots of reward.

Other reinforcement schedules provide rewards more intermittently: The ratio schedule is indexed to the child's ongoing success, say, every third time a correct piece is placed in the form board the child is rewarded. The variable reinforcement schedule is the trickiest: The child is never sure when the next reinforcer is coming, but it does. The idea is that if you have learned that working brings on the reinforcer, you will work harder hoping that producing more work will increase the likelihood that the next reward will come sooner. Which should be used in teaching children with autism?

It seems intuitively obvious that if you are doing something new and not particularly likeable, more frequent rewards should help. So, fixed-interval reinforcement is fine for the littlest kids, or kids doing new tasks—those needing lots of encouragement to stay with a learning activity. As the task becomes more familiar, though, and mastery of the task increases, fewer reinforcers tend to be needed to produce success. This is where the ratio reinforcement scheme comes in handy. "Success is its own reward," as they say. However, as it turns out, variable reinforcement schedules pull the best effort from people (and lab rats too). The art of using variable reinforcement is to know when to use the reward. Say a child started to learn to do a particular puzzle by getting a blueberry after each piece. Then, let's say he would do the puzzle even if he got a blueberry only after the fifth and tenth pieces. He has gone from ten blueberries a puzzle to two. Now, it's two weeks later, and this puzzle hasn't been out during that time. When it's taken out, the child seems uninterested in recapturing his earlier competency with this puzzle. What should the teacher do? Go back to ten blueberries, or stick it out with two, knowing he should be able to do it if he wants? It is at this point that a well-executed variable-reinforcement schedule can be of great value. If the child waves the first puzzle piece around, ignoring exhortations to "finish the puzzle," but finally places the piece, by all means, give the boy a blueberry right away. If he then places three more pieces quickly, but then flags, egg him on, and when the piece is in—another blueberry; maybe another blueberry after the next piece—just to ensure against further recidivism. The teacher needs to know when the child is applying himself, and when he is not really trying, and pace the blueberries accordingly. The real goal is to reward motivated behavoir.

Motivation: A Reward Hierachy for Reinforcement. Before teaching can begin, however, the first task is to think about what a particular child cares about most in order to develop a list of tangible reinforcers. The reinforcer could be a food, a toy, something the child likes to look at, or a sensory experience like bouncing on the bed. A reward hierarchy can be developed just by making a matrix. The list should have several headings; common ones are foods, toys, sensory activities. For each entry, there should be three columns: 1) what the reward is, 2) how the reward can be titrated, and 3) how rewarding the reward is.

Titration of Rewards. First, think about how small a particular item can be meaningfully titrated. For example, I personally do not have success with pretzel sticks broken into more than four segments. Baking M&Ms are about a quarter of the size of snack M&Ms and most kids do not seem to mind that the smaller ones are semi-sweet and not milk chocolate. Most children will be unhappy about a broken Pepperidge Farms Goldfish or a broken Oreo. Giving the child a bite and then taking the food away is too distracting. A spoonful of something is better.

A great alternative to food rewards, if it is desirable to the child is a more social sensory reward: For many children, a stroke on the face or arm, a kiss, or a "high-five" or clapping might work. In many instances, these are preferable so long as they still have high reinforcement value, because they are more naturalistic and more like what a child might receive along with praise in a regular classroom.

Non-social sensory reinforcers are often easier to use for children who respond in a more limited way to social sensory rewards. These non-social sensory reinforcers tend to be more reliable than food rewards, as the child will eventually become satiated if too much of a good edible thing is given. Not all children have sensory rewards that "fit" on their reward hierarchy. They may love to run through the drapes, but the drapes may be at home and the child may be at school. Similarly, a push on a swing requires a change of settings that might not be practical to the flow of instruction. However, a modified "swing," like rocking a child in his chair, may be fun for him. With sensory rewards, it is important to use enough to be rewarding, but not so much as to be distracting. When using a mechanical toy that the child finds exciting, it can help for the adult to maintain control of the object: Recently, I was to test a child during a school visit. I was handed a toy that looked like a pen-flashlight with a doodad to make it into a personal fan for hot days. This one though, didn't have a fan, but a clown with flashing eyes and a tinsel hula skirt that spun around when turned on. Then I was brought a child I was told would work for nothing else. I kept control of the flashing-eyed, hula-dancing clown, knowing that if I handed it over for the child to operate, testing would be finished.

Giving the child access to a sensory item or toy can be tricky because it will have to be taken away after a brief exposure; and which if it is really a reward, the child will be unhappy. The two things that can be done to mitigate this are 1) to make the particular item unavailable at other times so that playing with it for brief periods is the only alternative, and 2) to routinize the take-away with a countdown, or presentation of a "stop" symbol; then don't look back: Once it's gone, it's gone.

Judging the Salience of the Reward. The second column of the reward hierarchy for each item is a rating of how much this child really likes this item. For some children, this rating system will change daily; for others, never. There is no accounting for taste. Some children will do anything for a slice of raw onion; others want a ratty, chewed Ronald McDonald Happy Meals figurine. The important thing is how rewarding the item is to the child at that point in time. The point of this column is that the biggest rewards should be reserved for the greatest accomplishments such as completing a particularly long work session, doing something new and challenging for the first time, achieving a more self-guided completion of the task, or doing a task better than ever before. Also, when a child begins to flag and can be successfully redirected back to work, a higher value reward is called for as soon as a new activity is completed.

Motivation: A Reward Hierarchy for Teaching. So far, we have been talking in terms of how different kinds of rewards can be used at different times to mark the successful completion of a desired activity. We have talked about how the giving of these rewards should be a natural reflection of how hard the child has worked on each part of a task. One big piece is still missing: That piece can be described as "intrinsic" reinforcement or "direct" reinforcement. In an ideal situation, the task is its own reward. With typically developing children, they sit and listen carefully to a story because they find the story interesting. A child with autism may be active for an extended period precisely lining up objects—because it interests him. Getting it all "done" interests him. The motivation is there. The teaching challenge is to transfer that motivation onto new learning tasks that the adult, rather than the child, selects.

The best place to start in this endeavor is the child's reward hierarchy. Yes, banana slices can be a nice reward, but they can also be counted, making the eating of a banana slice into an activity that moves the child closer to understanding one-to-one correspondence (counting just one number for each object). In addition, the banana slices can be small and large. They can be on the red plate or on the blue plate. A new concept the child doesn't have (like size or color) can be paired with something he's interested in, like bananas. But, if the plate has round yellow disks that you can't put in your mouth, what's the point? The child with autism is much more interested when the materials, actions, or context include something that holds a high level of interest. "Down" is a much more meaningful concept when "we all fall down!" on the trampoline.

Instruction that integrates the child's interests is key for all children. Autistic children just tend to have different and narrower interests. By working from the child's specific interests, you play to that child's strengths—his greatest chance to be motivated and then to succeed at whatever the task.

"There's Nothing He Wants." Not everyone loves M&Ms, or pretzel sticks, or Cheetos. Sometimes I am told there is nothing this child will work for—the child likes nothing. He eats nothing. He plays with nothing. Well, I ask, what does this child spend his time doing? Every child has something he likes and prefers over other things. For some children reinforcers can be hard to identify. Among these children, there are usually repetitive sensory stimuli that are really enjoyed. In limited doses, these can be on the list of tangible reinforcers too.

Even the youngest, most severely withdrawn, or severely retarded children do some things rather than other things. Maybe I am told that this child likes to flick strings in the right-hand periphery of his vision. Fine. That can be an item on the reinforcement hierarchy. In fact, it can be several items. Some people worry that it is not good to reward the child with things that are used by the child in perseverative play, and which the child likes so much that they raise his level of arousal (inducing him to flap his arms, hop, etc.). There is in fact no good evidence to support this, but rather evidence to the contrary—that objects used for so-called self-stimulation *are* effective as reinforcers. Make a list of all the things the child commonly finds stringy in just that right way. At first, these can be used alternately as brief rewards. After a while, giving a choice of which string is preferred for each reinforcement break could be a whole activity unto itself. Then, things could be tied to the string as a bit of a handle or ballast. At reward time, choosing the allowable reward according to the identity of the ballast item could be a task unto itself. As the child develops preferences among his stringy things, he is helping you identify new things that might be related to the preferred stringy things that can go on the reinforcer list too. For example, a fan of strings with whom I worked came to really like a cheap helicopter party favor with a pull string that launched its propeller. Then came other helicopters, other planes, other vehicles. Stringing beads and assembling pop-bead chains became another "string"-related activity. The point is to integrate the reward and teaching functions where possible so that the child's curiosity and self-initiation are piqued to as great an extent as possible.

The Role of Choice in Motivation. The final and very important dimension of motivation is choice. Choice motivates everyone. If you made a list of the things you planned to do on a Saturday, which would you prefer—someone telling you the order in which you had to complete your activities, or your deciding for yourself? What if you didn't get to have a cup of coffee until after you'd done two car pools, watched a Pee-Wee soccer game, and gotten groceries? Even the mellowest person would prefer to have some choices. Most classrooms for typically developing younger children are set up so there is some choice. Free play time, roaming work stations, and recess are all examples. In older grades, pupils have choices about which book to read for a book report, what topic to choose for a science project, or whether to do their math or history homework first.

In working with children with autism, the same deference needs to be given to choice, too. Choice can be used to increase the motivation and interest level associated with any work. If a teacher has three puzzles for a child to do, letting the child successively choose which to do can be predicted to result in more on-time working, less time-avoiding work, and greater accuracy in completing the work. There are always choices a child can be given: where to sit, which pencil to use, what reward will be earned when the task is complete. For children who seem unmotivated, pairing a choice of a sometimes-preferred activity with a neutral activity, or even an undesirable activity can get the choosing process working.

One of the strengths of building choice activities into learning experiences for children with autism is that the child must take the initiative to make a choice. Being a "self-starter" when it comes to many learning activities is an area of weakness for many children with autism. Deciding on an activity is a way of making a commitment to your work, and choosing the reward he will receive encourages the child to make a commitment to the integrity of his effort to earn his reward.

Token Economies. One way children can be helped to begin to internalize the sense of working for a longer-term goal is by introducing the idea of what are sometimes described as "token economies." A token economy is where a reward is deferred until the end of activity, the end of the day, or the end of the school period. Children must first understand the simple cause-and-effect principles behind "doing something to get something," which is part of basic reinforcement, irrespective of whether they are being reinforced on a fixed or more variable schedule. Token economies work best when the child can be helped to have some sense of when the deferred reward will have been earned.

There are a couple of tricks that can be useful in introducing token economies and moving children away from more immediate and tangible reinforcers. First, simply allow reinforcers to accumulate in front of the child. Goldfish crackers can "dive" into a clear "pond" (a closed jar with a small opening) each time a reward is earned, with a snack time to eat them at the end of the teaching session. If the reward is not an easily titrated food (that is, it's hard to break into bits), a similar strategy is to have a picture of the reward (say, a computer screen with a favorite game displayed). The picture can be cut into parts and each can be Velcro-ed one at time to the token board as tasks are completed. When the whole screen is formed, the child knows the reward has been earned and can go independently to get his reward. This is a nice system because the child can constantly see how much of the needed progress has already been made.

For older children, these strategies can be more complex. Points can be earned or lost during the day, and specific lists can be posted showing which activities or behaviors earn points and which lose points. Some children have just one or two problem behaviors that really need to be under control before they can proceed with learning. This might include a child who jumps out of his seat and darts around the room, or a child who gets too loud and boisterous. In these situations, you can use a warning system in the form of a construction-paper traffic signal on the child's desk or a nearby wall. A green light indicates good behavior; a yellow light indicates the child is in a warning period, and points will be lost for the next infraction; a red light indicates that there is a permanent point loss and possibly a time-out or other consequence.

The purpose of each of these "tricks" is to help the child internalize self-monitoring strategies and learn to recognize what it feels like to be on task, almost done, almost losing privileges, or actually loosing them. The child with an autistic spectrum disorder is often very visually oriented, and so these visual strategies seem to be a particularly good way to convey a message that is otherwise likely to be lost in complex language the child may or may not fully comprehend.

FROM MOTIVATION TO
SOCIAL LEARNING AND PEER RELATIONS

So far, we've discussed the learning problems that arise from the fact that motivation is organized very differently for the child with autism. Although motivation comes from within for all children, for the child with autism, this drive more often than not centers on his interest in meeting his own needs rather than a drive to please others. Nowhere in development can this phenomenon seem more striking than when watching children with autism when they are among other children. Children of all ages have a natural affinity for one another and find the one another's activities endlessly fascinating. Not so for the child with autism. Often, the best approach for the child with autism is to draw him toward peers using activities that both the child with autism and the typically developing child find interesting. As the two can share the activity, the gratifying aspects of the play become associated with the playmate. This is the same learning strategy we use when we pair food reinforcers with social praise during direct teaching. After a while, the use of food can be phased out, and praise is motivating enough. Similarly, sharing preferred activities (as long as there are enough toys to go around) can build that same sort of positive association and acceptance. The development of peer relationships must be constructed from the bottom up, and, in this part of this chapter, we'll undertake to explore this topic.

PEERS

Is the child interested in peers? If not, does he actively avoid peers? Look away? Move away? Run away? Is he more avoidant of unfamiliar peers? Is he more avoidant in new places? More avoidant in crowded settings? If the child avoids some peers sometimes, does he take an interest in certain peers at other times? Is this an active interest? Will he approach? Will he try to be part of another child's or children's activities? Will he copy certain kinds of things he sees others doing? If he isn't likely to approach, will he watch passively? Can you tell how he feels about the play from the expression on his face (e.g., worried, excited)?

An assessment of where a child is in regard to all of these questions is important, as the teaching of social play skills needs to move forward from where the child is at to where, developmentally, the next step is. It is important to distinguish a child's "typical" level of social play from his "best" play. Many parents and teachers can produce a vignette or two about when a child with autism had some sustained contact with peers, but teaching play skills needs to take into account what usually happens. For example, Alex, a four-year-old boy with autism was at preschool. He called out to Liam, "What's your name?" Liam replied, "My name's Liam!" Alex said, "No, my name's Liam!" Liam said, "No, your name is Alex; my name is Liam!" A little girl sitting nearby chimed in that her name was Theresa. This sounded like a pretty typical preschool dialogue until a teacher told me that one of their concerns with Alex was that the only thing he seemed to know to say to peers was "What's your name?" Much of Alex's other language use was very repetitive, though he had no apparent difficulty understanding what people meant by what they said. In this case, we wouldn't want to start teaching peer interaction by involving Alex in rule-oriented games as this might feed repetitiveness but something simpler, like some things that you say after you approach such as "Want to go play bikes?" or "I've got a yellow crayon!"

DEVELOPMENTAL CONSIDERATION IN A PEER/PLAY PARTNER
Play Models for the Youngest Children with Autism

Play Partners by Developmental Level versus Chronological Level. One of the big socialization questions that should always come up when planning to introduce a child with an autistic spectrum disorder to more typical peers for the first time is how old should the peers be. The most intuitive response is to put the child with children his own chronological age, since the end goal is for the child to "act his age." However, if the question is asked from a developmental perspective, the answer is different: If the child has visual-motor, visual-spatial, and other problem-solving skills that are at the 18-month-level, put him with 18-month-olds. So, if an almost four-year-old-child with autism plays with toys in a simple, basic way—rolling cars down ramps, using shape sorters, making very basic tea parties—that child is playing like an 18-month-old. (For parents who aren't sure how to "stage" their child's play, I suggest they look at typical child development parenting books, which usually have plenty of charts and figures with illustrations of milestones like these.) The reason to put the autistic almost-four-year-old with one-and-a-half-year-olds is twofold: First, spontaneous peer interactions start when children see another child doing something they consider interesting. What a one-and-a-half-year-old considers interesting is anything he, personally, likes to do. By putting two children (one autistic, one typically developing) who are at the 18-month developmental level together for play, there is the greatest chance for them to have interests in common. By putting together two children (one autistic, one typically developing) who are both chronologically almost four, there will likely be little play because of few shared interests. The typically developing four-year-old might be assigning roles in play, stating rules, specifying an imaginary scenario, and so on. The autistic child would be lost and left out. He is being given an insurmountable challenge. Why would he want to join such play when he could go roll trucks with someone else rolling trucks?

Social and Play Skills of Three-Year-Olds. The second reason for more developmental and less chronologically based peer play opportunities is less obvious: Typically developing children under four or five are very poor at revising their social overtures for someone developmentally less adept than themselves. If a typical three-year-old says "Wanna play?" to a new kid on the playground, and the new kid doesn't look, smile, follow, or say "Yeah!" in about five seconds, the three-year-old will figure the other guy doesn't want to play and drift away. Preschool-aged children have very few skills to "repair" a social interaction. However, if a six-year-old sees a new (say, smaller) kid on the playground—and the new kid doesn't look, smile, follow, or say "Yeah!" in about five seconds, the six-year-old might bend over, grab at the other kid's shirt and say "C'mon!" or look for the child's parent to ask "Why doesn't he want to play?" This doesn't mean that autistic-four-year-olds should be in baby preschool classes with one-and-a-half-year-olds, but maybe in a mixed-age group in which there are opportunities for developmentally harmonious play as well as kids who can help "repair" any social-interaction snags that come up.

Mixed-Age Groups. Mixed-age groups have many advantages. Developmentally, there are many different skill levels. This means that an autistic seven-year-old who can play a little chess can do it with a ten-year-old but later go play monster dump trucks in the sandpit with the preschoolers. After-school day-care programs sometimes afford this opportunity. For many children with autism, a good resource can be family day care in which the group is fairly small, the setting is a home (and therefore smaller than a more school-like setting), and the peer group is a small, known set of peers. For some children, family day care can mean care with siblings or cousins—other children who are going to have a long-term relationship with the child, and with whom adults are going to be more likely to encourage cooperation and development of communalities in interests and activities. An ideal socialization setting for many children with autism who are under ten can be a family day-care arrangement with a couple of younger children at the same developmental level of play as the child with autism, and a couple of older ones to "scaffold" play. Girls tend to be more helpful caregivers than boys. But for boys with autism who need to burn a lot of physical energy, older boys can be a big help because the child with autism can roughhouse, and a bigger boy can be relied on to take care of himself if the child with autism gets a bit too revved up (and will likely respond by teaching rather functional consequences for overly revved behavior).

Play with Older Children. Another approach to implementing play arrangements is through neighborhood play dates or play dates with older children that the family knows. Often I ask parents if they have a neighbor or relative who is a few years older than their child with autism—maybe a seven- or eight-year-old for a four- or five-year-old, or a twelve- or thirteen-year-old for a nine- or ten-year-old. I refer to these slightly older children as "junior babysitters." The idea is to recruit such a child as a play helper, give them minimal instruction, and promise a small payment, like a dollar an hour. The payment is to make the child feel responsible and "in charge." I would go so far as to give the older child permission to be a bit "bossy." (When I explain this scenario to parents, they often look at each other—both having the same bossy eight or nine-year-old niece or neighbor in mind.) The idea is to get the "junior babysitter" to scaffold play and social interaction. (We will discuss the concept of scaffolded play in a minute.)

There is one element that all suggestions for developing peer play have in common: This is that the peer, by definition of his own interests, age, and skills, will try to find some way to interact with the child with autism, even with relatively little adult support. Access to such interaction is the single most powerful factor in any plan to develop play and social skills. It is important for adults to remember that no matter how good they may be at leading playing, or at playing along, they are never going to be as good in certain ways as a peer. The one caveat to this is that a typically developing peer (sometimes even if paid for his efforts) will have a hard time sticking to his play with the child with autism if there are many other children around who are much easier to play with, and who *want* to play with him. This means that play dates, reverse mainstreaming get-togethers (in which the typical child visits the special-education class), and play in small groups of peers will eliminate or lessen such competition for the interests and efforts of the autistic child's prospective playmate.

Integrated play may work very well when there is an activity both the autistic child and the typical child are interested in and when they can focus on their mutual interest without social competition being a factor for the typically developing child. For example, a parent showed me a video of her ten-year-old daughter Ashley, who has PDD,NOS, because she was concerned that her integrated play dates were not going as well as she had hoped. Ashley was playing in their swimming pool with three of the other girls from her class. The other girls willingly come over whenever invited to swim. However, they tend to play with one another and ignore Ashley who floats around with them but is usually a beat or two off the rhythm of their play. (By the time Ashley gets to their side of the pool, they've all gone to another side of the pool or dived under the water.)

Ashley's mother was struggling because she didn't want to remind the others to play with Ashley too often for fear they wouldn't want to come over in the future. I suggested she invite only one girl over at a time. This way, Ashley is the only other possible playmate. The girls know Ashley, understand her when she talks (a bit tangentially at times), and individually have each shown the capacity and interest to take things at her speed. It seems likely if there were only one girl over, it would increase the time that Ashley actually spent interacting, and both girls would still have fun in the pool.

Integrated Peer Play Groups. One model that has been studied to help children help one another learn to play and interact is the Integrated Peer Play Group model developed by Pamela Wolfberg and Adriana Schuler. In this model, typical, sometimes slightly older peers are selected as "expert players" to come together with a couple of children with autism—the "novice players." The "experts" receive only a small amount of coaching, but are formally made aware of their role as "scaffolders" for the play of the "novices." The activity could be a group drawing, other art project, or any cooperative activity. There should be enough "experts" so that they can take the lead without any one child's being forced into the role of "leader" rather than being allowed to be an equal participant. A 50-50 ratio can work well, as long as the adult facilitator encourages the "experts" to stick with the "novices" and not form their own group.

One school I visited did something quite similar but less contrived. At this elementary school, which had two model classes for pupils with autism, there was also a community "economy." Children could earn "dollars" helping around the school—bringing notes to the office, emptying the trash, helping in the school garden, and shadowing an autistic child on the playground at recess. In fact, there were three "shadows" for one eight-year-old-girl with autism, Ruby. The other girls vied to take her hands as they pulled her along to the water fountain, the bathroom, and a ball game. When Ruby's hands were free, she just sort of hung around this little klatch of girls, and when they decided where they'd go next, they took Ruby along. Having known Ruby since she was three, this was the first time I'd seen her aware of other children. It was great!

The goal is for the play among peers to be as self-initiated and internally sustained by the children as possible, though it will never be possible to achieve this one hundred percent. What will be described now are some techniques that move children with autism closer to more naturalistic peer play by using adults as the initial interactors in their play.

ADULT ROLES IN THE
DEVELOPMENT OF PLAY AND SOCIAL INTERACTION

Remember: Play Is Supposed To Be Fun. Sometimes when I watch adults play with children I get the feeling that adult standards of work productivity are being introduced. This can seem especially true when the child is playing with a paid tutor or therapist. More play is not necessarily better play. The challenge is for the adults to provide as much support as needed while actually doing as little as possible. When children play, it is the process not the goal that is the fun. The point is not what you get done, it's the doing of it. Parents tend to want to get all the trains on the track and linked up. They want the cars in the garage. If one dolly is fed, all the dollies must be fed. Just watch little kids, this is not what they do. Maybe some of the trains are included, may be some aren't. Maybe some are linked up on the carpet, separately, for no particular reason, going nowhere in particular, and are then forgotten. The point of play is not to bring law and order and the work ethic to playtime. The nonlinear way in which children play on their own is an abstract impressionist canvas, and the theme is dynamic. It is from drawing disparate elements together that the origins of abstract thinking and the ability to think in symbols emerges. Adults can easily muck this up by showing the child how to play, rather than letting the child be the innovator. Autistic children have a hard enough time with abstract reasoning as it is, without adults making things more concrete for them on the assumption that doing so will make the play more meaningful or fun.

On some level, parents know that fluidity in play is what makes it desirable to the child: When I watch parents play with their children with autism, each dyad has its own games. One child might like to be grabbed on the tummy and tickled with Barney. Another child might wait till the parent sits on the floor and then hop on her back, arms around her neck and jump off the floor to get a horsey ride. A third child might like to be turned upside down and held by his ankles. Somehow, in each parent-child pair, there has been a process through which this little routine has been worked out—and it is then often repeated because it's so fun. It might be hard to say how the routine started, but it's unlikely that it came from a book. Children add their own innovations, even to a fixed routine like ring-around-the-rosy, so that both parent and child know exactly when hands go up, legs go down, and so on. For this learning process to have occurred, the parent had to tune in to the child's signals and amplify them in a way that created a recognizable routine, expanding the best-liked parts, dropping attempts that were ignored. It is this type of responsiveness in play that is so important in developing play skills. Some parents and other adults working with children with autism do this naturally; others need to develop it.

Repetition in Play. Another way that adults sometimes intrude upon the natural rhythm of children's play is with their intolerance of repetition. If you watch small children, play will have a lot of repetitive elements. Toys designated for the youngest toddlers and preschoolers have the most repetitive operating features. Understandably, adults playing with children with autism are wary of encouraging repetitiveness. Some kind of developmental understanding of how much repetition is to be expected at a given stage needs to be built into the play so there is room for the child to experience the mastery that comes from repetition. Also, repetition is often reinforcing to children with autism, and so some repetitive elements can sustain participation in an activity that also contains novel elements from which the child can learn.

In the next few sections, we'll discuss some roles adults can take to facilitate play in children with autism. There is no one right approach. There is relatively little empirical research on the efficacy of any particular method of adult interaction to increase interaction with peers, or even to increase spontaneous interaction with adults. The various approaches that have been developed by people interested in autism treatment are based largely on clinical theory and observation. Since children with autistic spectrum disorders can be quite different with respect to approachability, active avoidance, and interest in imitation, it makes most sense to regard these different adult approaches to play dynamically, switching among them as the situation or child's mood seems to warrant, rather than rigidly adhering to any one approach.

ADULT AS INTERPRETER OF PLAY

Perhaps the most "traditional" therapeutic model for adults playing with children is the one in which the adult acts like an adult. In traditional play therapy, for example, the adult may interpret the child's actions ("Oh, Mr. Potato Head will be sad if he can't see!"), or build upon the child's actions ("Look, Mr. Potato Head has eyes now; he's so happy he can see what's happening!"). Sometimes in a more traditional play-therapy model, the adult goes in and out of this more adult role and plays along (as by announcing a parallel amputation on a second Potato Head).

For a child who is very adverse to being joined in his solitary activity, the adult's being in this sort of nonintrusive role may be effective in helping the child gain awareness that you exist in a next-door universe in which there are similar interests and activities. For the more socially avoidant child with autism, eventual observation of the adult and deferred imitation of the adult can arise from this type of low-pressure contact. It may be a particularly good way of introducing variations on repetitive themes in which the child with autism may have gotten stuck. Typically, this type of passive-modeling approach cannot be expected to work immediately. The first 20 times you put eyes on your Potato Head, claiming that Mr. Potato Head likes to see, the autistic child may rip the eyes off and fling them across the room because, in his mind, they do not belong there. A creative adult will put the eyes in different places, put the eyes in a Potato Head-looking clump of Play-doh, place the eyes as one of a number of facial features but not press the point too much at once, instead moving from this scenario to other play elaborations that can also be demonstrated with related toys.

This nonintrusive approach to play gives the child an opportunity to become more comfortable with having a play partner and may be his first step toward better accepting the presence of a peer who wants to be a play partner.

ADULT PLAY FOLLOWER

Closely related to the adult as interpreter and "adder" to play is the idea of the adult's functioning as a play follower. The idea is that a very avoidant child, or a very temperamentally sensitive child, can slowly be "joined" in his play if things are perceived as on his terms. As in the much older "Options" work of the early 1970s, the idea is to build a "bridge" between the child's autistic world and ours.

Today, this type of adult role in play is best represented in the work of Stanley Greenspan and Serena Weider in what they call "floor-time." The adult participates with the child in his space, often on the floor, and tries to enlarge the number of "circles" of engagement the child can sustain. In this model, the child's actions set the lead for actions upon which the adult can extend or elaborate. We can assume that since the child is doing something of interest to himself, adding to his self-selected activities will tend to be naturally very reinforcing. What is reinforced, then, is not just the activity, but acceptance of the adult's involvement in the activity. Over time, this can increase both play and interaction.

One of the really positive things about having opportunities for this type of play experience for children with autism is that it may stand in contrast to more adult- or routine-directed activities that may constitute significant parts of a child's direct-instruction day. Discrete trial training programs (discussed at length in chapter 10) are typically completely adult-led and TEACCH programs (discussed in chapter 11) are strongly directed by a combination of adult control, routines, and visual cues. Playtime activities that provide the child with an opportunity to free himself from instructional control but still remain engaged with the world of things and of people are an important counterpoint. This means that play in which the adult participates more as a follower can be used during "go-play" breaks in discrete trial programs and during time in the free-play center in a TEACCH classroom. A more "following" adult player, stationed in free-play areas, allows the child's self-selected activity to be used to practice emerging concepts or consolidate play schemes that the child already knows.

ADULT AS PLAY LEADER

Adults can also serve as the play leader to increase the child with autism's integration into peer play. Think of this as the playground monitor who all the children see as the adult who comes up with a lot of fun ideas. This is a model that works as well for four-year-olds playing Red Light Green Light as for nine-year-olds shooting hoops. The idea is that an adult who is organizing and structuring the play and the rules on a playground, at day care, during an art project, or during a gymnastics or judo class is also in charge of including the child with autism. This model usually works best when the adult is not the primary or only adult leading all the children, but rather an aide who is primarily focused on the child with autism. The goal of the adult's activity is to make it so that her charge just so happens to be at the center of the fun.

Recently, I observed John, age five, on the playground of his day-care program. His aide grabbed him with one arm and with the other held a three-foot-by-three-foot plastic wall piece, then called out, "Who wants to build a castle?" She invited certain children by name and, as they arrived, she assigned jobs like holding up a wall piece or intersecting it with the next piece, assigning jobs to John too, so that he did not wander off. She commented on what each child was doing and how well the castle was turning out, and asked each child, including John, things like "Where should we put the door? Should we make this our moat?" John was in the center of the action as two, then four or five other children joined in. When the castle was done, John and a couple others were "built" inside but had great fun figuring out how to get each other out. Another example was Amy who, with her aide, two other girls, and a teacher, began a game in which the children rolled a ball while sitting on the grass in a circle, legs extended, but with each child's feet touching those of the children on either side. Amy's aide sat behind her, her legs parallel to Amy's. This helped Amy stay with the activity and let the aide be there if Amy needed to be reminded to roll the ball back across the circle if it came to her. The teacher also sat with her legs parallel to those of another of the students (not a special-education pupil), so it did not look like Amy's contact with the adult was unusual.

The play leader has the opportunity to give the extra prompting and encouragement the child with autism may need to ask another child a question about the play, or to find out what to say when his basketball goes in the basket (such as "Slap me five!" accompanied by the visual prompt that is completely appropriate in that situation). If we think about the autism learning disability model, some of the best chances the play leader will have to facilitate this play will be when the play topic centers around a particular interest or area of expertise of the child with autism, like playing spaceship and asking the autistic child interested in constellations "Do you see Ursa Major yet?" Not only can the child with autism participate more readily in response to such a question, participation in the group is more rewarding for the opportunity it presents to talk about your favorite topics, and then perhaps be designated to take over the role of navigator and announce constellations as they appear.

SHADOW ADULT

Possibly the most common use of adults in facilitating play among peers for children with autism is as shadow aide. As the name implies, the function of a "shadow" is to stay close and be a near-invisible proxy for the child as he plays. The shadow aide should be there whenever needed to keep a "turn" in conversation or play from being missed, or to grab a natural opportunity to initiate an interaction. Shadowing is a term usually used to describe individualized one-to-one instructional support in an inclusion setting. Children can, of course, also have one-to-one aides who facilitate participation in special day classes, but the function of such an adult in that case is typically more direct rather than "shadowing."

Shadowing can be tremendously important in helping a child with autistic spectrum disorders join the mainstream. The shadow is essentially serving as a bridge between what the child knows and can do, and actually using those skills with peers. (A child may have learned to play Candyland with a tutor, but may still not know how to join in a game of Candyland being set up on the floor of his classroom.) These situations involve the shadow's helping the child develop successful social initiative, learn when and how to engage in imitation, and learn to read the words, gestures, and faces of peers—basically to compensate for the ways in which his autistic learning disabilities make it so hard for him to understand what is going on in the worlds of other children. For example, a child with autism may need to be told that his action is about to make (or has made) another child cry, because the child with autism will likely not notice or understood the pouting face or worried look of the other child who was concerned that a preferred toy was about to be taken away from him.

Shadowing and "Over-shadowing." Shadow aides who don't really understand what they are supposed to be doing are sometimes rather derisively referred to as "Velcro" aides (a term undoubtedly coined by a teacher using TEACCH, PECS, or both). Such an aide doesn't know when she has done enough and when it is time to back off. For example, I observed four-year-old Charles, a preschooler with a PDD,NOS diagnosis who was included in a typical preschool. He was doing so well that he and his buddy spent much of snack sitting side by side, ogling one another through the toilet paper roll "binoculars" they'd just made as art projects, giggling uproariously. The aide, desperate to be useful and keep Charles on task snack-wise, opened his juice box for him, the first thing in an hour she had found to do to inject herself into Charles's activities. In this case, the child did not really need a "shadow," but his progress was still new and felt tenuous to his Mom, and she was understandably reluctant to give up either the aide (or the diagnosis) lest all supports and progress disappear.

For children like Charles, especially school-aged children with milder autistic symptoms and substantially age-appropriate academic functioning, new issues about shadows come up. One is that the presence of the shadow as "his" teacher is going to be stigmatizing to some extent. By the end of kindergarten other children start asking, "Why does Isaiah have his own teacher?" and this will certainly be talked about among the children by second grade. The shadow's presence can easily come to set the child with autism apart from his peers so that classmates treat him like a baby brother or mascot, not one of the crew.

This does not have to be the case, however. I visited a fifth-grade class in which Brennan, a boy with high-functioning autism, was placed along with his shadow aide. The children sat in cooperative work groups with desks pushed into formations of six. Brennan's desk was the closest to the side wall of the class, but at the front, while his aide had her own little seating area at a counter along this side wall. During individual seat work, the aide spent time circulating among the cooperative work groups, but focused about 40 percent of her time on Brennan's table, and more time on Brennan's work than that of his peers, if he seemed to need help. At no time did the teacher indicate that the aide was Brennan's. The teacher called on Brennan as often as other students, and he performed similarly. When asked to recite a memorized poem out loud in front of the class, Brennan hesitated and stopped part way through, but he wasn't the only one. He was prompted to resume by the teacher—just as she had prompted other pupils in that situation. A sign that this shadow worked perfectly was that when Brennan couldn't think of the next line of the poem, he looked at the teacher, not his aide, just like everyone else who'd forgotten a line.

One way to make shadow aides more invisible to the kids they serve is simply not tell child that the aide is *his* aide, make sure that the aide does not transport the child to or from school (no matter how convenient), or always be curbside to meet Mom and escort the child to his classroom (unless she does this for other pupils who arrive by car as well). The general-education teacher needs to take equal responsibility for calling on the child when there is a whole-group response type of lesson. Since most children with autism who have one-to-one shadows will need some one-to-one work, the shadow can do this less obtrusively if there is either another child who she also shadows or if other children receive other types of in-class one-to-one, like a speech and language therapist who works with kids on an in-class "push-in" basis.

One of the real shortcomings of the shadow-aide system is that when individualized support is assigned at all, it is usually assigned full time, while in reality the child and the school would probably be better off if the child had some time to be less shadowed and more independent, but with an adult in the room charged with serving two or three special needs children among whom she divided her time.

A big concern with "overshadowing" is that an aide may try to make more happen than she should: Sometimes, a child will have a better-quality learning experience if less happens, but the things that do happen aren't so prompted. When children learn to play on their own, they start with just fleeting interactions with one another that over time are repeated and become sustained and more diverse in content. When children with autism start to play on their own, they too can be expected to start with very fleeting contacts. Imagine that you needed a translator to talk to a colleague who spoke a different language. If the translator assumed you understood at least a little of what was being said based on key words common to both languages, body language, and facial expression, the translator might keep her translations brief, and stop translating as soon as she saw you understood. If the translator seemed to move past the translation of your exact question and talked on and on to your colleague, adding her own clarifications, you might become increasingly disengaged or even uncomfortable with their interaction. The shadow aide is a kind of translator. By only partly interpreting and being sensitive to the child with autism's comprehension of the situation, she does a better job of increasing the likelihood that the child with autism will remain interested in the interaction. If the child with autism is having a hard time reading body language, facial expression, and tone of voice, or understanding words, just the right dose of "translation" provides assistance, but also promotes the need for the child to apply himself to understanding the words being spoken, the tone of voice being used, and so on. The adult does not want to be so interesting that the typically developing child ends up playing with the adult rather than making a bit of an extra effort to get a socially interesting response from the child with autism.

Developmentally Appropriate Expectations. Another possible pitfall for shadow aides is that they may not have a good sense of the ways in which interactions are developmentally appropriate for children of a certain age. A "shadow" has ceased shadowing when she tries to get two-and-a-half-year-olds to tell one another their names. Two-and-a-half-year-olds do not start play by introducing themselves to one another. An aide who thinks they do does not know what is important to a two-and-a-half-year-old in a play partner. An effective shadow can help a child with autism by placing her in play near a peer engaged in something she too finds interesting—and then wait until further suggestions are needed. For example, Molly was a six-year-old autistic Barbie fan. She loved to flick Barbie's hair, but would also undress Barbies, put them in the dollhouse, and do other more typical things. Her shadow in kindergarten saw Molly pick up a Barbie and start flicking it around and gently moved her to an area in which two other girls were playing Barbies, then asked whether Molly could play Barbies too. The shadow then asked the girls what their Barbies were doing, all the while keeping Molly around to watch, and eventually Molly made some brief eye contact with one of the peers as she grabbed for some Barbie clothes for her Barbie.

Shadow-Aide Training and Transitions. Who is likely to make a good shadow aide? Often, a tutor from a child's home-based program seems a logical choice. Usually, this would not be my first choice. The child has expectations for one-to-one interaction with this person. It is an expectation of direct reward for compliance and attention to this person. It's going to be confusing for the child to shift from that relationship with his tutor to one in which she is a shadow and where there should be little one-to-one interaction between them. It's like going to a preschool where your mommy is the teacher and suddenly having to share her with everyone else (and having her treat you no differently from anyone else.)

Home-based tutors and their supervisors should play an important role in transition to an inclusion setting but not be shadows for any substantial period of time for this reason. The school's shadow might get to know the child by making several observations of his home program, and/or being watched by a home program staff as she begins to shadow the child at school. This allows a sensible and gradual transition based on how the child adjusts as they go along. The shadow should learn enough of the teaching techniques that the child is accustomed to that she can use them herself, while acknowledging that a classroom is a different setting from a one-to-one home program and will be less intensive in certain ways, though newly challenging for the child. The shadow will need to learn from the child's current teachers or tutors any specific behavior-management techniques and targeted maladaptive behaviors a particular child has and how she will need to handle them. Another important transitional task is for the school-based shadow to learn from the home tutors exactly what it is that the child knows: the words she can say, the directions she can follow, toys she prefers, and so on.

The shadow should be someone who understands what to expect of children at different ages, especially in play. This might involve the shadow's serving as a general classroom aide for a couple of weeks before beginning to shadow the child with autism so that she can learn the culture of the classroom and the developmental capacities and predilections of the students. This strategy will give her an opportunity to learn the classroom routine, the kind of work the children do, and something about each child, and get ideas who might be good play or work partners, and who should be avoided. Similarly, the classroom teacher should have an opportunity to get to know the autistic child before he comes to her class, as well as to see what his current levels of achievement are by observing him in his home program. As the education expert in the classroom, she will be one of the people supervising the shadow and so must have some understanding of the contingencies to which the child is accustomed. This is also true for any child who transitions from a special-education class to an inclusion setting, though this is often easier to accomplish, since these transitions are often within one physical school, and the child can gradually increase regular-education hours while decreasing special-education hours.

Sometimes, parents request that a child who is being included with a shadow aide receive direct one-to-one service from this aide as well. In an ideal world, this would be worth avoiding so that the shadow could maintain some degree of anonymity. In this ideal case, different adults would provide shadowing and one-to-one service. If it is not practical for the child to receive these services from different adults, then moving the child to a separate room for the one-to-one service is a sensible compromise. This mimics the model used with other pupils who are pulled out for resource help or speech therapy—something that most likely will be happening to others in the class. In chapter 12, we will discuss inclusive educational models more and will discuss further why inclusion in the form of a curriculum-within-a-curriculum in which the child with autism engages in rather different assignments on a one-to-one basis instead of doing class work is not recommended as an inclusion model.

TEEN "EXPERT" PLAYER

One more way in which adults, teenagers actually, can facilitate play and social interaction among children is by functioning in the role of the "expert" player. Teenagers are old enough to be perceived as "near-adults" by younger children, but are much closer to their own childhoods and what it means to just hang out and play around. They themselves have often not fully incorporated the adult work ethic that organizes so much of our behavior into a goal-oriented focus. The idea is that the teen expert player is quite like the adult play leader but uses a much less formal and structured manner. If you can think of the adult play leader as a camp counselor, then think of the teen expert player as your best babysitter. In fact, high school-aged babysitters should be considered the main pool of candidates for this job. Think of the most fun babysitter that non-autistic siblings want to have come over when parents go out, the high school student who thinks she wants to major in education, child development, or psychology in college. One or two such young people each of whom comes for a couple of hours once or twice a week can become the cornerstone of a play date treatment component.

Special Consideration in Promoting Play in the Autistic Toddler. The teen expert player can be most useful in the "downtime" between more structured teaching activities. Toddlers (20- to 30-month-olds) and young preschoolers with autism usually tolerate no more than two to four hours per day of direct instruction, but parents rightfully do not want them engaged in repetitive "downtime" activities the rest of the time. At this age, the teen expert player can play a critical role in preventing the young child with autism from developing increasingly repetitive patterns of behavior that are self-satisfying and self-reinforcing and can lead to an increase in autistic behaviors. Instead, a very good babysitter who simply redirects repetitive behavior and introduces new, varied, and simple sensory and motor activities can be just the ticket. We are not speaking here of behaviorally trained aides, but rather babysitters who get the going rate for babysitting—maybe less if they are on the younger (pre-teen) side. Historically, cross-culturally, after all, this is the age of caregivers for many toddlers. A willing, eager young person will intuitively know what to do. Providing this sort of "guided playtime" can be good for the young caregiver as well as the toddler, building a 13- or 14-year-old's credentials for nighttime babysitting without a parent at home. The teen expert player simply needs to be told to "play" with the child, to keep him busy, to not let him engage in whatever repetitive behaviors he might otherwise engage in if the parent were on the phone, preparing a meal, or in the bathroom. If he is a very active little guy, let the teen chase him around in the backyard and wear him out. Better her than you. This can provide meaningful, non-repetitious activity that can be a counterpoint to the hours devoted to the autistic preschooler's adult-led, formal instruction. We need to remember that typically developing toddlers and young preschoolers almost never experience adult-led, structured activity of the intensity and directiveness of early autism therapies. Creating opportunities for self-initiated play lets autistic toddlers and preschoolers be just toddlers and preschoolers part of their day. Like typically developing children, there is potential to learn from self-initiated activity that is exploratory.

Nowhere is it written that direct one-to-one adult-led instruction is the only activity that can pass muster as "stimulation." Simply keeping the very young child with autism from retreating into social isolation is an important goal. Temple Grandin, an adult with autism, has written about her nanny who would "yank" her from her autism, simply forcing her to play and be "here" rather than "there." She will tell you she didn't like it much at the time but now credits such informal activity with helping her establish more expected functioning. In Temple's days as a preschooler (in the early 1950s) there were no effective treatments, and this is just what her mother decided to do instinctively. Even today, this approach seems consistent with what we know about how autistic children who have been highly responsive to treatment had what mental health service providers might call a "wraparound" life—something that was designed to be helpful one way or another almost all the time.

Of course, the idea of teen expert players can be extended beyond preschoolers and can be equally useful for the elementary school-aged child who has a few spare after-school hours in her schedule. For children with autism who are included in some regular education, supervision of some play dates by a teen expert player—rather than just letting the kids play alone together around the house—may be a helpful adjunct, even when the main playmate is a younger or older sibling. Even very "parentified," well-intended, well-motivated older siblings can benefit from a pre-teen or teenager who introduces new themes into the play repertoire and can give some encouragement in keeping the siblings playing together. Giving the teen a list of songs, favorite videos, or favorite toys is about all the instruction that should be required in this situation—along with a mandate to redirect as much social withdrawal as possible.

SOCIAL INTERACTION AND PLAY

In this chapter, we have covered some key aspects of the social-interaction difficulties experienced by children with autistic spectrum disorders, especially in terms of their motivation to be part of social exchange. Lack of interest in peer relations compounds social isolation. Approaches to developing greater interest in peers is fundamental to facilitating play, which is fundamental to exploring and self-initiated learning, as will be discussed more in chapter 8. In this chapter, we discussed ways of starting social exchange with adults, as well as starting peer interactions. In chapter 8, as we talk more specifically about problems in exploring the world of objects. Then we will return to the topic of peer play in the context of the developing stages of toy play and how the child with autism can be helped to achieve and move through those stages.

CHAPTER CONCLUSIONS

In this chapter, we discussed social autistic learning disabilities. Discussion centered on the learning and relating problems that children with autistic spectrum disorders develop when they aren't interested in observing and imitating others. This affects informal social-observational learning, spontaneous and formal imitative learning, and the ability to acquire the underpinnings needed to develop friendships with others—not just as source of fun, but to learn how the world of human interactions works.

In the next three chapters, we examine communicative autistic learning disabilities—probably the most complex area to understand and in which to develop tailored interventions. Since we often communicate to be social, or as part of being social, the domain of communication impairments in autism is overlapping rather than distinct from social autistic learning disabilities. However, given the tremendous range and types of communication deficits within the autistic spectrum—from mute to overly loquacious, from performing poorly in receptive understanding to being pedantic, as well as the tremendous range of interventions—from strategies to developing initial communication skills and speech in the preverbal child to developing higher-level abstract thinking and theory of mind, the topic will be covered in three chapters. Chapter 5 will define communication problems in the autistic spectrum in terms of the autistic learning disabilities model. Chapter 6 will deal with treatment for the preverbal and persistently nonverbal child with autism. Chapter 7 will deal with developing better language and communication in the verbal child with autism.

Autistic Learning Disabilities of Communication: Identifying the Components of Communication

This chapter will deal with defining the ways in which the earliest stages of language development in children with ASDs differ from children with other reasons for their communication difficulties. Communication-based autistic learning disabilities can be seen as emerging from successive failures to normally develop skills like the use of communicative gaze, gestures, and body language. It is these pre-language, paralinguistic failures that eventually lead to a failure to develop any or much spoken language. Receptive and expressive language relies on these earlier-emerging paralinguistic skills as a foundation. This chapter will take a very developmental perspective, laying out a rationale for building these foundational skills when treating communication disabilities in ASDs.

Then, in chapter 6, we will focus on treatment approaches that move the child from the nonverbal or preverbal stages to communicating with visual augmentative approaches that emphasize these foundational paralinguistic skills and that, therefore, should serve to potentiate capacity for development of spoken language. In chapter 7, we will deal with issues in the development of communication skills for the verbal child with autism.

LEARNING AND COMMUNICATION ARE BOTH TWO-WAY STREETS

It is clear that children with autistic spectrum disorders have a very differently organized social world from that of others. In this world, *they* count more than anyone else. Messy emotions like empathy, sympathy, shame, and guilt do not exist as we know them. They certainly don't get in the way of self-interest. This very different organization of emotional life has a lot to do with a sanguine satisfaction with aloneness and self-generated action and activity. But, some of it has to do with being cut off from pathways that might otherwise allow a child to process and make different sense of the world around him. A big part of being cut off has to do with having difficulty in receiving, processing, and sending communicative signals.

Receptive and Expressive Difficulties. Communication, and autistic learning disabilities of communication, can be described in two dimensions: First, children with autism often have problems in both of the key aspects of auditory processing, namely, receiving and sending communicative signals. Of course, if auditory information is not properly or fully received, any sense that might be made of that information, or any response to it, will be limited, too. Second, children with autism often have problems not only on the auditory processing "channel," but on the nonverbal communicative "channels" as well. There are often also problems in receiving (and therefore, further "downstream," in sending) information using body language as well as words. Each of these signaling modalities (auditory and paralinguistic) needs to be considered with respect to how it influences the perceptions of the world that will be formed by a child with autism. Whatever communicative signaling systems are missing need to be built, or enhanced to set the stage for spoken language development. In typical development, the paralinguistic capacities associated with the use of communicative gaze (like eye contact), facial expression, and gestures (or body language) serve as backup systems when comprehension of auditory signals does not work. By assuring that these paralinguistic capacities are developed in children with ASDs too, we increase their chances of picking up the auditory "signal" more readily and more fully.

UNDERSTANDING THE
LANGUAGE OF THE EYES, FACE, AND BODY

Facial Expression. Often the child with autism seems not to comprehend or even notice the most basic and unconscious gestures that all parents use to regulate the behavior of their children. This includes things like a mother's wary facial expression after calling her child's name sharply—intended to indicate that he should keep his hand away from something sharp, hot, or otherwise dangerous. Gesture is used frequently, especially with preverbal children, to let them know what we are thinking. Gesture, then, is a very apparent and early manifestation of the parent's theory of mind that they are exhibiting to the baby when they virtually say, "Look at me! Read my mind by reading my face! I know what you are doing is dangerous! Don't do that!" By this kind of unconscious act, something most parents will do to babies by the time they are eight to ten months old, the parent assumes the baby has a theory of mind.

Facial gesture is probably the most automatic form of communication used with babies to communicate something with a high level of positive or negative emotional "signal." Parents will use a very mad or frightened face if they wish to communicate that the child really needs to inhibit his behavior. They'll use a smile, nod, and twinkle of the eye to indicate pleasure or encouragement. Especially when a baby is still preverbal, expressive facial gesture is the channel for getting some of the most urgent or exciting signals across to the baby. Along with tone of voice, it is what parents are most likely to use when they most want to be sure their message is being received.

When Should Learning through Communication Begin? It is not surprising then that one of the first problems that parents notice, or realize in retrospect, is that the baby doesn't make eye contact. What lack of eye contact implies is that the baby is not receiving signals. In fact, it may appear as if the transponder is simply turned off. During a diagnostic interview I was doing through a translator, the child's mother suddenly broke into English, expressing her concern about her son's failure to learn from her, very elegantly saying it all: "He does not look at my eyes!"

Typically, when a parent sees a baby doesn't "get" the message she is sending, the parent will amplify that message—adding a congruent (happy, sad, worried, excited) tone of voice, using whole-body language, or even making physical contact with the child to enhance the original signal.

Sometimes a parent talks and the baby looks fleetingly. This may thwart the parent's perception that the signal is *not* being received, because the baby *has* looked her way, even though it may have been just long enough to decide that there was a signal, but that it was unintelligible. Logically, many parents come to the conclusion that this must mean that the child has a hearing problem, in other words, that the signal isn't being clearly received. After all, if the child could hear well, why wouldn't the child look for more information, or try to "read" the situation some other way?

Paralinguistic Deficits and Innate Disabilities. Lack of understanding of the paralinguistic signals, like facial expression and gesture, is an autistic learning disability that can be thought of as a "virtual" disability as we discussed in chapter 2. It arises from earlier, more basic innate processing problems that create a secondary notable problem for the child, one that contributes directly to the diagnosis of an autistic spectrum disorder. Possible components of lack of understanding of gesture may relate to a lack of theory of mind, a lack of affiliative orientation, and a preference for stimuli that are very proximal (happening physically close to the child), among other things.

It is important to think about which innate deficits may contribute to a particular child's failure to pick up these paralinguistic signals so that the deficit in reading facial expression or gesture can be remediated. As one contemplates teaching the child how to respond to important messages in facial expressions and gestures, it is necessary to deconstruct these virtual disabilities: In other words, strategies like holding a desirable food item between the eyes to "teach" eye contact is, on its own, pretty useless. It's like turning on the transponder when there is no signal to be received, a waste of energy and certainly of no meaningful communicative value. One must think about *why* you want the child to look. The goal is for the child to "read" a signal (like the communicative partner's facial expression) because it is a cue for what may happen next—it requires decoding the meaning of the facial expression (the "signal"). If what will happen next is something the child sees as meaningful, he will learn to look into your eyes for a cue in the future when he desires the same consequences.

This is why some children with autism do use communicative gaze when *they* want something, but don't use it when the message originates with you.

Building Natural Reasons to "Look at Me." Getting the child to look is not as simple as giving a hearing-impaired child a hearing aide. Once he looks, he may say to himself, "So what?" Meaningful associations and consequences, in terms of something meaningful to the child, must be paired with the request for eye contact and the appropriate gestural signal to help the child know there is a message there. His inability to understand that you think the way he thinks (his "mindblindness") may otherwise render making eye contact communicatively meaningless. So, if a child looked toward an M&M held between the eyes, but was taught to reach for the M&M when the face was smiling and not when the face wasn't smiling, the child would be learning something about what smiling signals.

Misinterpretation of Absent Signals. Sometimes the child's lack of reception of gestural signals gets the child with autism into trouble: One way the lack of assumed understanding can backfire is when an adult is convinced that the child has looked, has understood and is paying attention, but is intentionally, defiantly deciding not to respond. I have always worried that children with autistic spectrum disorders are probably at a higher risk of being abused when reared by stressed, unattuned parents who may be the ones most often to make this sort of error. The parent or other caregiver who is a little paranoid, or a little depressed, may be at greater risk to attribute negative intentions to the child with autism when in fact there is non-comprehension, not defiance. Maybe non-comprehension is harder to accept in some ways than is defiance.

More commonly, the child with autism's lack of gestural understanding, especially paired with a low affiliative orientation may promote the occurrence of self-endangering situations: Many parents talk about fearless climbers. Teachers talk about fearless escapers. (I'd like to try to get someone to sell child-sized skateboarder T-shirts at the national autism meetings with the "No Fear" logo on one side and the ASA logo on the other.)

Why does it often seem that autistic children have no fear? A group of classic developmental psychology experiments explains this in terms that are highly relevant for understanding the implications of not "reading" parent warning signals: In studies done with crawling babies (eight to ten months old), babies are placed on a "visual cliff." A visual cliff is essentially a big clear box (think of a box that would hold a refrigerator turned on its side) that has a thick layer of clear Plexiglas for the top, and a black-and-white parquet floor, half laid out on the bottom of the box and half laid out directly under the Plexiglas top. A friendly examiner holds the infant at one end of the Plexiglas top surface so that the infant is over the higher of the two parquet floors and it looks like he is crawling right on the floor. The mother stands at the other side, smiling, nodding, cooing to the infant to come to her. The baby typically crawls forward, but stops when the floor appears to drop off (the visual "cliff"). At this point in the experiment, the typical baby looks to her mother's face with a worried expression. If the mother continues to smile, nod, and coo, the baby proceeds, unworried that she will "fall" off the "cliff." But, if the mother suddenly looks frightened, looks fearful, and shouts, "No, stop!" (or any of these), the baby will freeze—and often start crying. If the mother keeps a neutral face, says nothing and does not gesture, the baby will also cry—the baby is looking for a needed signal and does not know what to do without one. This experiment has been repeated many ways—with positive or negative gestures, with positive or negative tones of voice, and so on, with much the same results. Typically a baby will try to find a parental signal to "read" and will proceed accordingly. No one has ever had a group of autistic eight-month-olds to run this procedure with, but we can imagine that most babies with autism would not pause to look for a parent's signal to "read" but, rather, would just keep going.

The infant relies on the parent to make judgments when all that the infant knows is that he doesn't know what is safe to do. It is understandably much easier to feel you have a better chance of successfully protecting your baby when he does look for your signals than when he does not. When the baby does not look to you, you have to do the work for both parties. No wonder parents of children with autism feel so exhausted by the child's care demands. Others might not understand what's so demanding about a child who isn't constantly seeking your attention—instead seeing a child who is extra "good" and very able to be on his own. Babies are *supposed* to nag and demand attention—so they're not forgotten, left behind, and eaten by wolves!

In typical development, the baby very automatically relies on the parent for what he senses are questionable or potentially dangerous situations. Babies rely on parents to learn interesting new, fun things, too. This why when autistic babies lack these receptive and expressive signaling systems, they are not only at a safety disadvantage, but at disadvantage in accumulating information about how the world around them is put together. So, it is critical that as we move into an examination of the auditory signaling systems we remember that nonverbal, paralinguistic signaling should have developed first and that typically developing babies rely on such systems to learn about their worlds long before words make sense. In designing treatment, therefore, we will need to provide some way to key children with ASDs into the value of nonverbal signals so that just like typically developing children, they can use that information to begin to understand spoken words.

By following a gaze, reading a face, or perceiving the intention of a gesture, a child can narrow in on possible word meanings associated with the communicative context. Not being able to read paralinguistic signals can, therefore, make it harder (certainly not easier) to understand spoken language. Since there are all sorts of reasons that children with ASDs may not do well with spoken language, it is all the more important that we try to enhance paralinguistic signaling as part of an overall plan to teach verbal communication.

SPEAKING THE
LANGUAGE OF THE EYES, BODY, AND FACE

One thing that places a child's receptive difficulties beyond a more simple aphasia and into autism or an autistic aphasia is the concomitant inability to use gesture, eye gaze, or facial expression to clarify meaning. What if you understood nothing of what was being said around you? Say you'd just stepped off the plane in a foreign country where you spoke none of the language and were dying of thirst. You might tap someone, try a hand gesture like tipping a cup to your mouth, point to possible places to get a drink and shrug your shoulders, and so on. You might lack an oral vocabulary, but you would have a more universal nonverbal vocabulary to fall back on—as would a deaf child.

Some gestures are universal, like many facial expression such as disgust, shame, empathy, grief, kindness, and so on. The child with autism often appears not to comprehend the social communicative value of these, and therefore often does not use these expressions communicatively. It seems that the innate lack of an affiliative orientation is key to facial gestures not being used *communicatively*—because most autistic children can show a range of emotional responses on their face (for example, disgust, if a new and horrible food is stuck in the child's mouth. This response is correctly "read" by parents, though not necessarily intentionally "sent" by the child to the adult.

Many parents do note however that their child with autism more often has a solemn, serious (unemotional) look on his face and tends not to display as wide a range of more subtle emotions clearly (such as shame, guilt, empathy, or sympathy), or know the difference between emotional states that are closely related).

Autistic children tend to be very slow to acquire conventionally taught gestures such as waving bye-bye. Natural gestures (ones that develop without being taught—though they *can* be taught) are delayed in most children with autistic spectrum disorders: These include shaking the head in refusal (as a baby does when he's finished eating), following a gaze, and, most notably, pointing.

The Importance of Pointing. The absence of pointing may be our earliest and most universal identifier for autism. When a ten-month-old points, he is essentially telling us that he understands that your optical system works the same as his and he knows that you will see what he sees if you gaze in the same direction as he is pointing. Pretty complicated for ten months old! This is the core of theory of mind—the idea that babies should quickly come to understand that parents can "read their mind." Sometimes, the lack of ability to understand this is actually referred to as "mindblindness," a term that is really quite a bit more descriptive than "theory of mind."

The lack of ability to point, in particular, and to express in gestures, in general, has a profound effect on the child's ability to get information about his world: When a baby looks at something and vocalizes, a parent typically follows the baby's gaze and then can give him information about what he's showing interest in. Similarly, babies usually begin to point when they are about ten months old. Pointing is really a more notable elaboration of gaze: The baby will typically point, vocalize, and look between the parent and the object of interest until the parent talks to him about the object or gets it for him. What is really happening during such an interaction is that the baby is virtually saying, "What is this? It's interesting. Give me a lesson about it." The baby's "receivers" for information about this object of interest are fully turned on, and this probably means that he is in a state in which he is more likely to retain the information he's then given, than if the parent had randomly told him about something he wasn't pointing to. The autistic baby doesn't point, and he doesn't get these lessons. I remember interviewing one mother who was describing her four-year-old son with autism, Joey, when he was a 16-month-old, the current age of his younger sister, Elizabeth, who was clearly very bright. The mother suddenly realized that she was always teaching Elizabeth new things—every time Elizabeth pointed to something. She then said, "Joey never pointed. I never taught him the way I teach Elizabeth. That must be why he doesn't understand so many things." She started to cry. I said, "No, that's not why. Joey never *asked*. It isn't anything *you* didn't do."

Communicating in Natural versus Conventional Gestures. It follows that children who do not easily develop spontaneous use of natural gesture, like following a parent's gaze or pointing at something themselves, are going to have a hard time expanding this repertoire with conventional (taught) gestures, which are essentially an elaboration and codification of natural gestures. The best example of this might be how, in our culture, shaking the head from side to side means "no." A baby naturally moves his head to avoid or refuse things he does not want. Quite naturally, a parent will elaborate on the baby's spontaneous gesture by shaking her head "no" and querying the baby, "No?" This should help the baby come to understand the "formal" meaning of the side to side head shake "no." (It also explains why "yes" comes in later—it is conventionalized, but not from a natural gesture the way "no" is.) Similarly, in American culture, babies are taught quite early that clenching and releasing the hand when it faces outward usually means "bye-bye" (but can also be used toward them in greeting). Waving is harder to learn than shaking the head "no" because it is a conventionalized gesture rather than an adaptation of a spontaneous one. (It also partly explains why many children with autism, who are taught, at great effort, to wave "bye-bye," will say "bye-bye" when prompted to wave "hello." The child with autism tends to learn waving as a behavioral routine with one specific meaning, typically, "bye-bye." This unitary under-standing of just one meaning is compounded by a frequent desire *not* to indicate "hello," but to indicate "good-bye" upon meeting up with a new and friendly person (because of lack of affiliative drive). If I had a hundred dollars for every time a child with autism has waved and said "good-bye" to me when I've waved and said "hello," I could retire now.

What all this means is that children with autism who don't understand language can't fall back on getting or giving information by gesturing their intentions as "mindblindness" has left those signalling systems impaired with respect to communicating intent. So, autism compounds the difficulties of a language disorder alone and can leave the child very cut off from any of the usual ways of getting information about his world when he can niether speak nor gesture. (It also speaks to why teaching sign language to children with autism is often an uphill battle and certainly is not likely to play to strengths. This will be discussed more in the chapter on remediation of communication deficits associated with autism.)

Tantrums: Results of Communication Failures. The result of being cut off and unable to communicate by either gestures or words can result in a variety of tertiary symptoms as described in chapter 2. Tantrums are the expressed frustration of a child who knows what he wants, but doesn't know that others understand his intentions or can "read his mind." Tantrums come from the child's failure to express himself in gestures or words so that others understand him directly and efficiently. This is the core of the most frustrating kind of failure that children with autism can experience, but it is also the root of their rehabilitation: While making children with autism "more social" can be a tough nut to crack—because you have to make the child *want* to be more social first— it is usually easier to make communication skills inroads, because the child usually wants to communicate, at least to have his needs met expeditiously. So, the motivation to communicate needs is usually there, even though the motivation to engage in more purely social exchange is likely not at the forefront.

INITIAL AWARENESS OF COMMUNICATION DIFFICULTIES

For most parents, the first thing that seems clearly wrong in a child's development is that he isn't talking or isn't talking as much as expected. This is usually clearer to the parent who has had a typically developing child first. It is usually more ambiguous to a parent who hasn't parented before. Complicating this is the folk wisdom that boys talk later; the first born son is the king of the family and everyone acts like his slave; the baby of the family doesn't need to talk, just cry; middle children are used being ignored, and quickly learn to do for themselves; and little girls are treated like princesses and everyone caters to them too much. That about covers the bases for delayed language irrespective of birth order and gender. Sometimes it takes an experienced "outsider" like an aunt with older children, a grandma, a neighbor who is a teacher, or a day-care provider whose life is filled with nothing but 24-month-olds to point out that a child's language development is definitely off track.

When this realization occurs, different children may be in different places in terms of language development, but there tend to be some things young autistic children share in common in their language development problems. These communalities provide a window into what may be wrong.

Babbling. First of all, many autistic children either don't babble *and* don't talk, or don't babble much, or babble oddly, or never really babbled before they talked. So what? Babbling is a fascinating thing. Now, some parents will say they believe their baby never babbled because they never talked baby talk to the child as a baby—because they wanted him to talk right, and not like a baby. An interesting idea, but very unlikely to explain why a child didn't babble. Babbling is language practice. If you don't practice, you are not getting the experience needed to speak in a way that will be understood. A very obvious example of this is deaf babies—who babble for a while—and then stop. It is as though the apparatus to talk is there; it exercises and flexes itself a bit and then goes dormant because there is no apparent need for it.

The earliest kind of babbling is sometimes call "prelocutionary," meaning prior to locution or words. It's just sound practice, like a symphony tuning up and each instrument testing its range of sounds so each musician can tune an instrument. Babies younger than six to nine months gurgle, coo, and produce all the odd sounds that are possible in the human vocal repertoire. By about seven to nine months, babbling changes in response to what is heard: This is when babies start to control and "reduplicate" common sounds in their personal language environment such as "de-de-de," "ma-ma-ma," "pa-pa-pa," easy-to-produce sounds (that just happen to serve as words to label "mother" and "father" in many different languages).

Sometimes toddlers with ASDs persist too long in this first stage of prelocutionary babbling, and so what parents notice at 12, 14, or 18 months is that their child still sounds like an infant, and the sounds don't seem to mean anything yet. Since all parents naturally are listening for first words that mean "mom" and "dad," the absence of regularly reoccurring sounds that seem to mean something can be quite striking.

Clinically, this persistence of prelocutionary babbling (or a virtual absence of sound production) and a failure to develop reduplicated, more meaningful babbling may mean that the child is not getting the auditory signal, just like a child with deafness can't get the auditory signal. However, there is a key difference: The deaf child does not get the auditory "signal" because he can't hear. The child with an ASD may not be getting the "signal" because it is not clear, or there is too much "noise," or there seems no reason to attend to this kind of signal.

"SIGNAL" AND "NOISE" DIFFICULTIES

Let's explore these alternative explanations for "signal" and "noise" difficulties one at a time: First, the signal may not be clear. A child who often has ear infections and fluid in his ears may be getting an unclear signal. However, when this happens to otherwise typically developing children, there is usually a fairly impressive rebound onto the expected trajectory of language acquisition within days or weeks after drainage tubes are inserted. But there are other reasons that the signal may not be clear: If the brain is not ready to pick up and recognize repeated patterns of speech the way it should, language may sound more like "noise" or static than a sensible signal. It may be as if you found yourself in a new foreign country every morning and were hearing a new language every day for the first time.

Second in the list of reasons a child may seem "word-deaf" is that he "hears" too much "noise" instead of signal. This may be the case in children who cover their ears when a sound is loud or when things just seem too much to handle. For most of us, hearing sound we can't make sense of is more annoying than hearing sound we can make sense of (think of loud music with incomprehensible lyrics versus a song you enjoying singing along with, played just as loud). "Too loud" or too much "noise" is partly a function of the sense we can make of what we are hearing.

Third is the problem of picking up the language "signal" because you just don't know there is any reason to attend to it. Many young children with autism lack basic cause-and-effect understanding until explicitly taught. They lack a sense of the intentionality in the actions of those around them. Again, the brain may not yet be ready to see the link between a circumstance and the one that tends to follow. Some theorize that seeing such cause-and-effect links is how language learning typically begins: For typically developing infants, this would be the powerful result they get when they repeat "ma-ma-ma" or "da-da-da" on cue and everyone pays attention. For the autistic child for whom the social attention is not particularly a desired end, the potential value of figuring out which sound produces the most social result may simply not be that interesting.

Making "Noise" into a "Signal." So what can be done if a child seems "word-deaf," seems to regard language as "noise" rather than a "signal," or seems not even to understand why language should be attended to in the first place? Let's go back to the example of being in a new foreign country every day. It would take a while to pick up patterns in the things people were saying. You could expect to be able to pick up the patterns if you stayed in the new country long enough.

The way you would accomplish the task of figuring out what people meant by what they said can give us some insight into how to teach language to a child with autism who seems "word-deaf" in the different ways that have been described: First of all, in a new country, you would "read" the nonverbal communication of a speaker whose words seemed of interest. You would ask yourself, "Who did he look at as he spoke? Did he smile or look upset? Did the person being looked at respond with the same kind of facial expression? How far apart were the people? Did they seem related to one another in some way? Were certain words said by one person and repeated by the other (maybe for clarification of a main point)? Were there objects being looked at, touched, or used as these people talked? What did the tone of voice used by each person in the conversation tend to say about the emotions or social status of each?"

Of course, we know that many of these questions that you or I might ask ourselves in the "foreign country/foreign language" situation, would *not* be asked by most young children with ASDs because, as we've discussed, specific areas of autistic learning disability often include a lack of ability to read faces or gestures, to follow gaze, or to decode tone of voice. So how would the child proceed to figure things out as best he could? To answer this question for a particular child, one must inventory the child's non-verbal communicative autistic learning disabilities and figure out how natural "self-accommodations" (natural abilities compensating for disabilities) might be best shaped to help this particular child learn language efficiently.

KNOWING COMMUNICATION STRENGTHS AND WEAKNESSES

Typically developing young children figure out what is being said to them by relying on as many "signals" as they can get. This includes not only words, but also the speaker's tone of voice, the physical context, who is speaking, and the paralinguistic clues—what the speaker looks at, what gestures he or she uses, and his or her facial expression. Without thinking about it, most of us communicate on all these channels at the same time, giving a great deal of well-coordinated (and usually somewhat redundant) "signal." In developing communication skills in a child with an autistic spectrum disorder, it is important to inventory all of these and to know which kinds of signals are being processed and which are not. Understanding how to teach communication will depend on what existing channels (relative learning strengths) the child can rely upon.

The first thing is to carefully think about, and even informally "test," what information a child is processing. Often parents have the impression—and report—that the child understands more than he really does. Why is this? When we think about it, most of what we say to children, especially children who don't seem too interested in hearing us talk at them, is fairly routine—"Come on, let's go! Get your shoes!" or "Get your sippy cup, I'll give you more juice." When a child can't fully understand words, the child will fall back on other cues, such as a key word and what we might broadly think of as contextual cues. Many young children with autism are relatively more advanced in their "visual maps" of their worlds than they are in vocabulary. So when the child hears "shoes" and sees that his mother has *her* shoes on and is holding her purse and car keys, he knows it's time to go out and that he doesn't leave the house without shoes on. That child may be able to visualize perfectly well where his shoes are and get them, so the scene he is picturing can take place—shoes on—get in car—go for a ride somewhere. To the parent, this may look like one hundred percent comprehension, because functionally it is, but it is not necessarily comprehension of all the words that have been said. To test comprehension, a parent might try moving the shoes to a novel location—say, the bathtub—and saying, "Let's go! Go get your shoes from the tub." Quite likely, the child, who can "understand" a sentence with the word "tub" when it's bath time and the water in the tub is running, may be stymied when it comes to "shoes" in the "tub" when everyone looks like they are ready for a ride in the car.

If a child is understanding language in the way that has just been described, and "fails" the "tub" test, you have learned something important about his learning style. Namely, that this child with autism (like all of us) figures things out the easiest way possible. In this case, paying close attention to visual context makes sense of the action needed for "shoes." This pattern of natural compensation is fairly typical for young children with autism and tells us that they are "thinking in pictures," and not so much in words. It's a different use of the child's intellectual capacities, not an absence of capacity. The next important step is to systematically figure out which paralinguistic 'signals' the child may or may not be 'receiving' so each can be compensated for and explicitly taught.

Reading the Face to Decode Speech. When a child does not have an ASD, and he does not fully understand what you are saying, the child is likely to look at the speaker's face for clues as to what is meant by what is being said. Without thinking, most of us will move our head and eyes toward an object we are talking about if that object is present. The mother who says, "Let's go! Get your shoes." Will probably look at the shoes as she says those words, if the shoes are in sight. Further, if the child looks at the mother's face, the mother might nod, and direct her head and gaze toward the shoes once the child looks at her. This is a subconscious way of saying without words—"The shoes are right there. Look!"

As we've already discussed, many children with autism don't automatically look to a speaker's face for information. If the child does not look, this type of "signal" cannot be received. Over time, lack of response to such signals may even modify how a parent communicates with a child with autism, and the parent may stop expecting that a gaze or nod can clarify the meaning of what has been said. (This may mean that the parent gets in the habit of just getting the shoes for the child.) Later, as parents head down the road to diagnosis, they may be told that the reason the child doesn't talk is that he doesn't have to, that everyone just babies him and caters to him and doesn't expect him to do for himself. In fact, the parent is being "conditioned" by the child's response and habitually comes to do things for the child because the child can't read the parent's signals. It may however feel intuitively right to acknowledge that this child is more babied because the parent realizes that she does do more for this child than for her others.

Understanding Body Language to Decode Speech. Similarly, the child may not comprehend the signal that comes from various types of body language. It would be quite natural for a parent who is indicating the need to get shoes to point to them, if they are right in front of her and the child. If the parent is indicating that the shoes are in the bathtub, she might point at the bathroom door, which would provide needed clarification when the child needs to understand something out of the ordinary. A language-impaired child who was not autistic might follow the point, go in the bathroom, look around, glance into the tub, and see his shoes.

Similarly, body language might be used to modify what is being said, without any words to go along with it: The parent might point repeated and rapidly to indicate that the shoes were right in front of the child's nose and would be seen, if only the child would look. This would be a slightly different kind of signal than gaze direction, but also one that the child with autism would be likely to miss.

If a particular child with autism does not follow a point or respond to other common forms of body language often used to modify speech ("come here," "sit down") then the need to teach a response to body language must go on the list of communicative deficits that need to be remediated.

Listening to Tone of Voice. Yet another channel of information, another kind of signal, resides in tone of voice. If a request to "get shoes" was being spoken as a purely optional hide-and-seek type game, the parent might use a playful, even silly, lilting voice. If getting shoes was part of a routine, a checklist of things that needed to be accomplished to walk out the door, the tone of voice might be matter-of-fact. If the parent were running late and realized at the last moment that the child had taken his shoes off moments after they'd been put on, the tone of voice might convey the parent's feeling that she was in no mood for messing around. Sometimes, all these variations are lost on the child with autism. From the parent's point of view, the child may be seen as very obstreperous and defiant if an irritated tone of voice doesn't seem to make a difference. From the point of view of a parent who was feeling a bit depressed and confused about why this child seemed so uninterested in playing with his mom and pleasing his mom than an older sibling was, the child's ignoring of a playful tone of voice might feel like rejection.

In any case, if the child appears not to modify behavior according to tone of voice, or only does so when the volume knob on this sort of "signal" is turned up really loud (like when the child is being yelled at), this is yet another channel of communication that is not yet to be relied upon to help "amplify" the meaning of spoken words. When this is the case, response to tone of voice may also need to go on the list of difficulties that needs to be addressed. Many children with autism respond appropriately to a very loud, negative tone of voice ("Stop! No!") used as they are about to dart into the street or stick a wet finger in a light socket. However, most do not respond uniformly to a range of affective tones of voice, such as by acting differently in response to a cajoling versus a more straight-out requesting tone of voice, or a sad tone of voice versus a disappointed tone of voice.

INTERVENTION: USING LANGUAGE SO THE CHILD "HEARS"

What Needs To Be Included
in a Communication Program for Autism?

Visual Interaction Augmentation (VIA). In the next chapter, we will begin to discuss the mechanics of what are sometimes referred to as visually augmentative communication systems, or picture communication systems. These involve physical materials that can be used to teach language and language concepts to children with ASDs. While it is critical to use such systems in intervention with preverbal and nonverbal children, it is also important to use these more contrived communication strategies along with training the child to pick up what should be natural and augmentative paralinguistic signals, like gaze, point, body gesture, and tone of voice, as we have just discussed. In planning treatment, we need to be as aware of paralinguistic deficits as of those in spoken language, as both types of skills together give the child the best tool kit for decoding what those around him mean by what they say. To this end, we will discuss an integrative approach to visually augmented communication that will be referred to as VIA, for Visual Interaction Augmentation. The VIA system was designed as a developmentally based integration of existing picture-based communication approaches and the need to teach paralinguistic signaling.

Sign Language and ASDs. Any strategy that a non-ASD nonverbal or preverbal child would use would rely on paralinguistic strengths to help develop a strategy of compensations. For example, teaching sign language to deaf children teaches them to compensate by using a relatively strongly attended to "channel"—body gesture. That's all sign language is—codified and elaborated body language. As long as a child reads gesture and body language poorly, teaching sign language plays to weaknesses, not strengths. In the absence of a functional understanding of what is meant by what is being "said" with the eyes, the face, gesture, and tone of voice, any signs the child learns are "behaviors," not the communicative functions they would be for a deaf child. For example, it is common in infant-stimulation programs to teach the sign for "more" to pre-verbal, language-delayed toddlers. With autistic toddlers, the sign "more" means, "I've done something; now you do something! Figure out what I want!" While such a behavior is more functional than shrieking, it is not semantically specific the way, for example, pointing to a particular object would be.

Putting Nonverbal and Verbal Communication in Place Developmentally.
We know that the paralinguistic signaling systems largely develop before the
linguistic ones in typically developing children. Typically developing children
follow a gaze even before they point. They point well before they talk well. If
our remediation strategies are to be developmentally based there needs to be
a way to develop these paralinguistic skills for children with autism so that
they can rely on gaze, point, body gesture, and tone of voice to amplify the
meaning of words, too. Children with autism need all the help they can get
decoding words. So, teaching paralinguistic communication strategies makes
sense as part of an overall communication program if it is thought about
developmentally and in terms of available compensatory communication
strategies.

We've mentioned how parents and other caregivers subconsciously provide redundant information when communicating, saying the same things
with words, facial expression, body language, and tone of voice. In the case of
typically developing children, we tend to amplify each of these signals to make
the overall "volume" of the signal as "loud" (comprehensible) as needed. The
whole field of developmental psycholinguistics is aimed at understanding the
various components that turn the "noise" that is initially perceived by infants
into increasingly sensible "signals." By applying research from developmental
psycholinguistics to the treatment of autism, we can come up with a few
guiding principles for modifying our (adult) communication to the child with
autism that can serve to make different kinds of communication signals more
sensible.

DETERMINING LEVEL OF LANGUAGE DEVELOPMENT

When autism is first detected, most of these children are not understanding
and using language as well as expected for someone their age. Some parents
have an excellent sense of just what level their child's language is at while others
do not. An infant educator, or a parent who has another child a year or so
older, usually has a very good idea of the stage at which language understanding
and use should develop. If the level of a child's language understanding
(receptive) and use (expressive) is in question, it may be helpful to have
language testing.

Testing Language. First, of course, we want to know if the child can hear. If the child responds to some sounds, but not others of equal loudness, he very likely can hear just fine—but may not yet be making sense of what he hears (that is, it's still mostly "noise" and little "signal"). Once there is a good degree of certainty that the child can hear, then language testing can proceed. Even if the child has had a "conductive hearing loss," meaning that fluid in his ears may temporarily have blocked some sound for a while, it is important to measure at what stage language development is once the blockage has been alleviated. For many children, standard language testing such as the Preschool Language Scales or Peabody Picture Vocabulary Test can be administered to see how much the child can understand and say. This, however, assumes that the child participates reasonably cooperatively in the activities that the tester chooses. This is often not possible for young children with autism, as they still lack any understanding of a system of incentives that would make participation seem worth their effort. In fact, just being coerced to sit at a table and do anything of someone else's choosing may seem hateful sui generis. In this case, it is always possible to give a parent-administered measure of communication skills like the MacArthur Communication Development Index or the Communication Domain questions from the Vineland Adaptive Behavior Scales to get an estimate of the level to which language understanding and use has developed. If testing is done, it is important not to get hung up on any one test being the exact or only "right" test, or the test result being the absolutely true measure of the child's abilities. Any test is just one imperfectly clear window into the child's development at one point in time.

Test results are subject to all sorts of errors that have to do with how well the tester can relate to the child or parent, how nervous the parent is, and how interested or uninterested in the testing the child is. This does not mean, however, that results are meaningless. There is a lot of space between "meaningless" and "perfect." Early language testing should simply seek to establish if there seems to be a significant difference between what the child understands and can say, and whether the child is still mainly understanding and/or using single words, phrases, or sentences. For the purposes of the earliest ways of treating language problems in children with autistic spectrum disorders, it is important to know whether the child is still essentially preverbal, meaning he mainly understands a handful of key words that have been explicitly taught or that are frequently used, or whether the child can pick up words incidentally—just from hearing them and/or seeing others use them.

Inventorying Communicative Autistic Learning Disabilities. The task of developing language as it has been defined so far is to first identify which channels of communication work and which don't work. This consists of appraising the child's abilities to understand, as well as his abilities to express. The channels of communication that need to be considered include the child's ability to understand things from the context in which he sees them, the ability to understand words, the ability to read faces, the ability to understand hand gestures and body language, and the ability to get information from tone of voice. The next step is to think about ways to rely on the existing and stronger channels for understanding and expression and devise ways that these strengths can support the channels of communication that are either turned off or just full of static. To begin this process, refer to the Autism Learning Disabilities Inventory (ALDI) in Appendix A that was talked about in chapter 2. Four of the scales from the ALDI (Receptive Gesture & Body Language, Expressive Gesture & Body Language, Comprehension of Spoken Language, and Use of Spoken Language) contain items that deal with specific deficits associated with these areas of autistic learning disability. The scales are intended to help organize your observations about a child's functioning in each of these areas and clarify which kinds of linguistic and paralinguistic, and verbal and nonverbal skills development need to be included in developing a treatment plan.

USING SLOWED SPEECH, PROSODY, AND REPETITION TO MARK MEANING

We talked about how mother-ese can be used to help the youngest children tune into the fact that they are being talked to and to make it interesting and easier to listen to the most relevant parts of what is being said. As a child's language develops far enough along that it is no longer necessary to use baby talk with them, it may still be necessary to keep in mind the mother-ese strategies for making speech intelligible. This can include slowing speech, using marked inflection with key words, and repeating the key words to get them into that part of auditory memory where the child can make repeated attempts to decode them.

Putting Yourself in the Child's Shoes. The easiest way to think about this is to think about what it would be like for you to go on vacation armed only with high school Spanish and a Berlitz phrase book that you read on the plane, and then have to ask how to get to the bathroom in a noisy Mazatlán restaurant. You might glance at your phrase book and temporarily memorize "Please, where is the bathroom?" If you did it really well, and with a good accent, and the restaurant was noisy enough, the waiter might mistake you for a more competent speaker of Spanish than you are, and rapidly answer, "Down that hall to the right." You might have rehearsed the respective words for "right" and "left" in Spanish before you asked—so your brain would be listening for those words—but maybe would have missed the other words or simply didn't know how to translate them. When you don't know two words in a row in another language it can be pretty hard to tell where the one word stops and another begins. However, if you finally figured out which word was "left" and lo-and-behold, the waiter pointed to a hall to his left, you could feel pretty confident you'd find the toilet at the end of the hall. If there was no pointing, and there was too much noise in the room for you to be confident that you heard all the words distinctly, what would you want to have happen next? For one, you'd want the waiter to repeat himself. For another, you want him to speak slowly. Or you might want to find a quieter place. Saying the key word, "left," repeatedly might help. Finally, having the good fortune to have the waiter using nonlanguage cues—pointing or looking toward the bathroom really would help.

All of these criteria apply when talking to the child with autism. All of these things may help. Knowing the child's communication strengths and weaknesses so you have a sense of which of these adaptations will help and which will not is also useful. If the child doesn't follow a gaze or point, teaching those is important insofar as it opens another channel the child can use to construct meaning. This will be discussed in the next chapter under strategies for utilizing existing augmentative communication systems like PECS (Picture Exchange Communication) or another enhanced augmentative communication system (like VIA) that also incorporates paralinguistic signaling.

The Bilingual Challenge. Sometimes when I am talking to parents about how children with autism learn language and the problems they have learning it, I use an example like the Mexican restaurant. Since most Americans are not truly bilingual, but have taken a foreign language for a while in high school, this example can work adequately. However, for families that are bilingual, it raises a whole new set of questions. More than a quarter, and close to half, of the families I see use more than one language at home. Not infrequently, it is also the case that the child is cared for by a non-English-speaking monolingual Chinese or Spanish-speaking grandmother. Other times, the father works outside the home and speaks English, but the mother is at home and does not. Increasingly, there are young professional families who want to pass on the advantages they feel they accrued by growing up in a bilingual home and make it a point to speak only the mother tongue at home, with the assumption that the child will learn English from preschool, peers, television, and videos. Sometimes, monolingual English-speaking families choose (or can only find) a child care provider who is non-English-speaking, so the child's daytime hours are filled with a language he does not otherwise hear.

When a child who is in one of the situations just described is diagnosed with autism, questions always come up about the benefits or liabilities presented by exposure to more than one language. The first thing is that the reality of the situation is that special-education instruction, be it a special day class, speech therapy, or a home-based program, is going to be all or primarily in English. To find qualified bilingual special-education professionals who just happen to have the skills to work with a particular child with autism is a real long shot. If the parents reside in the United States or any other English-speaking country, it is likely that resources available for the child will be in English.

I take the position that if vocabulary acquisition and language use are going slowly, why multiply the difficulty by two (or three)? Not everyone agrees with this position one hundred percent and the research is both sparse and a bit ambiguous. Even if a three-year-old autistic child with a ten-word receptive vocabulary is being cared for by his monolingual Mandarin-speaking grandma, it can be argued that she should be able to learn English at least as fast as he can. In addition, of course, such a child will need many additional services to develop language capacity, but if a part of the day is spent with Grandma, she should be able to use and reinforce new emerging vocabulary, in English, which is the language we can expect 95 percent of special-education specialists to teach. The important principle is that as a child learns new word meanings in one setting, he or she should be helped to use those words in all settings, so that the word is a true word and not just a trick performed for one person in one place to accomplish some particular desired end (like getting a pretzel stick or Cheeto).

That said, there is also the question of whether parents should then try to cut the child off from all exposure to the mother tongue. If the conversation is not one being directed to the child, there is no clear rationale for taking things to such an extreme. In fact, most children with autism continue to learn at least some language incidentally (without being explicitly taught the words), and incidental learning will increase as flexibility of language use develops. This means that most parents report that by the time the child is eight to ten years old, he may understand basic requests and statements equally well in both languages but may only speak in English. This is actually not much different from what many bilingual families report—that by the time their typically developing children are eight to ten years old, they understand the mother tongue perfectly well and can speak it, but preferentially speak English, resorting to the first language only when confronted with a monolingual family member or when they really, really want to get a parent's attention, and the parent is conversing in the first language. Interestingly, children with autism do this too, with parents also reporting that they incidentally learn bits of the first language. However, when this happens there is usually much more receptive than expressive language in the mother tongue, and any expression is heard only in those rare circumstances when the child really wants something and other modalities of communication have failed.

OPENING ALL THE COMMUNICATION CHANNELS

So far, we've talked a lot about the preverbal or nonverbal aspects of communication; all the tools the typically developing child would have in his toolbox before really tackling spoken language. In the remainder of this chapter, we'll focus more on how these earlier skills integrate with the development of receptive language understanding and the emergence of spoken words.

Understanding the Spoken Word. We know that one of the key ways of differentiating children with autistic spectrum disorders from children with other kinds of difficulties is that in children with ASDs there is a lack of coordination between gaze, verbalizing, and gesture during communication. All three of these are signal systems that we expect to send congruent messages. Not only should a child look to her parent's face for signs of encouragement or warning, she should follow up by listening to the parent's tone of voice and, if possible, what is being said. A deaf child misses the verbal signal, but compensates by directing exceedingly close attention to the facial expression and gestures.

Similarly, a language-disordered child may not be able to make sense of what is being said to him, but will react according to the tone of voice and will pay special attention to facial expression and gestures.

Communication is built as a kind of fail-safe system. In the examples I gave a few minutes ago about how children with autism appear to have no fear and would likely fail a visual-cliff experiment, the reason is not just a failure to look at and read faces and other gestures, it is also that the "backup" system of signals—words and sometimes even tone of voice—are being missed, too. Parents are often the best observers of their children. Parents may be puzzled because they can see that a sharp tone of voice "works," but the child needs to hear that sharp tone of voice before he inhibits his behavior. This is because he is responding to tone of voice and not specifically to the words.

Tone of voice is our most primary, primitive, perhaps earliest arising means of communicating and corresponds to the way animals use different tones of voice to signal fear or danger to members of their group. Nobody likes to yell at a child, and nobody likes to be ignored by their child, so it can be frustrating when the child doesn't respond *until* a sharp, disciplinary tone is used. What is really happening is that tone of voice may be the only part of the system that works, and so later-developing signals—words, facial expressions, and body gestures—go unheeded, and the first meaningful signal the child receives is through the parent's tone of voice. When we talk about tone of voice here, we are referring to something different from "prosody," the melody of speech, which is often also atypical in children with autism. Abnormal prosody occurs when the child cannot *use* tone of voice to amplify meaning the way you and I can. Expressively, tone of voice refers to the way language can be "punctuated" by a sharp or particularly loud word designed to convey prohibition associated with the word. Prosody is the cadence of speech, often singsong or monotonic in individuals with autism, that indicates problems in linking the emotional content of what is being said—such as warning, excitement, disappointment, and so on—with the content of the words being spoken. We will continue to discuss prosody later.

WHAT RECEPTIVE DEFICITS MEAN FOR LEARNING

It is critical to have a full description of the child's receptive deficits and strengths for three reasons: First, we must know what kinds of information (or signals) are likely being received or not. Second, we must deconstruct the nature of those deficits in order to understand the underlying innate processing problems that may have contributed to why the child seems not to understand what is being said. (In the case of receptive language, there are likely contributions from the autistic child's lack of affiliative orientation, his lack of theory of mind, and his difficulties with the speed at which auditory information can be processed.) Third, knowing which of these basic, innate problems underlies a particular child's processing problems gives a focus when structuring remediation.

Not All Have the Same Kinds of Receptive Language Problems. At this point in developing an understanding of where learning difficulties in autism come from, it is simply important to understand that a lack of receptive understanding of speech is not a unitary problem, but rather something made of the primary components listed in the previous paragraph. In addition, some children's ability to learn language may be influenced by attentional factors, perseverative tendencies, memory difficulties, etc. This means there may be a slightly different kind of receptive language problem in each child. From the point of view of an educator, the fact that each child learns language a bit differently shouldn't mean a zillion tests to examine all these factors before individualizing a treatment plan. All that is needed is careful observation, parent reporting, and interaction with the child. (Of course, some formal assessment gets you looking in the right place.) Children with similar levels of language disability may have different underlying problems and therefore will benefit from different teaching modifications. For one child, language may go by too fast and need to be slowed down. For a child with theory of mind difficulties, building initial vocabulary around object labels works much better than building them around vocabulary about social or emotional attributes. For a child whose desire to listen and attend is not socially driven, reading about a topic of the child's interest may be much more effective at building vocabulary than teaching a topic of no special personal interest. For another child who has very limited comprehension of the emotional inflection of speech (say, during a dramatic reading of a fairy tale), there is little reason to be drawn in, and little language decoding comes from the affective tone, while for some typically-dveloping children, affective tone might aide in word decoding. (Interestingly, some parents note how their children with autism, who apparently can't understand the dialogue, will get scared at the appropriate parts of a video, even running out of the room or averting their eyes from the TV. It may be that such children do perceive emotional tone or tension when it is musical (since musicality resides in a different part of the brain than language) and are reacting appropriately, because they intuitively understand. What a great compensatory strategy!)

Taking Care Not to Assume the Child Understands When He Doesn't. In the case of the youngest children with autistic spectrum disorders, they may not be receiving the language signal for more than one of the reasons we just mentioned. Therefore, treating lack of response as defiance and not as a comprehension problem is likely to get you nowhere. For example, sometimes in behavioral programs a directive is repeated until the child complies. The child may really just be guessing from subtle cues rather than words. In this case, it is possible to miss that what is needed is a breakdown of the language, not repeated prompts. If mastery is easier, motivation will be higher.

Similarly, selecting a "talking therapy" treatment such as "floor time" (discussed in chapter 4) may assume that the child can understand what is being said to him. Again, if the child is not understanding words, but just reacting to actions and objects, language learning is not being promoted.

KNOWING WHAT TO SAY AND HOW TO SAY IT: EXPRESSIVE IMPAIRMENTS

Receptive/Expressive Language Disorder and Aphasia. Whenever we consider a child's expressive language problem, we must realize that output will not be better than input: Sometimes I am told that a child has been previously diagnosed with a receptive language disorder. Then I'm asked, "But don't you think he has an *expressive* language disorder—because he can't talk?" If the child does have problems receiving language, the child will inevitably have expressive difficulties of a comparable or greater magnitude. Sometimes I am told, "I know my child isn't autistic because he's aphasic." But one does not rule out the other. An aphasic child is one who cannot speak, cannot understand, or both. It is the processing difficulties that occur in unison with the aphasia, the subsequently arising matrix of disability, that defines how the aphasic symptoms interact with other strengths and weaknesses the child has, which may result in a pattern that represents an "autistic" aphasia—what we may more simply call autism.

Use of the Spoken Word to Communicate with Others. Children with autism often have such a profound impairment in gestural comprehension that words actually may appear before any gestures do. It is not unusual for there to be key communicative words (or parts of words) for highly desired or highly interesting things even before basic natural gestures like looking between a parent and an object or pointing to an object. When a child uses words before gestures, it is a good example of how what was earlier described as a "fail-safe" system works: A relative cognitive strength (ability to process spoken words) can automatically step in and fulfill the same function as should have been fulfilled by an earlier-developing function (gesture)—for the purpose of communication. Many children with autism use first words that are labels for favorite foods, or that are words for their narrowly focused, highly interesting objects (like "F-a-f!" for "fan"). When a child does something like talking but not gesturing, which should have come first, his behavior is serving to lead us to his strengths—to the natural self-accommodation he is trying to make. This can then be capitalized on as an apparent readiness to learn words and word meanings, even in the absence of expected earlier skills like using gestures.

This idea of accommodating to the child's disability can also be put to use to help the child compensate for weaknesses in what should have been earlier-developing skills by using strengths in areas that seem less affected, like word memory. An example of this would be helping a child point at an object as he learns to label it verbally so that he can come to view pointing as a parallel signaling system to speaking.

Building a Communication Foundation. Finally, there is one more point worth making about working to identify accommodations that can be used to teach earlier "missing" skills the way words can be used to teach gestures: From a developmental perspective it is critical not to skip steps in development. A solid developmental foundation eventually will be needed for self-generative learning to arise. A child cannot skip learning to point, nod, or otherwise gesture because "it would be better for him to know the words." There will always be times when a child must know how to ask for information when he *doesn't* know the word, or when something new is being explained to him, and the use of gestures is part of the explanation or feedback on his behavior intended to reflect his understanding.

CHAPTER SUMMARY

In this chapter, we have exhaustively reviewed the problems that children with autism may have in developing basic communication skills. You need to know what's wrong with something before you can fix it. The two take-home messages from this chapter should be: Remember that nonverbal communication is supposed to develop before verbal communication, and if it doesn't, that's a problem that needs to be addressed, too; and there are many different reasons and combinations of reasons that expressive language can be impaired. These must be assessed along with nonverbal communication problems so that we know where the child gets the "signal," what is "noise," and how the signals being received can be amplified to develop an individualized intervention. In the next chapter, we will discuss strategies for augmenting communicative understanding in the preverbal and nonverbal child with autistic spectrum disorder.

Autistic Learning Disabilities of Communication: Treatments for the Preverbal and Nonverbal Child

In the last chapter we discussed the many ways in which the autistic child's world and what he perceives of it can be altered by specific communication-based autistic learning disabilities. These difficulties, a well as the common compensations children with autism make when they have such difficulties are a road map to treatment. The approach taken here is a developmental one. Children with autism can be seen as having communicative difficulties that may begin with the earliest emerging aspects of nonverbal communication, including difficulties understanding and using paralinguistic systems that should provide amplification to spoken language via the message embedded in gaze, gesture, body language, and vocal tone. Since these deficits, when they exist, are notable even before spoken language should be emerging, I take the point of view that construction of communication skills needs to start from the bottom up and must include teaching these paralinguistic skills as well as words. We start this chapter, therefore, with understanding what typically supports the earliest emerging aspects of communication in typically developing children and how we can use that information to inform therapeutic efforts with children with autism.

MOTHER-ESE/PARENT-ESE

Language "Age." How do we make our attempts to communicate with a young child with autism a developmental fit? The answer, very simply is to talk to the child at his or her language "age." The way we talk to most children when we first are wanting them to understand language (that is, from birth onward) is to begin using a manner of speaking to infants that was first called "mother-ese" in the research literature and is now increasingly referred to as (the more "politically correct") "parent-ese." This manner of speaking to children has two key advantages that persist for the child with autism long after the chronological age at which it is still usually employed for typically developing children. "Mother-ese" slows down language and provides repetition to increase the time available to process what is being said, and it uses highly inflected cadence to mark what is the key thing being said to help the child focus on the most core aspect of what is being communicated. Let's go through some examples of what you see when you watch an adult (or even an older child) talk to someone younger than them; the using of different words, tones of voice, vocal speeds, and vocal inflections, depending on whether the speech is being directed to an infant, a toddler, or a five-year-old.

If the adult is talking to a child he or she has never met, that adult quite automatically makes a certain adjustment based on the size (or known age) of the child and speaks in a particular manner. If an adult encounters a friend's cute three-month-old in a stroller at the mall, she may lean into the stroller and coo, "Are you a pre-t-t-y girl?? What a swe-e-t baby!" If the baby is awake, and in a good mood, the baby might fix her gaze on the new person and give a big smile. The adult's voice rises and falls with a prolonged "pretty" and a high-pitched "girl." The key words "pretty" and "girl" might have been repeated a few times until it looked like the baby comprehended and was about to take her "turn" in the conversation and smile in response.

Why do people talk this sort of "baby talk" to babies? We talk to babies this way because babies respond to it. What's the point of talking to someone who is not likely to respond? (Some parents say they didn't talk "baby talk" to their baby because they wanted him to learn to talk like a grown-up, not like a baby. This is actually not the way it works. It's like wanting someone to learn to drive a car before they can walk because they're going to cover a lot more miles in a car than on foot.) Of course, some people are better at talking to babies than others. Some people simply feel foolish talking baby talk to a baby. Some solve the dilemma by often talking *at* the baby rather than *to* the baby ("Well let's put on those little Baby Moschino overalls that Grandma sent because she's coming over this afternoon.") It's not that typically developing children who get talked *at* like that and don't get much baby talk aren't going to learn to talk, but they simply may not end up taking the most direct route to decoding language. They may rely more on other channels of "signal." For the autistic child, this could be a particularly bad problem, especially since these alternative channels are mostly the ones that are very "noisy" or have a lot of static.

In teaching language to children with autism, we want to take a direct route (or any route that's open), and that's where talking baby talk or "mother-ese" comes in. We want to appraise the developmental level where the child's language understanding is at, and talk to him at that level. That's what we would be doing with a typically developing baby.

Even with a 12- to 14-month-old, parents will use more mother-ese than usual when introducing a new concept ("L-o-o-k, Grandma brought you new big-girl pan-t-i-e-s!"). The speech will be drawn out, the key words "panties" and "big girl" repeated to drum up attention and interest in what is being said. These same principles can be used to teach a child with an autistic spectrum disorder to listen to language and decode its meaning.

Talking to a young child with autism by limiting conversation to topics that interest (or might interest) him, and using mother-ese can provide the opportunity for the slowed input that allows for delays in auditory processing, and also marks the important part of what is being said by highly inflected prosody (tone of voice). In my clinic, I often demonstrate to parents how to do this, by talking about some food or toy the child has shown interest in and demonstrating how mother-ese can be used to gain the child's attention when they want to talk about that item with him: If the child is interested in Pepperidge Farms Goldfish crackers, I might say "An-dr-e-w, do you want g-ol-d-fish!? G-ol-d-fish!?" (I go ahead and use that silly voice that those of us who love playing with babies use with nine-month-olds.) Many times if the child is just wandering around the room unengaged when I do this, he'll pause and mill over to where his parents and I are seated—scanning the table—presumably for goldfish. It's almost like a parlor trick. . . . I really just want to teach how to use mother-ese and how it may be effective, but even such a demo not specifically directed at the child often gets a reaction from the child the first time I try it.

If we assume that the maturation processes governing the child's ability to extract meaning from speech are delayed in developing, it makes a lot of sense to give the child access to the same kind of speech we would use with any child at the same language level, even though the child with autism may be chronologically older. Later in this chapter, I will talk more about VIA, a way of adapting existing picture-communication methods to place more emphasis on developing paralinguistic communication skills. One aspect of this is teaching the child to look for semantic cues through the use of mother-ese inflected speech.

Telegraphic Speech and the "Lovaas" Accent. Many people these days are familiar with the work of Ivar Lovaas and how he has pioneered the use of discrete trial training to use methods of applied behavior analysis to teach young children with autism. There are both advantages and disadvantages to this method—as there are to all methods of teaching children with autism because it is not a "one-size-fits-all" disorder. In chapter 10 we discuss the strengths and contributions of this approach in detail, but for now it is relevant to focus on an informal tradition of teaching language that has grown along with the widespread use of discrete trials.

Often, I encounter discrete trial trainers or tutors (as well as parents who have been so trained) who talk to young autistic children with what I sometimes call "the Lovaas accent." For those who may know Dr. Lovaas—or those who have heard him lecture—I do not mean a slight Norwegian accent. What I mean is a tone of voice that has a fixed use of prosody, with the instruction uttered in a flat voice followed by a louder volume at a similar pitch which is reserved for the "SD" (discriminative stimulus) or objective of the instruction (such as "Touch C-O-W!" or "Touch N-O-S-E!"). Articles, adjectives, and adverbs are not used unless they are the SD, in which case the article, adjective, or adverb is uttered using the same fixed pattern "Touch B-I-G Cow!" Touch M-Y Nose!" The child is exposed to a very simplified telegraphic form of speech that instead of including the filler words (that is the articles, etc.), has the filler words deleted so that the child has no exposure to them until they are explicitly taught. By contrast, the more developmental, mother-ese model includes filler words, though they are spoken faster and more softly so that they don't attract the bulk of the auditory-processing time or effort. However, the filler words are there for typically developing children so that as soon as the child comprehends the key words, he can begin to understand the filler words, too. The underlying goal implicit with mother-ese is to build the internal structures that ultimately support syntax and what is called "generative grammar" (the ability to use word combinations that have not been explicitly taught) so the child can form new word combinations that he has never actually heard. (By contrast, SD talk omits grammar and thereby ensures that natural speech that the child hears outside of specific teaching situations remains mostly incomprehensible "noise.")

There is no real reason why developmentally geared speech like mother-ese can't be used with discrete trials. The reason that it is not is that in the 1960s Lovaas was one of the behaviorists who postulated that language was a complex series of conditioned behaviors—that there was no uniquely "human" quality to language such as the capacity for "deep grammar" as others, like linguist Noam Chomsky, called it. (In the intervening 40 years, virtually all developmental psycholinguists would agree that the data support Chomsky's position more than the position of behaviorists like Lovaas on this point. While it is easier to conceptualize how to teach language as a long series of "discrete" conditioned behaviors, it does not appear to be how real "language" is learned. However, it is clear that for some children, language that is learned via discrete trial teaching kick-starts more generative language learning that the child can continue to elaborate on on his own.

Features of a Communication Program. Irrespective of what specific treatment methods are selected to help a child with autism develop communication skills, some basic principles apply. These include an awareness that slowed language gives more time to overcome possible processing speed difficulties. A highly inflected tone of voice and/or increased volume directs attention to key words. Repetition of key words provides compensatory help for any short-term memory difficulties. Repetition of key words should help comprehension by giving more chances for the key word to be noted. Pairing auditory information like object labels with the corresponding objects helps since so many children with autism are more visual than auditory learners.

This is not to say that, as a child with autism develops, we should continue to talk to him like a nine-month-old, even if that worked well at first. We don't keep talking to nine-month-olds like nine-month-olds, we naturally modify our language to children and make it more sophisticated as the child demonstrates increasingly mature capacities. So while it is fine to overly inflect and to repeat and slow speech, as the child responds, these should be naturally pulled back. The adult should rather move toward a model more closely resembling speech directed to typically developing children of the same age. Sometimes more formal testing and retesting of language can help a teacher or parent keep a pace of where language abilities currently are.

PICTURES AS COMMUNICATION

Many children with autistic spectrum disorders are much stronger visually than they are verbally. This is almost universally true of children with diagnoses of autistic disorder and PDD,NOS. (For children with Asperger's disorder, the reverse is often true: The world of words is complex and interesting, even if at first it consists of large chunks of only partly digested and not fully comprehended content. While children with Asperger's share many other autistic spectrum social and behavioral traits, they tend not to share the same language learning style. Thinking primarily visually is often not a strength for children with Asperger's that it can be for other ASD children.)   We will focus in this chapter on the teaching needs of children with ASDs who are nonverbal, preverbal, or minimally verbal. (In chapter 7, we will focus on enhancing verbal communication.)

Visual Icons. Here we will focus on teaching communication skills through the use of visual icons. For those children who are visually strong, who take much information from context, and who are preverbal, low verbal, or poorly understood because of oral-motor apraxia (which we will discuss), visual icons can be almost like a Rosetta stone to making sense of all that is being said in the world around them. It is wonderful to give such kids their first icons and see them finally develop some sense of control over the world around them.

VIA (Visual Interaction Augmentation). The major approach that will be discussed in this section is the use of a strategy in which pictures of desired objects are exchanged by the child for the desired object itself. The best-known method for doing this is a curriculum model known as the Picture Exchange Communication System or PECS. Here, we will talk about principles of PECS as a foundation for visually augmented communication. Then, we will introduce VIA, developed as part of my clinical research program, a newer-generation model that is a modification to existing picture-communication approaches like PECS.

First we need to understand where the idea of pictures fits in. The term "picture-communication systems" (PCS) or, even more broadly, "alternative augmentative communication" (AAC), can be thought of as more generic than PECS and is largely what I will speak about here. While the PECS method has many strengths, here we will rethink visually based communication strategies more developmentally and more specifically with respect to how autistic children, in particular, learn, adopting some aspects of the PECS method, eschewing other aspects, and modifying implementation for certain children.

THE IDEAS BEHIND AUGMENTATIVE COMMUNICATION

What Does Augmentative Communication Mean? One of the main concepts in helping children with ASDs learn to talk is the idea of augmentative communication. Augmentative communication includes pictures, talking machines, video displays, or any device that provides the child with a way of representing a word or idea he wishes to express. Ideas about augmentative communication originated in work with children who had primarily physical barriers to talking, such as children with cerebral palsy or severe oral-motor apraxia that left them with little control over oral-motor (mouth, tongue, lips) movements. Not all children with these problems have developmental disorders as well, but many do. This meant that devices that were intended to circumvent motor problems in order to permit communication also often allowed for adaptations that could start the child with simple language concepts and proceed to more complex ones. (Even physically disabled children without substantial cognitive handicaps can become delayed in language just because of the absence of a way to practice and refine emerging language concepts.) An important part of learning to talk consists of someone's trying to understand you and helping you modifying your efforts until they do understand.

So the field of augmentative communication developed with two goals: first, to help children who could not physically produce audible or comprehensible speech, and second, to help children who might also need special assistance to learn, practice, and refine the ideas they wanted to express. Obviously, most children with ASDs do not need the benefits conferred by physically adaptive devices to overcome any motor aspects of communication problems. Many produce sound just fine. There is, however, a small number of children with ASDs with oral-motor apraxia or other more "central" auditory processing problems who at times seem to have better understanding of language than can be reflected in their ability to express. For these children, sounds come out poorly or are incompletely articulated, garbled, or not made at all. The use of some mechanical or physical apparatus allows us to know what they want to say. This group includes some children who are clearly saying something (the same sentence over and over), but no one knows what it is. It is almost as though each phoneme (letter sound) is going through a scrambler, and we would need a secret decoder ring to understand it. Other children may verbalize in a similarly garbled manner, but with one key word intelligible. For children such as these, augmentative communication devices can be very important because they allow communicative attempts to be understood. When we can respond to such attempts, we are reinforcing the whole (difficult) communicative effort, which is critical when we want the child to want to talk. If a child has a hard time formulating the words and then isn't well understood when he says them, you can expect less, rather than more, speech over time.

Does Augmentative Communication Interfere with Development of Spoken Language? A big controversy about the use of augmentative communication devices is whether their use will slow down or even replace spoken language in a child who *can* learn to talk. There is no evidence for this. In fact, what little empirical evidence there is suggests that it may prime spoken language development.

From a developmental point of view, it makes sense that visually augmentative communication should help spoken language get started: Children learn to recognize things as familiar and functional before they can label them (for example, a baby knows a "bottle" is a "bottle" long before he has a word for "bottle"). Children also learn to understand words before they speak them. It therefore makes sense to rely on these earlier-developing systems that don't require the production of spoken words to help the child make the move from what's on his mind to what he wants others to know is on his mind.

The "Speaking" Child. We also know that about a third of children with autism never develop spoken language. A smaller percentage of this third become what is sometimes called "speaking" (rather than using language in a truly generative way). This means that some children with much training learn to vocalize a small number of words that are associated with well-rehearsed meanings. Usually, "speaking" children have five to 15 words or short whole phrases that are used with varying regularity and usually relate to strong needs or wants, including preferred objects. Sometimes these words are understood mainly by familiar caregivers. Sometimes they are more universally understood. Some children have words that are heard only rarely, under unpredictable circumstances. Being in this "speaking" category has some substantial advantages over being completely nonverbal or mute. "Speaking" serves as a universal way for your caregivers to know what you want, albeit for a limited (though probably core) set of needs. A final and key point to consider in the use of augmentative communication is that it can be difficult to know with certainty if a preverbal, or nonverbal child with autism has the capacity to learn to communicate well orally. So, one hedges one's bets using augmentative communication: Maturation or neurodevelopmental processes in the brain needed for language may be delayed, or spoken language may not be in the cards for a particular child. All children deserve the best opportunity to be able to communicate to the best of their ability now, to not be frustrated, and from an educational point of view, not get turned off to learning communication skills because talking is too hard or impossible.

When to Start Augmentative Communication. All children deserve to succeed rather than fail whenever that is possible. Language instruction approaches that begin with an "oral-only" approach for nonverbal autistic children run the risk of asking a child to do things he can't do, or can't do yet. A more conservative approach is to start with a visually augmentative communication approach for every nonverbal child with an ASD and teach spoken language side by side with the visually based communication system. This way both systems have a chance to develop, complement one another, and provide a foundation of communication success from which a drive to communicate can arise.

Sometimes I talk with parents who don't want their child to work with any kind of an augmentative communication system because they think he will get lazy and won't bother to speak if he can touch a picture or push a button. This really shouldn't be much of a worry with children with autism, because above all else, children with autism are instrumental: They want what they want when they want it, and they want it five minutes ago. It will always be quicker to utter a word (or even word approximation) than to go get a picture or a device that requires that you press a button to "say" the word for your need. Autistic children can be counted on to consistently prefer to have their needs met sooner rather than later, so if the child can utter a word, he will. As long as spoken-language models are appropriately used alongside any augmentative-communication device, spoken language will emerge if it can, because it will always be a more efficient adaptation.

Augmentative Communication Electronic Devices. Starting with the section below, we will focus discussion of augmentative communication on the use of pictures and some three-dimensional objects as icons or symbols for what the child may want. However, in addition to the major thrust into picture-based communication for autistic children in recent years, there are sporadic efforts to have children with autism use a variety of electronic devices to communicate. These have several practical disadvantages for the child with autism that are often not a concern for the wheelchair-bound child for whom such devices were developed: 1) They can run out of batteries. 2) They are fragile and typically don't do well being dropped (or put in the toilet, sink, or swimming pool). 3) They are expensive to replace. 4) And, most importantly, any fixed device makes it difficult to use with simultaneous training of the social aspects of communication, such as gaze or gesture. Typically, a non-ambulatory child will have a voice or picture-communication device affixed to his or her wheelchair. When the child pushes a button to indicate a choice or need, a non-autistic child will typically look, make eye contact, smile, or in some other way, socially acknowledge the adult's response "Oh, you want a cookie?" The device is one actor in the full script of the joined social and linguistic activities that together are the child's communication. An autistic child may readily push a button, but is less likely to spontaneously add the social part of the communication—looking to see if he's understood and smiling in acknowledgment that he is. Really, the device is just a convenient excuse to continue to act autistic. It's all "bells and whistles" compared to a picture or three-dimensional icon—as it does not provide positive opportunities for the child to meaningfully add more nonverbal social aspects of the communicative act.

CREATING THE MOTIVATION TO COMMUNICATE

So far, we have introduced the idea of augmentative communication. We've discussed the idea that some communication is better than no communication. I've suggested that children with autism are often thinking in short videotapes. Children with autism often have organized a visual recognition of activities and objects in their world before they have a "sound track" (namely words) on their videotapes, let alone higher-level abstractions like intentions.

The Picture Exchange Communication System (PECS). In recent years, a big innovation in the development of communication skills for children with autism is the use of a curriculum model called the "Picture Exchange Communication System" (PECS) developed by Andy Bondy and Laurie Frost when at the Delaware Autism Program. This curriculum model takes advantage of understanding that children with autism often "think in pictures." PECS uses pictures to teach a communication system based on stronger visual than auditory skills. Then, using principles of applied behavior analysis and discrete trial training methods, children are taught to exchange pictures for the things about which they might want to communicate. This has been an excellent and pioneering model that has moved special education for the communication needs of children with autism way beyond the often futile use of sign language, and beyond "communication boards" or "communication books" in which icons were often numerous, overwhelming, fixed, and used in a way that did nothing to address the social deficits in communication.

PRINCIPLES OF VIA

Here, we will consider how the principles of PECS can be further informed by a more developmental approach and by our understanding of autistic learning disabilities and autistic learning styles. The goal here is to come up with ideas that can be used to individualize a PECS-like approach to make it as relevant, and thereby as motivating, as possible for each child. Because we will be discussing additions and modifications to the basic PECS methodology as it was initially developed, I will not refer to these modifications as PECS, out of respect for the original work. Rather, I am acknowledging PECS as a starting point, and refer to modifications and additions as constituting "visual interaction augmentation" or VIA.

FINDING THE CHILD'S "NATURAL" ICONS

Does this child think in pictures? If the answer to this question is "yes," then some sort of a visual icon-based system should probably be part of teaching communication skills. As we've already said, "thinking in pictures" for most children with autism means that it is as if they possess a large collection of short videocassettes, each containing a narrative of a routine that helps them achieve a frequently desired goal. If Chips Ahoy cookies are beloved and Mom keeps them on the second shelf of the cabinet to the left of the fridge, the Chips Ahoy "video" may consist of pushing a kitchen chair to the counter, climbing onto the counter, triggering the childproof latch, pulling down the bag of cookies, and chowing down. One problem that has also been mentioned is that this videocassette has no sound track. Another problem is that these videos most often star objects, not people, who at best play supporting roles, like the hand opening the fridge door. It is very usual for children with autism to memorize complex routines such as this one, well before they have acquired the use of words for any of the stars of their movie (like the Chips Ahoy cookies), let alone words for the supporting actress (like "Mommy, help me!"). A central challenge of a picture-based teaching approach is to lay down a sound track. Over time, the sound track as well as pictures can be shared, and what's in the child's mind can readily be made known to others.

Theory of Mind and the Use of Visual Icons. If we take this videocassette analogy a step further, we can think about how a picture-based communication system should essentially "freeze" a key scene from the video. This is important for a couple of reasons. First, as we discussed in chapter 4, most younger children with autism lack a theory of mind, meaning that they don't know that others have thoughts (and feelings) the way they do. Unlike the typically egocentric two-and-a-half- to three- year-old who thinks mommy has nothing better to do every minute of the day than to read his mind and anticipate (and meet) his every need, the autistic two-and-a-half- to three-year-old has no clue that mommy can "see" what he is thinking when he is pushing the chair up to the cabinet to get to the cookies, or when he dives into her purse to extract forbidden chewing gum. This is because the two-and-a-half-year-old with autism lacks a theory of mind—the idea that others can reason to the same conclusions he does based on the same evidence. This means the two-and-a-half-year-old with autism doesn't know that you know that the reason he is digging in your purse is to find the gum. And, since he doesn't know that you know, he isn't deceptive; he does it in plain sight. Cute as this is at two-and-a-half, it is less cute at six-and-a-half when the boy with autism, still lacking a theory of mind, takes down his sweatpants and masturbates in front of polite company. When typically developing children learn communication skills, it is based on their ability to understand that we can tell what they are thinking. When we teach communication skills to children with autism, they too need to come to understand that we can tell what they are thinking. This "mind reading" is the bedrock of communication.

The single, most powerful early advantages of a picture-communication strategy is to be able to take a "freeze-framed" shot from one the child's favorite mental videos and essentially say, "Here, Chips Ahoy! Is this what you have in mind?" By taking the exact image the child "has in mind," you are making a de facto statement to the child about your capacity for "reading his mind." This is where development of theory of mind needs to begin.

This is also where VIA and PECS diverge. With PECS, a more generic cookie picture will typically be used if possible, with the idea that you are teaching a conceptual prototype for cookie. With disabilities other than autism, in which theory of mind is not a core deficit, this type of approach makes a great deal of sense. However, we know that children with autism may have what is sometimes termed stimulus over-selectivity or perceptual inconstancy (as discussed in chapter 2). This means that with a child with autism, we cannot assume what it is visually that makes a Chips Ahoy cookie recognizable. It may be the size, the texture, or the particular smell. The child may not believe it's a Chips Ahoy if it doesn't come from a blue package. If the parent can see that a Chips Ahoy cookie *is* what the child has in mind, the parent is taking the first step in teaching the child that she can indeed "see" what he has "in mind," by using a very literal icon such as a photo of the cookie, the packaging, the cookie and the packaging, whatever the parent thinks the child has "in mind." This means that even if a child can recognize the drawn icon of a chocolate chip cookie used in PECS, it is not as developmentally useful an approach as a photo or other literal icon—since we also need to develop theory of mind.

It is very useful for a child with autism to know that others can know exactly what he wants. This, from the point of view of the autistic child, means his needs will be met sooner, and more precisely. What could make communication more motivating?

3-D Icons. When we use the analogy of a freeze-framed videotape, adults naturally picture two dimensions. Yet, if I were to ask you to picture or "mentalize" a basketball as you see it on a TV screen, and then mentalize a basketball that was sitting on a table in front of you, you would actually have two different kinds of images in your head. The way we do this is completely automatic. However, it is an ability that was developed somewhere along the line. For some children, the use of picture-based communication gets bogged down when the child has not yet made that developmental shift where he automatically recognizes the difference between a TV basketball and a basketball on a table and knows that they are exactly the same thing.

When children are still not able to conclude that two-dimensional and three-dimensional representations of an object are the same thing, it can be very helpful to start using a visually augmented communication system in which the visual icon is three-dimensional. How can this be done in a way that is true to the principle of "freezing" the mentalized representation of the object (what the child sees in his head)? The challenge is to devise an icon that represents what it is that the child wishes to communicate about, but make sure that the object is indeed an icon, a symbol, and not so real or functional as to replace the item itself. So, for example, there are classrooms in which a child can choose a pear or an apple for his snack by touching a plastic pear or apple. Many times the child will reach for one of these and try to bite it. It's *too* real. Biting the plastic pear becomes a second activity that may be nearly as interesting, or possibly even more interesting, than eating a pear slice. Then, getting the plastic pear away from the child and replacing it with a real pear slice may seem like a booby prize rather than an accomplished goal. The act of "communication" is, in that case, no longer communication, but a series of activities—seeing a plastic pear and plastic apple, deciding to play with the plastic pear, having it taken away, and being placated with a pear slice that actually doesn't look like the whole pear anyway.

Another difference between the VIA and PECS approaches is related to the selecting of literal three-dimensional icons: What is needed is an icon that stands for the thing it portrays, but does not become something unto itself (like the plastic pear being something fun on its own). The item needs to remain a completely clear three-dimensional representation or symbol, just the way a word is a symbol for the thing to which it corresponds. The best strategy I have seen for this is using clear cassette boxes that can be used to hold a sample of the desired object. A cassette box (sealed with superglue) might contain a few goldfish crackers, a mini-Oreo, or a couple of pretzel sticks. Items that are perishable or too big for a cassette box might go in a small screw-lid plastic container that has an actual pear slice in it that can be replaced at each snack time, or a small rubber snake (if that's what the child craves for play). (The PECS approach recommends laying the desired object on a two-by-two-inch piece of oak tag and covering it with clear contact paper. Sometimes this works fine, too, but sometimes you have a small square card of goldfish crumbs after one use—not very helpful, as almost all of the literal qualities have been lost.)

A visually based exchange strategy can then be followed using the literal three-dimensional icon that comes as close as possible to what the child has "in mind." Using the prompting strategies from discrete trial training (described more in chapter 10), the child is then supported in handing over an icon such as a goldfish cracker sealed in a cassette box to get a real goldfish cracker in exchange.

2-D Icons. For children who have developmentally passed about a 12-month level of overall visual understanding of their world, two-dimensional icons are likely to work well. You can tell if a child has reached this stage in one of a few different ways: One sign of readiness for a two-dimensional approach is when the child has achieved "object permanence"—knowing where to look for a desired object when it is covered up in their plain sight. Another sign of readiness for a two-dimensional VIA approach is if the child can watch TV and consistently recognize people or things on the TV. A variant of this would be the ability to recognize different examples of the same objects in a book, such as Barney seen in different poses.

If the child does not yet have clear signs of readiness for a two-dimensional approach to augmented communication, separate activities can promote readiness: The child can match pictures to actual objects. This will establish that the child has a way of understanding that the two-dimensional and three-dimensional representations of something have strong similarities. Again, the same discrete trial prompting methods can be used to promote three-dimensional to two-dimensional recognition of key desirable objects and activities.

What Should the 2-D Icon Be? A big question is what kind of two-dimensional icon to use. All sorts of things have been tried, including photos of the object, photos of the child with the desired object, magazine cutouts of the desired object, and pieces of the box or wrapper depicting the desired object. However, when a child matches a mental image of a desired object or activity to a photo, he is not going to be seeing himself in that image. So, he should not be part of the picture. But, as we talked about earlier, there is no one right icon. The goal is to select an icon that comes as close as you think you can come to what each particular child has "in mind." That will be most motivating because it will help the child develop an understanding that you can see what he has "in mind," increasing the probability of future attempts to communicate.

Making Icons Material and Literal. These days, the easiest thing for a teacher, certainly, and for most parents as well, is to create two-dimensional icons from digital photos. These can be saved, reprinted, and resized. Parents and teachers and other therapists can readily share icons, increasing the power of the icon as visually based augmentation to interaction that is universally useful to the child.

Despite the sensibility of using literal, personal icons, most children I meet in my clinic, and most children whose classrooms I visit, are primarily or exclusively using Mayer-Johnson icons from the Board Maker software. These are either simple black-and-white line drawings of generic forms of objects or colored-line drawings. Some are figural (like a three-sided trapezoid topped by an oblong to represent a "cup"). Some are metaphorical (like a simple smiling face with upturned eyes gazing at a halo to represent "good"). There are several potential disadvantages to the use of such icons. First, they do not "freeze" what the child has in mind. Children think in terms of very material images, not in Mayer-Johnson icons. Second, the mental effort involved in associating the more abstract Mayer-Johnson icon with the more material mental image has nothing to do with furthering communication by establishing a foundation for the development of theory of mind. Third, many icons are so abstract as to be incomprehensible to, say, a nonverbal five-year-old who is quite unlikely to have a frame of reference for understanding a halo. Fourth, the lack of material, literal quality to such icons detracts from how immediately recognizable, and therefore how motivating, they are likely to be to the child. For example, if you could not think of the name of the type of sushi you wished to order in a Japanese restaurant and the names of the various sushi on the menu did not help you either, what do you think would most assure you that you would get the one you had in mind: a Mayer-Johnson icon of a rectangle colored pink, or a color photo of sashimi? The color photo of real sashimi not only would closely match your mental image of sashimi, but would likely motivate you to order sashimi more than a picture of a pink rectangle would. (Yes, this means we can assume that all those sushi photos and realistic plastic sushi are in Japanese restaurants both as a communicative aid, and for marketing purposes.)

Certainly, children can come to recognize simplified drawn icons like Mayer-Johnson icons (which are what are most often used with PECS).

However, the whole point of using a visually based strategy with children with autism should be to *motivate* communication and then create a lexicon of icons that the child can use as easily and effectively as possible. This argues for using the icons that most closely represent the child's mental image of what he wants. From the conceptual framework of the VIA approach, there is no real value in a more abstracted icon. The icon is a step on the way to talking. Wasting effort on promoting recognition of abstract line-drawing type icons is tantamount to promoting reading in five-year-olds using Gothic script one day, and cursive the next. It requires a level of abstraction that detracts from the child's real task— getting what's in his head into your head.

Getting Started with Icons. Once it is clear whether a two-dimensional or three-dimensional icon should be used, the next question is content. What should the icons depict? There is an unfortunate tendency to overdo things at this stage, what with there being 24 or 36 exposures on most rolls of film. (Hopefully, the dawn of digital photography will end this particular problem.) Starting with just a few pictures to teach the rules of this visually based communication "culture" stacks the odds in favor of quick success. Having a list of things the child wants, and introducing icons from the top of the list down is the way to go. Each picture should be an image of what the child is likely to have in mind. Next, you must think about how this object can be doled out piecemeal to give the child many opportunities to make a request for that thing. The method of using discrete trials to give the child an opportunity to make many successive requests for a desired object via the exchange of the icon for a desired object was innovated by the PECS curriculum. This technique involves placing the icon of the desired object in front of the child, and having an adult take the child's hand, placing the child's hand on the icon, and placing the icon into the waiting, outstretched hands of the adult who is there to receive the icon and immediately supply a response in the form of a small amount of the indicated item (like one goldfish cracker, or half a goldfish for a slow eater). If the child seems to be pleased indeed to get a goldfish, this procedure is repeated several times, each time with slightly less assistance in getting the icon into the child's hand and in transferring it to the waiting adult.

As far as the mechanics of constructing icons, photographs or easily recognized logos can be glued to a piece of oak tag (or cut-up file folders) and then laminated. Most schools have laminating machines, and parents can purchase a smaller home version for under $50. Each icon (two by two inches is a good size to gain attention, but still fit in tinier hands) should have a small square of Velcro attached to the back, with the corresponding half of the Velcro square affixed to the place to which the icon should be attached. By using colored poster boards or file folders as backgrounds, icons can be made so that all foods are mounted on one color, all toys on another color, all places to go on another, etc. This should help both children and adults locate icons when they are wanted. Each icon should have a small caption with the appropriate word in a clear font attached to the front of the icon, the use of which will be discussed below.

VIA: Developmental Linking of the Visual and the Auditory. Earlier, it was noted that some parents express concern that a picture-based communication approach such as PECS might move a child away from efforts and opportunities to learn to communicate in spoken words. This should never be. Visually augmented communication should be viewed as a strategy to prime and enhance spoken language capacity. One way to do this is to ensure that teachers and speech and language professionals using visually based approaches understand the importance of pairing spoken *language* with the use of icons.

Because children with autism are so visual, they should always be given visual and auditory equivalents together. One way to do this is for all icons to have clearly visible words on the icon's label. The presence of the label is not so much for the child to look at as for the teaching adults. Each use of an icon is an opportunity to link the visual icon, the mental image of the icon, and a specific auditory input.

In addition to simply pairing the visual and auditory, it is also important to gear the auditory (the words) to how the child is able to hear them, developmentally speaking: As we discussed, "mother-ese" is basically a slowed, highly inflected, repeated way of talking that flags the key word or words in a statement. The purpose of mother-ese is to gain the auditory attention of someone who is just starting to decode auditory "signal." Mother-ese doesn't have to sound like baby talk, but should be geared to getting the child to listen more attentively. To make it as easy as possible for the child eventually to learn to respond to a word (without the icon), every opportunity should be taken to say the word for the object repeatedly. If the child hands over a cassette box with goldfish in it, that box should have the word "goldfish" written on it. The teacher should prompt, "Oh, do you want G-O-L-DFISH for snack today? G-O-L-DFISH???"

If the child then picks up the goldfish cracker cassette, when taking it from the child, the teacher should say, "Oh, you DO want G-O-L-DFISH!" and then, when producing the goldfish, say, "Here's your G-O-L-DFISH!" The purpose of the word "goldfish" on the box is to ensure that the teacher doesn't say "goldfish" while an aide calls them "crackers," and a second aide forgets to label them at all.

Any icons a child uses at school or at speech therapy should be duplicated at home, or in any other care or teaching setting the child is in, so that there can be consistent reinforcement of emerging concepts across all these learning situations.

VIA: Reading the Nonverbal Communication "Signal." Why look someone in the face when you want to talk to her? Part of normal discourse is not just knowing what is being said and to whom, but how it is *meant*. Much of this latter part of the meaning comes from how we look, where we look, and how we gesture as we say something. Mostly, as we discussed in the last chapter, the communicative use of gaze, gesture, and facial expression are used very little, if at all, by children with autism. Not only do they use it little, but they understand it little. But, we also talked about how these paralinguistic communication strategies are, in typical development, the ones the child comes to rely on first. Also, understanding the paralinguistic part of what is being said should bolster and clarify the meaning of words. So, from a developmental perspective, visually based augmentation of communication *must* include a way of teaching paralinguistic communication too. It is in this way that VIA departs strongly from PECS by putting major emphasis on simultaneous use of a paralinguistic "mother-ese" alongside (semantic) mother-ese speech.

VIA: Speaking "Mother-ese" with the Body. Communication is a two-way street, so if a visually based communication strategy is used, it must be set up as a two-way street as well. If it is more simply a system of "I (the teacher/ parent) ask," and "You (the child) reply," we are still stuck in the same place at which most communication with children with autism is stuck. There is a lack of reciprocity.

To generate reciprocity, the child must have opportunities to communicate spontaneously what is on his mind and what he wants, *and* he must learn how to "read" what others are telling him. This begins with reading the face of the person with whom you are communicating. Let's go back to the initial, basic interaction using a picture or icon exchange strategy. The child has a picture placed in front of him. He is motor-prompted to give the picture to a person ready to receive the picture, who will then supply the pictured item.

The person receiving the picture or icon is on the edge of a great teaching opportunity: The icon, once received, should be held to the face of the speaker to get the child to direct his gaze to her face. If the child doesn't spontaneously look at where his icon is going, the speaker may have to adjust herself into the child's visual range, or the prompting person may have to help the child continue to look in the direction of his icon and the speaker's face. If this is begun after the child has the basic idea that the icon's disappearance precedes the corresponding desired object's appearance, continuing to look at the object is a natural response. The adult holding the icon now has the opportunity to hold the icon to her face and repeat the word printed on the icon a few times in an emphatic manner ("BA-A-R-NEY? Do you want to see BA-A-R-NEY?"), holding the icon near her mouth so that the child has the opportunity to not only hear the object label, but also to "see" what the word looks like when it is spoken. Then the adult should use a positive facial expression that conveys that she indeed recognizes what the child wants (Barney), and then present the desired object (Barney). This is cuing the child to learn to look at the adult's face to know whether his request is being processed. A smiling face, a head nodding "yes," will then come to signify that the child has acted in a way that tells him that his needs are about to be met. From the autistic child's point of view, he now, finally, has a reason to look at a face as part of communication, namely, to see if he is about to get what he wants. This lays the foundation for the child's understanding the successful rudiments of a communicative act that involves both verbal and nonverbal elements used in a coordinated manner.

Conversely, if the child attends poorly and picks up an icon at random, handing over a picture of an undesirable object (like a raw broccoli floret), then the adult can use a puzzled face, shake her head "no" and say in a questioning voice, "BR-O-CC-OLI? You don't want BR-O-CC-OLI, do you?" During these interactions, the adult who is helping the child give the icon can also help the child mirror the adult's nonverbal response—such as by helping the child shake his head "yes" or "no."

Whether the communication involves having needs met or refused, the point here is that the child will come to look at the face of someone speaking to him when he has reason to believe that he will find some information that will help him understand what's about to happen. Children with autism value predictability, and this builds a system that ensures predictability through action, words, gestures, and tone of voice. This makes VIA an augmentative communication approach that is more autism-specific as a teaching method. It addresses a range of possible autistic learning disabilities—lack of facial expressiveness, lack of gestural communication, and lack of verbal language.

In the VIA process, the child begins to develop a lexicon for the meaning of different facial expressions, gestures, and tones of voice. To miss out on these teaching opportunities when using a picture-based exchange system is essentially to reinforce a more autistic method of communicating that obviates the need for coordinated nonverbal communication alongside words used to communicate. Without an emphasis on gaze, gesture, and tone of voice, the "exchange" is just that—a transaction, not an interaction. It is important to contrast the VIA procedures that have just been outlined to what is often used in PECS as well as in the discrete trials—the applied behavior analysis curriculum that will be described in chapter 10, in which the child may be trained to look into the teacher's face, using an unrelated reinforcer prior to initiation of an instruction. Using this method, the child is indeed being taught to look at the face of the teacher, but is not being taught anything about *why* he should look or what kind of information he should be seeking from that face.

Making Choices from Two. As long as the icons are ones that represent desired physical objects, this procedure can be slowly elaborated to include several icons. The object doesn't have to be food. If the picture is of a favorite toy, like a rubber snake, the child can be given 15 or 20 seconds to play with it, or to have someone play with it with him before it is put away. Once the child understands the paradigm of giving something to get something quite like it, and understands he must pick up and hand over the icon on his own, it is time to begin with a choice of two things.

Something new is happening at this stage at which a choice between two things is being made: When a child gets to make a choice, he is essentially choosing what he sees as the more rewarding or reinforcing of the two items. This is where the system starts to become self-sustaining and the act of communication becomes truly meaningful in terms of controlling what can happen in one's own life.

Sometimes, when the concept of making a choice is introduced, the power of choice making doesn't hit the child right away. There may be a sense on the part of the teacher, parent, or therapist that the child is just responding by rote, or at random, especially when substantial prompting is still needed. This is more likely to occur when the child is presented with icons that represent a choice between two rather desirable things. If you showed me, personally, pictures that gave me a choice between a semisweet chocolate bar and a bittersweet chocolate bar, I might well plop my hand down on an icon at random. Either would be fine. However, if you gave me a choice between a chocolate bar and a raw broccoli floret, you'd have my full attention; I would be very motivated to indicate the chocolate bar lest I be bitterly disappointed by raw broccoli.

VIA versus PECS. There are many classrooms in which the use of PECS is routinized. It may only be used at snack time to get snack items. It may only be used in explicit training sessions, and the icons might not be put in functional contexts for the child. In this case, PECS is not really being used as a strategy for teaching a child about communication. Using PECS only at specific times (i.e., during class) is like taking a foreign language that is never practiced anywhere outside the classroom. How motivated would you be to study that language? This is what happens when PECS is only used at snack time at school, not at other times, and not at home. The reason we want to introduce the idea of picture communication is to give the child an understandable bridge into the world of our communications. If the child has a way of communicating, he is more in the mainstream. There is both a reason and a way to interact.

Teachers can get caught up in the mechanics of a picture-based communication system and forget the "exchange" or social interaction goals that are intrinsic to developing spontaneous communication. For children with autism, the need to learn the social rules of communicating is at least as important as knowing what the objects are called.

During initial training using a visual-communication strategy, the child will need many trials just to learn the concept of exchange and choice making. This certainly needs to be done in direct didactic sessions, initially with two adults, and then one adult and the child. At these times, it makes sense to have a booklet with copies of all of the child's pictures or icons available and organized by topic—for the teacher or therapist—not the child, as in the PECS method. Making the child go through a catalogue just to say something interrupts the spontaneity and contextual relevance of the social interaction part of communication. Similarly, it makes little sense from a social development or language development point of view to include in these sessions the use of a "sentence strip" or other place to attach the icon rather than directly handing it to the adult. (This would be like having to write a word down before a teacher would consider a request a pupil was making.) Further, the use of a card that says "I want ____," is not so much grammar as a routine—the way a child who can't get his mother to get his father to buy him the toy he wants might first add "Please," then "Pretty please," etc. The "I want ____" card is just part of a routine, not an independent part of a flexible use of grammar with unique meanings to "I" and "want." As such it just gets in the way of the content of the communication, making it longer and probably less motivating for the child to engage in this form of communication.

DEVELOPING AN ABILITY
TO UNDERSTAND WORDS: WORDS AS OBJECTS

When most children with ASDs begin to talk there are two strikingly different things about the words they say: One, children with autism mostly use words for things they want. They tend not to use words to share attention ("Look!"), or to share concern ("Ut-oh!"). The second thing is that almost all first words are for objects that are important to them. While some will develop instrumental words for help that is needed ("Up"), this is less common. This is yet another indicator that the early linguistic world of the autistic child maps words for objects with higher contrast than words for actions or feelings. So, object labels are a good place to start teaching words.

Sometimes, though, there is emphasis on object labels to the exclusion of other less salient parts of speech. Earlier, we talked about the disadvantages of the simplified, telegraphic utterances often associated with SDs used in discrete trial training. Talking to children with autism using only very simplified phrases containing mostly the object label ("Touch nose!") may indeed provide higher visibility to the part of speech that can be seen (the noun). However, sustaining this way of talking may play into autistic learning weaknesses by allowing other parts of speech to remain "noise" rather than trying to remediate their not being "heard" and incorporated into emerging grammatical understanding. A child will eventually need exposure to natural grammar if he is to acquire it for himself.

Sensory-Motor Learning of Word Meaning. One of the strengths of a visually based communication system is that it gives the child things to do physically as he engages in the process of communicating. Little children are like machines that charge up from their own activity. As the child can touch, look at, and physically move an icon, he is representing the acts of "giving" and "getting" through his own actions. This makes it important that the physical activity of the "interaction" or "exchange" part of using visual icons is not ignored, as when the child can indicate a need by simply touching a picture, but not having to move it or do anything else with it. There is too little communicative effort in such requesting, too little self-initiated, self-guided, self-monitored behavior. For young children, autistic or typically developing, doing is learning.

Sequencing Pictures. Sometimes, however, it makes sense for a child to have available the opportunity to generate his own sequences with pictures so that the use of visually-based communication can begin to form a visual "grammar": Omar, a three-and-a-half-year-old boy to whom I'd just introduced picture communication was working on single icon requests, and had learned that the picture of his favorite rubber beach ball got him the ball, and that the picture of the doorknob of his treatment room got him a chance to go out in the hall for a few minutes. The room was carpeted; the hall was not. The beach ball actually didn't bounce very well in the carpeted room, and so when Omar would give me the icon for his ball, it wasn't that much fun to play with, because he couldn't bounce it. Then one day (on about the third day of using pictures), he gave me the ball icon, and as I went to get the ball, he also grabbed the doorknob icon off the doorjamb and gave me that too. I gave him the ball, opened the door, and out he went into the hall to bounce his ball. Omar was "thinking in pictures," and the two critical "freeze frames" he needed me to see in his bouncing the beach ball videocassette were getting the ball and getting out the door. Being aware that what the child has in mind may involve more than one step opens the use of a picture system to greater flexibility and the emergence of a sort of visually based grammar or action sequencing.

Of related importance is that pictures, just like the objects they stand for, may not (should not) always be available. While it may be fine to request going out the door once, even twice (just to see if this system really works), there will also be times when going out the door will need to be removed as an option for a while. When this is the case, the icon can be placed in an envelope with a universal "No" sign (circle with a diagonal slash), an opaque container with a slit just big enough to deposit the icon, or some other similar device. The child may scream and protest upon being told "No" in this manner, but then all young children need to learn to respond to the limits set by adults.

VIA: Placing Pictures in Context. Going back to the "thinking in pictures" concept, we know that context imbues a great deal of meaning to children with autism. Therefore it is important to use context to function as part of the visual "grammar" for the icon. The context in which the icon is likely to be thought about is part of the natural understanding the child has about the meaning of any icon. So how can we use context as "grammar" for picture icons? The most logical answer is to place the pictures in the context in which the thoughts about the thing that the icon represents are likely to occur. A photo of an individual serving of Tree Top apple juice should be attached to the door of the refrigerator if that is where the boxes of juice are kept. In this manner, the photo represents the "freeze frame," and the placement of the photo represents the preceding and subsequent frames of the video about apple juice. (This is a departure from the basic PECS procedures that place icons together in thematic groups in a binder.) Of course, when an icon is first being introduced, it needs to be taught in a teaching context, just as when a student in an intensive foreign-language course might have one section a week on vocabulary and grammar, and another three for conversational practice. Keeping the pictures in contextually relevant locations is more like the conversation section of the course.

Children should have access to the same icons at home as at school, just the way we use the same words to mean the same things, irrespective of where we are. There should be a copy of each icon or picture in its functional context. This means some pictures might go on kitchen cabinets, some on the refrigerator. Pictures of favorite videotapes should be placed near the VCR (and even if the child can select a desired video and operate the machine for himself, the tapes should be locked away so the child has an opportunity to practice "asking"). Pictures of toys and equipment in the backyard should be placed on the doorjamb to the outside so that a choice of what to do first can be made. Other pictures can be taken outside, and successive choices for subsequent activities can be made by having a longer strip of Velcro to attach pictures to so the child can construct a plan of what he will do. In the bathroom, tub-toy pictures can be attached to a plastic bin so that the child can make a choice of toys to take in the tub. Everyday routines present teaching opportunities when having a way to communicate should become most meaningful, thereby reinforcing communicative effort.

Putting pictures in needed contexts is an excellent way of building them into a communication system and making them meaningful in everyday life. But sometimes the child is at McDonald's, Grandma's, or the park and wants to express a desire or preference. It obviously won't work to have one parent run ahead to McDonald's and post icons throughout the place. What's an alternative strategy? The best one I've seen (and this depends on the temperament and age of the child), is to have one of those key chains on a retractable cord that attaches to a belt or belt loop. A big key ring can be attached, and small-sized versions of possibly needed icons can be attached, one to each of several cards. The strategy of color coding by topic (foods, toys, places) can help organize this, perhaps with different key rings for different experiences, like restaurant foods, playground toys, etc. The child then has a more portable communication system than using the blue PECS binder. It is just too much work to go through mom's baby bag looking for an icon book in order to say what you want. In this case, screaming is much more likely to be the most expeditious way to get your needs met.

USING PICTURES TO TELL, NOT JUST ASK

The applications of picture- or icon-based communication that have been discussed so far all are based on the idea of the child's asking for something and the adult's giving the something. This is just one reason children use communication. It is just one reason that adults communicate to children. It is the best place to start, since in many children with ASDs, prior to any treatment, communicative initiations are nearly one hundred percent "instrumental"— designed to get something the child wants for himself.

Visually Based Communication and Insistence on Routines. If a child has some means of expressing preferences through pictures (if not words), routines that may have seemed like irrational insistence on having something a certain way, or having something right away are directly addressed because the child now has a way of controlling what happens and doesn't have to rely solely on things being exactly the same from one time to the next.

Many children with autism (and most children with poor language under-standing) are likely to prefer a routine as a way of having some predictability. This is why we can say that being fixated on routines is an autistic learning disability—it is so common in autism. We can also say that taking advantage of the desire for routines can be an autistic learning strength, style, or manner of positive adaptation: Using a picture icon of familiar objects (the dinner table, the bathtub full of water and toys, pajamas laid out on the bed with a book), a parent can "tell" the child things (as opposed to the child using them to tell the parent). So if the child usually eats dinner, takes a bath, and gets in his pajamas for a story, the parent can announce a change in routine by showing that tonight the child will have his bath, get in his pajamas, and then eat dinner. This can help the child be flexible by assuring him he is not losing predictability. It allows the parents a possible change in routine if friends are coming over, and allows them to get the bath done before the child's dinner hour.

Similarly, many children with ASDs can be very insistent about where they go when in a car. But sometimes, a new route may need to be taken because of the need to get gas or pick up a prescription at the pharmacy. Many parents of children with autism are terrified of such moments. Use of a visual schedule can really help in this sort of situation: A strip of Velcro across the seat back in front of the child can be used to order pictures of the stops that will be made. The procedure helps establish predictability about where the car will be going next. The visual ordering of the stops also can accompany conversation the parent makes about where the next stop will be, taking down each picture as the stop is completed.

MAKING PICTURES WORK AS COMMUNICATION

The foregoing examples illustrated how pictures can become a starting point, not just for teaching vocabulary, but also for supporting communication around everyday events. The emphasis in the VIA approach is to make visually based augmentation of communication as natural a form of interaction as possible—the way sign language is. While sign can be great for children with a natural comprehension of gesture, the opposite is true of children with autism. When there is no comprehension of gestures or gaze or facial expression or tone of voice, those must be paired with the thing that is understood—pictures. To me, this is very different from many classrooms with PECS programs, which can feel like a place where the only kind of communication going on is a banking transaction: The autistic child is the customer, and the teacher is the bank teller at her kiosk, ensconced behind a couple of inches of bulletproof glass with almost no interaction, just pieces of paper passing back and forth. It can be easy to fall into this with children with autism because, given their druthers, most are happy enough to keep social interaction to a minimum. However, the activity of a picture or icon exchange is the ideal moment to work on integration of social interaction and language using the para-linguistic and verbal "motherese" methods we've covered.

PICTURE COMMUNICATION FOR VERBAL CHILDREN

Fading Picture Communication. Once a child can say a word or use a reasonably intelligible and consistent word approximation for an icon, it is time to stop using the icon. The use of icons is simply a bridge to the next stage—talking. (I remember visiting a class where a popcorn icon was being used at snack. One little girl, impatient to wait her turn for the popcorn icon to be available again so that she could get another serving, started saying "Puh-crn! Puh-crn!" The teacher turned to her and said, "Show me!" I wanted to scoop up the popcorn and give it to the little girl myself.)

Fading the use of a visually based system is likely to be a gradual process, with some icons being taken away as the child demonstrates the ability to verbalize instead. Verbalization should always be differentially positively reinforced. When an icon is removed from a child's "vocabulary list," it might be substituted with a blank icon containing just the word to remind all teaching staff that the child should now be able to give a word or word approximation. (The child should not be required to do the exchange in this case, but simply say what he wants—as long as the adult knows that "bu-u" is a request for bubbles and not for a Buzz Light Year action figure.) While some icons may be faded as words emerge, icons can still be useful to indicate new things that the child is just learning about and may understand and recognize, but not yet have developed a receptive vocabulary for.

Using Pictures with Children with Severe Oral-Motor Apraxia. Some children with autism have notable problems with articulation. While most children do not have this kind of difficulty, perhaps 10 to 20 percent of children with ASDs do. Even after ASD children with articulation difficulties begin to try to talk, speech may be indistinct, garbled, or missing initial or final sounds or certain specific sound blends. Speech therapy and other specialized treatments like Fast ForWord aimed at articulation can address this and will be covered further in the next chapter. However, unclear speech can be a particular barrier for the child with autism who has a low communicative drive anyway. Pictures can be used to help him indicate what he wants, amplifying the communicative "signal" he puts out and raise communicative drive by increasing expressive successes.

There are a couple of advantages to continuing to use pictures as a partial support after initial attempts to say a word starts: First, even if the child does not engage in an exchange of an icon for an item, he can learn that once a picture is indicated, you do know what he wants and you will be able to respond contingently. If the child has learned his paralinguistic communications lessons in the early stages of a VIA program, he will look to see if his utterance is being understood, and if it is met with a blank or questioning expression, will follow up with a point to the picture until he sees a facial expression to show that his communicative effort *has* been understood and will be acknowledged. Second, once you know what the child is trying to say, you as the teaching adult are in a much better position to understand what specific articulation errors are being made. A list of missing sounds, positions within a word in which a sound may be dropped, and blends in which one sound is missing or another sound altogether appears can be a road map to articulation therapy. An experienced speech and language professional in collaboration with a classroom teacher or parent can help develop remedial strategies and priorities for teaching successions of sounds that the child will need to master.

CHAPTER SUMMARY

In this chapter we have focused on putting together a systematic understanding of the developmental stages of language development in children with ASDs. The VIA (Visual Interaction Augmentation) approach was introduced as a more autism-specific way of working with picture-communication systems such as PECS. We discussed approaches for developing communication skills in preverbal and nonverbal children. Emphasis was on using visually augmented strategies, since most young autistic children, as well as many older children with ASDs, have stronger visual skills than verbal ones, and the visual strengths can be employed in a number of ways to bolster and build language. The VIA system was introduced as a developmentally structured method for teaching the child to read and ultimately use both paralinguistic as well as spoken word strategies to communicate. The motivation of children with autism to learn and use language is closely tied to coexisting difficulties in social understanding, and the chapter showed how development of communication skills must exist within a framework of instrumental purpose for the child. In the next and final chapter on communication skills in individuals with autistic spectrum disorders, we will address specific strategies for development of language skills for the verbal child.

Autistic Learning Disabilities of Communication: Treatments for the Verbal Child

"LESS IS (NOT) MORE": GETTING THE CHILD TO USE HIS WORDS

Some children with ASDs have words all along, but do not use those words as much as others their age, or use expressive speech in peculiar ways. Others are very delayed in initial language development, but with speech therapy at two, three, and four years of age develop functional speech and grammar by age five or six. In this chapter, we will focus on verbal children with ASDs and the challenges of improving their language use. This chapter is intended for parents and teachers who focus on children who have moved beyond the "preverbal" or limited verbal "speaking" stage and are speaking in phrases and sentences. By kindergarten or first grade age, these children are often in separate and different educational placements from the children who continue to need the support of visual icon communication curricula. For parents, children at this stage usually present new challenges, like that of getting the child to talk more.

Instrumental Language. Most early language expression in ASD children who have been delayed in language development starts out as limited to instrumental functions—words for things they want, or words for how the child wants things

("Lights off!" or "No juice!"). Often, even when the parent knows the child has responded to a particular question or direction in the past, the child may seemingly not comprehend what is being said on a different occasion. It can be hard to tell whether the child is not responding because he truly doesn't understand (maybe he has forgotten what a particular word means because he hasn't used it in a while); is being avoidant or defiant; or whether the "who," "what," or "where" of the question is just different enough that the child is put off from answering for some other reason.

When a child doesn't understand, it is important to know why. Analyzing when the child does not respond can tell a great deal about his learning deficits. With children with autism, these deficits usually fall into one or more categories of what are being called autistic learning disabilities, meaning that the child is missing tone of voice, gestural, or affective cues that might help another child understand the meaning of what has been said. Children with autism may not answer simply because they lack the social drive to respond. Usually, a child with autism is not interested in responding just because someone is paying attention to him or because he wishes to remain the focus of attention.

IF HE UNDERSTANDS, WHY WON'T HE ANSWER?

Autistic children need a reason to answer. "Just because I asked" is usually not a good enough reason, as that would be a more purely social reason. The probability that a child with autism *will* answer, or appear to comprehend or comply increases as the "instrumental press" increases. This means if the child can see that there are clearly desirable consequences to answering, and he knows how to answer, he will respond. Just as is the case when using visually based communication, it is necessary to create a situation in which the child wants to answer, or wants to ask a question because in his mind, it will get him something he wants or wants to know.

Upping the Communicative "Press." When the child really wants something, it is a good opportunity to increase your communication demands just a bit. If the child has just seen you open a bag of Cheetos, and he said, "Cheetos" while approaching your bag with what looks like an intention to grab the bag, this is a good time to tighten your grip on the bag and say, "Kevin, do you want

Cheetos?" If Kevin replies, "Cheetos!" prompt him by touching his chest lightly with your forefinger (I'm assuming Kevin is almost on top of you by now) and saying "I want Cheetos." If he says, "I want Cheetos," thank him for asking, and give him a few Cheetos. I prefer "Thank you for asking!" to "Good saying 'I want Cheetos!'" since the latter is not a grammatical sentence and can only serve to confound any emerging sense of grammatical rules. Adult responses that result in the child's possibly echoing grammatical formulations that are not correct fails to provide available opportunity to reherse meaning.

Depending on how many Cheetos you have, and how much Kevin likes them, this could be a good time to practice related conversational gambits like "I want more Cheetos," and "Mom, I want more Cheetos, please." Take advantage of the tendency to echo by developing a way of prompting an echo like touching his chest, (or cheek or lips, or touching your own lips then pointing to the child's mouth). The prompt should model appropriate speech with just a bit more elaboration of the statement the child has generated on his own.

A common error in prompting speech revisions, however, is to take the conversation lesson too far. If the adult starts to prompt the child to "say it better," add "please" *and* use a proper noun to address the person with the Cheetos, and keeps withholding the Cheetos until all these additional demands are met, it is no longer a conversation or even a conversational lesson, but just too-hard a lesson. The child is likely to give up and just walk away. The chance to prove the idea that spontaneous requesting is useful is lost. The child will have learned nothing about rules of language pragmatics, which is that you clarify an utterance only until the listener understands. It is also a key teaching opportunity in these kinds of situations for the adult to add real, natural conversational responses, like the "Kevin, do you want Cheetos?" response to an initially nonverbal communicative initiative on the child's part (trying to grab the bag). This exposes the child to natural language models at a time when his receptivity to what is being said will be high—because he wants something.

THE FUNCTIONS OF ECHOLALIA

The first type of noninstrumental spontaneous speech to emerge that does not pertain to needs and wants is often echolalic. There are two basic forms of echolalia: immediate echolalia and delayed echolalia. The presence of these tells us something about how the child is trying to process language.

Immediate Echolalia. Usually the first type of echolalia to develop is immediate echolalia. Sometimes the child just echos something he hears, for no particular reason. This shows us that the child can hear it and that he can keep it in short-term auditory memory long enough to reproduce it. So, this says that two of the mechanisms necessary for production of language are functioning. But is the child comprehending? Probably not, or maybe only partly.

The next step in processing language input is comprehending. If language gets stuck at this point, it could be said that the child has a "central auditory processing disorder" (CAPD). This is a term favored by some speech and language pathologists. Saying that an autistic child with echolalia has a central auditory processing disorder is fine, but it doesn't tell the whole story. Children with "mixed receptive-expressive language disorders" (a more medical term originating from the field of psychiatry) have central auditory processing disorders, too. To be accurate, CAPD describes where language processing first gets stuck (that is, at the point at which the child tries to construct meaning). Having a CAPD does not mean that the child *cannot* also have an ASD, and it does not mean the child *has* an ASD. However "CAPD" in an echolalic autistic child is about as common as sneezing in someone with a head cold.

Functions of Immediate Echolalia. If very little meaning is extracted from language that a child hears, the child may produce immediate echolalia. This serves a number of functions. Often it serves to show the adult that the child *is* trying to respond, and that he is attempting to give a topical answer. When the teacher asks, "Xavier, do you want graham crackers for snack?" and Xavier replies, ". . . graham crackers for snack." The reply is generally taken to be an affirmative reply. If the snack had not yet been set up, and the teacher had said, "Xavier, do you want popcorn or graham crackers for snack?" and Xavier had replied, ". . . graham crackers for snack," the teacher might have concluded that Xavier *was* interested in a snack but was not getting the idea that he was to make a choice, or that the choice today was between popcorn and graham crackers. (She could confirm this hypothesis by switching her question and asking Xavier if he wanted graham crackers or popcorn for snack and seeing if this time he replied ". . . popcorn for snack.") In this case, the teacher might have produced icons for each of these or filled bowls with the snack items and repeated her question in the presence of a physical prompt, which may have aided comprehension and produced a definitive, non-echolalic reply. Immediate echolalia, then, can serve as a placeholder in a conversation. It is a "partial self-accommodation" as discussed in chapters 2 and 5. It partly it works and partly doesn't, but it shows us where the room for improvement is.

When a child gives a verbal response that is sparser than he is capable of producing, he may need a little prompting to produce fuller expression (as in the foregoing "Kevin and the Cheetos" example). It is the same for an echolalic child. The important thing is to acknowledge that even the echolalic response is an attempt to be in the conversation. The modifications you push for should not become so overwhelming for the child that the conversation becomes just a lesson. Everyone needs to make clarifications in a conversation, but it is important to have a sense of the boundary between conversational clarification and an academic exercise. If the interaction is no longer a conversation to get information and reach a goal, the autistic child is not being shown why he should be using his words functionally. Since motivation to speak spontaneously is so low in most children with autism, reinforcing attempts to use language to communicate must take into account that motivating language is usually at least as important as speaking better—and sometimes more important.

This approach to working with immediate echolalia is based on a developmental understanding of how conversation skill develops. It is different from what a teacher with a behavioral orientation would do, which would be to ignore the echolalia, re-prompt and wait for an appropriate reply, or step back further, practice the reply utterance, and then re-prompt with the question. This is not recommended here because, while such an approach may be used to create the desired response, the response is rotely elicited and is de-contextualized from its conversational meaning. In the more behavioral approaches the opportunity to let the child know that his attempt to respond with echolalia has got him part way there is taken away from the child, so there is no contextually-meaningful reinforcement of his emerging attempt to take his turn in a conversation.

For most children, immediate echolalia is a developmental phase that occurs when they begin to understand the function of words but can't always decode what a word means soon enough to give a specific and relevant reply. Typically developing children do this to some extent as well, at about two to two-and-a-half years old. In children with autism it is usually a more prolonged phase because they are not able to use the additional paralinguistic cues (following gaze, following gesture, listening to tone of voice) to figure out meaning the way a typical two-year-old can. Similarly, children with non-autistic language development difficulties (which might result in diagnoses such as "expressive aphasia," "expressive dysphasia," "developmental language disorder," "expressive language disorder," or "central auditory processing disorder") might also show echolalia for some of the same reasons, although such children can usually achieve better self-accommodations or compensations over time by relying on the paralinguistic signals that do come in more clearly.

Delayed Echolalia. Delayed echolalia is the other half of what happens when a child has some sort of difficulty with extracting meaning from language (or what may have been described as a central auditory processing disorder). Delayed echolalia occurs when the child repeats whole chunks of something that has been heard in the past. Sometimes, delayed echolalia functions in a way that a whole phrase or statement stands for a simpler word: Recently, I asked a mom to take away her child's giant cookie, so that the cookie could be broken in pieces and used as reinforcers in a testing session. She took the big cookie, leaving Ezekiel (her three-and-a half-year-old with likely Asperger's syndrome) just a small piece. This was a mild-mannered college professor mom, who often gave her child elaborate verbal explanations for things, often kindly prefacing or ending her requests to him with "Sweetie" or "Honey." Upon having the cookie pried gently from his fingers, Ezekiel, without turning around to look at his mother, said, "That's really very annoying, Sweetie!"   Another example, starring Thomas: "We're not going to Grandma's house today" meant "No" (for any reason) after having once been told that although his father had taken the freeway exit for Grandma's house, that was not where they were headed that day. "We're not going to Grandma's house today" subsequently came up in many non-driving contexts.

Often the delayed echolalic phrase that is used in this partly functional way was initially heard in a context with a degree of somewhat negative affect attached to it. So, a child in my clinic interviewing room who is trying to open the door may say "Don't turn the lights out!" after being told to leave the doorknob alone. The proximity of the light switch to the doorknob, and the fact that a half hour ago, he may have been flicking the lights and was told to stop that too, makes it obvious why this particular phrase has emerged at this moment. Not infrequently, a child may respond to a prohibition by repeating it in other situations in which other prohibitions apply. It seems likely that the child is able to understand the meaning intended by the parent's tone of voice, as well as some of the words in "Don't turn the lights out!" when he later reuses that phrase in a related situation. What that tells us about that child's learning style is that he is getting some paralinguistic information in the form of understanding the meaning of at least certain tones of voice. This would be an indicator that this type of "signal" on this "channel" (as it was described in chapters 5 and 6) is functioning for this child, and language development work could take advantage of that by accentuating tone of voice congruent with word meaning. In both of these examples of delayed echolalia, the delayed echolalic phrase is just one way of saying what the child is trying to say, but the child overuses the phrase and overextends its meaning.

In some ways, delayed echolalia is not so different from what typical children do. Typical children use "overextensions" when they are first acquiring words— "ga-gee" (meaning "doggie") may be used whenever the child sees an animal. Over time, as the child's vocabulary grows, only indoor animals are "ga-gees," and later, only dogs are. The difference is that this stage typically comes later (at three or four years old) for autistic children, while it may be in evidence as early as 12 to 18 months in typically developing children. The autistic children, being older, may have more mature capacities for auditory memory and employ that capacity to compensate for lack of specific understanding.

TV Talk. As children spend more time watching the same videos over and over, more of delayed echolalia consists of "TV talk," repeating very long portions of dialogue from children's programs like *Blues Clues* or Disney movies. Not surprisingly, there is much more movie echolalia today than there was before the mid-1980s when the VCR became ubiquitous. A historical note: What kind of delayed echolalia did we see in children with autism before VCRs? Mostly, they sang songs from audiocassettes or from school. I know one Russian immigrant boy with autism who can recite 70 poems but cannot use the vocabulary in them. And, that's the first thing to know about this type of delayed echolalia: The child usually does not understand most of what he is saying— though he may well get the gist of the dialogue. Some children produce delayed echolalia with no clue as to meaning, especially in the case of songs. Parents may be puzzled as to how their child could memorize 20 or 30 songs, but still can't talk. However, when questioned, such parents realize that this seemingly-bright child does not know what she is singing about. Nevertheless, storing such vast numbers of words is an impressive feat, *especially* considering that little is understood. In such cases, the child may be showing us that melodic cues are more comprehensible and memorable than words. Teaching object-label vocabulary through song (nothing fancy, try doing the "Hokey Pokey" or "Head,

Shoulders, Knees, and Toes") may be a viable way of employing compensatory strategies from which this type of child can particularly benefit.

Are Videos Bad for Children with Autism? Some parents are very impressed by delayed echolalia at first because it seems to suggest that the child not only has the capacity to develop spoken language, but to speak in sentences and even paragraphs. However, there is a threshold at which delayed echolalia can start to sound frightfully odd, even to the most optimistic parent. The child may engage in long recitations of entire scripts, becoming quite agitated when interrupted. Other children take to mimicking the voices of different cartoon characters so well that when they are not "doing dialogue," they still sound like Barney and have to be reminded to "use your real voice, not your Barney voice." Jessy, a 28-month-old girl with autism has no functional language, but during a play session she sang the ABCs in a Baby Elmo voice so well that we could not tell at first whether it was her or the singing ABC Baby Elmo on the floor nearby. Parents of children like these don't know whether to love or hate TV and videos. Some resort to banning videos, while others let the child watch them ad litem. Other parents may ban videos on the simple principle that television rots young minds and stifles creativity.

So, are videos bad for all children with autism? Are videos bad for delayed echolalic "dialoguers"? The answer is not cut and dried. When we think about helping a child with autism learn language, there are many advantages to videos: They can be viewed repetitively. If an adult watched a foreign film in a poorly understood, or not at all understood language and sat through it once a day for a week, by the end of the week, that adult, and certainly most typically developing children, would have memorized some words, figured out some words, and begun to "hear" some of the words more distinctly. This suggests that the autistic child with a strong auditory memory and a good ability to match words to visuals would be helped by repeated viewing too.

When you watch a video, the tone of voice used to utter a given phrase or segment of dialogue is exactly the same every time you play the video. For children with autism with prosody processing difficulties, this can be great. (The ones with prosody processing problems are usually the ones who talk in a monotone or in a lilting, or "deaf-sounding" prosody themselves.) Each time the child watches, the same words appear with the same scenes. Over time, and with the aide of a good visual and auditory memory, this kind of experience allows the child to predict what will happen next—and understand better what is being said. There are other reasons that videos can be a good way to decode some language: Autistic children who enjoy anticipating a routine and enjoy repetition know they can completely rely on the predictability of a repeated video viewing. If you like repetition more than novelty, what could be more rewarding? This means that repeated viewing can be its own reinforcer in the course of being a language-learning strategy.

There are many advantages to improving language comprehension through the strong pairing of repeated words and repeated visuals. Anticipation of causal actions and developing an ability to predict (following a story line) is one advantage. In chapter 8, we will return to this topic to discuss how videos can be used to provoke imaginative play.

What can be bad about videos is that watching the same one, especially a very simplistic one that is completely memorized, can introduce too much mental downtime. Time spent watching familiar videos is time not spent doing something newly informative. When the video becomes such a routine that the child is highly agitated when it is turned off, or when the child only wants to watch one small segment repeatedly, then it is a problem and needs to be curtailed. (We will discuss more about avoiding mental downtime and curtailing routines in chapter 9.) The bottom line on videos for children with ASDs is really no different than for typically developing children: If it is appropriate for the child's level of development and language understanding, and he is getting something out of it (learning new words, colloquialisms, getting play ideas), it's fine. If he's not, it's not. This means that for children with ASDs videos should not become an unsupervised electronic babysitter. Parents need to keep tabs on what the child watches and how often it is watched.

Functional Delayed Echolalia. At times, whole chunks of memorized script can get injected where just a single word or phrase belongs, but the child is clearly echoing this to try to convey a meaning that is idiosyncratically associated with the memorized chunk. This pattern of delayed echolalia is actually quite similar to immediate echolalia in terms of language pragmatics—the thing the child echoes is an attempt to take a turn in the conversation without fully comprehending the content of the conversation. As is the case with overly brief responses and immediate echolalic responses, a child producing a functional delayed echolalic response can be prompted to be more specific. So, if Thomas is asked whether he'd like a turn putting the car down the ramp in the play parking garage and he says "We're not going to grandma's house today," the adult might respond by cuing Thomas with a touch or a quietly vocalized "You say . . . " followed by a louder "I don't want to play with the garage!" Of course, if Thomas repeated the prompted speech successfully, it would be an excellent time to move the garage out of the way and offer another toy, rewarding the effort he used to pull together the needed vocabulary for a relevant, non-idiosyncratic response.

Non-Functional Delayed Echolalia. There also are times when a child repeats a phrase incessantly for no apparent purpose except for the satisfaction he gets in hearing it over and over, much as you or I might hum or whistle a tune "stuck" in our heads after hearing it on the car radio. When a child does this in a way that interferes with trying to talk to him or instruct him, that definitely may be a good time to use a more behavioral approach to reduce the echolalia, which in this case is certainly a behavior incompatible with learning. If what you want to say or tell the child at that moment is something of interest to him (and it should be if you want the repetitive speech to stop), you should cue the child to be quiet (such as by putting fingers to your lips or his) and then quickly issue the statement of interest in order to redirect his interest. So, if Calvin is repeating, "Nickelodeon is brought to you by . . . " over and over, he can be cued to be quiet, and then immediately asked if he would like to do a puzzle or a worksheet (assuming he enjoys at least one of these).

I'm always surprised that many parents (and some teachers) think that interfering with the delayed echolalia might be harmful to the child, that he "needs" to do it. Not true. Do you "need" to "hear" in your mind's ear, some insipid Christmas carol three hundred times after you heard it in the mall? It does nothing for you, and non-functional delayed echolalia does nothing for the child. He needs help stopping. Working to eliminate annoyance echolalia in children with autism need not be like military school, and so a few seconds of perfect silence on Calvin's part need not precede the adult's offer of a choice of functional preferred activities designed to redirect focus away from the echolalic speech. When this sort of approach is taken, much more time is spent on power struggles than instruction; it doesn't have to be this way.

Another example: Taylor, a six-year-old boy with high-functioning autism drove his family crazy on the five-hour ride to my office, repeatedly announcing some bit of something he'd picked up in school. His parents, dreading the ride home, gave this kind of echolalia as one example of the disruptiveness of what they saw as his uncontrollable behavior. (The gorgeous little 18-month-old sister would start to shriek after listening to him for a while, I was told.) Taylor's parents were afraid to insist he stop because they thought it would somehow hurt him to do so. We devised a plan in which he would be asked twice to stop, and on the third request, they would pull the car over and give him an accompanied time-out at the road side to the count of 60, with as many repetitions as was needed. Since it was clear to parents that Taylor's agitation had to do, at least in part, with a desire to end the car trip, prolonging the trip seemed an appropriate deterrent.

The Link between Music and Language. We have already talked a bit about how some delayed echolalia is the repetition of songs. Some children with autism gravitate to music particularly, and this may have started with their being soothed by nighttime music cassettes, or a particular attraction to the lyrical repertoire of Winnie-the-Pooh. What implications might this have for the child's learning?

It is understood that musicality occupies a different area of the brain from most language function. (We can know things like this because of studies in which different parts of the brain show activity when different sorts of stimulation are given.) If the child is viewed as having a selective pattern of impairments (like good auditory memory but not-as-good central auditory processing), it may be that the child has the wiring for relative musical talent. It is not known whether autistic children with exceptional auditory memories and significant echolalic tendencies are also the ones with greater music skills. It certainly seems possible that this is the case for the subset of highly echolalic children who repeat from videos and are able to imitate the original voices extraordinarily well.

For many children with ASDs, just as for many typically developing children, music is elemental and inherently attractive. Music is another way to build sensory motor involvement in a learning task. If it allows the child to move, touch, look as well as listen, the child is more fully engaged. In the case of ASDs, there is an increased chance that when information is being delivered in modalities other than a purely linguistic one, one of those modalities will be able to receive a stronger "signal," one that the child can more readily understand.

Sometimes it is difficult to know which children with autism will do the best in terms of being able to learn things musically. It can also be difficult to know whether music enhances language development in the most musically gifted of children with autism. Typically, parents discover these talents inadvertently. Casey, a blind boy with Asperger's syndrome, was discovered to have perfect pitch when he began to announce "B-flat" when the doorbell rang. Finally, his father, a music producer, realized that Casey was consistently right. Other parents who are musicians themselves start to teach their children and soon discover that the child can readily replicate any note given. There does not seem to be anything about autism that would mean that there would be more musically talented children among the autistic than among typically developing children. In fact, most of the time, musically talented children with autism seem to come from a musically gifted family, just as is true of typical children.

Musical talent can also be important not just in an instructional modality, but in terms of helping the child define himself over time: Six-year-old Trevor came from a very well-off family who bought him a fancy electronic keyboard after he quickly learned "Twinkle Twinkle" on a toy xylophone. A piano teacher was hired, and she began with "I've Been Working on the Railroad." During lessons, Trevor soon learned that flipping some of the other switches on the keyboard produced interesting sounds, too. In his spare time, it became a minor life goal for Trevor to get to the keyboard and flip some of those other switches. After a couple of weeks he seemed to hone in on the switch that played the theme music from "Star Wars." One morning, his teachers heard the "Star Wars" music and figured Trevor had once again made it to the keyboard before they had. The music sounded a little slow, and one teacher worried that Trevor had finally managed to break the keyboard. When they arrived in the room with the keyboard, they found it was Trevor sounding out the "Star Wars" theme by himself on the keyboard.

One of the great things about musicality in a child with autism is that it can give the child a sense of success and pleasure at the same time. In Trevor's case, he performed "I've Been Working on the Railroad" at his first piano recital. Being six, it did not seem all that unusual that an adult had to help him to his seat in front of the piano to begin, and then retrieve him when it was over. When his mother told me this story, I could tell that this was her proudest moment with her son. For the first time I felt she was able to measure him—in one way—on the same meter of achievement she used for his siblings.

Music Therapy? So are Trevor and or other autistic children like him good candidates for music "therapy"? Should all children with autism have music therapy? It all depends on how you define "therapy." If anything a child can learn from is therapeutic, then music can be therapy. However, I would suggest that for most people, "therapy" implies remediation of a specific deficit. Learning, as in the case of learning to play an instrument, is the result of "teaching," not "therapy." If the child shows an aptitude or interest in music, it will be more intrinsically motivating to learn than other things. Getting a child with autism to apply himself to learning something is always better than letting him avoid learning experiences. So, if a child with autism shows aptitude or interest in music, by all means, help him pursue it. Just don't call it therapy.

Music as a Tool for Teaching Language in Autism. Music is processed on the right side of the brain; the opposite side of the brain from language. Many children with autism can hum, mumble, or babble songs before they can produce any clear speech. Some higher-functioning children with autism sing songs and use delayed echolalia before much functional speech, probably processing this type of output with the right sides of their brains too. If right-sided functioning is unimpaired compared to left-sided functioning, it makes sense that the child will begin to show skills that utilize the right side of his brain before regular speech, which uses the left. It also means that language-teaching strategies that rely on right-sided abilities (like singing) may really help a child compensate. Embedding speech in music and pairing it with strong visuals (like dances with gestures designed for young children), may utilize all the stronger areas of cognitive capacity surrounding the relatively weaker areas that should support language. Pairing music with words may be may be one way of inducing the autistic brain to listen better. "Better" listening in this context can be measured by increased word comprehension. In using music, it is important for teachers and therapists to remember that the language learner is typically at a very sensory-motor stage of development. This means that language should be taught in a way that enables the child's participation as he listens, for example, by clapping his hands, banging an instrument, or blowing a kazoo.

Fast ForWord and Earobics. Another way to provide a higher level of engagement in language learning may be through visually attractive teaching methods that use computers. While the computer does not offer the same kind of sensory-motor experience that a drum or a kazoo does, it can incorporate multisensory responses to stimuli by use of constantly moving graphics and incorporating special means of data entry such as touch screens, power pads (very simplified keyboards that may have only four, eight, or twelve very large keys), as well as keyboards, and a mouse.

This category of intervention may include a couple of recently developed methods that slow speech down for children with autism by digitizing speech. The two best known of these are the charmingly named Fast ForWord and Earobics. How are these programs supposed to work?

There is evidence that children with autism know that there is a sound to be heard (which is why they pass hearing tests); the problem begins when the child tries to make sense of sounds and words in sequence. When the brain begins the process of decoding what it is listening to, it may stop paying attention to new things coming in on the heels of the words not yet decoded. In chapter 5, we discussed how this is like listening to a foreign language, getting hung up on translating the first part of the sentence, and losing the rest of what gets said. There is some research that suggests that as speech is slowed down, the child can understand more of what he hears. The most sophisticated of the methods that have been developed to "retrain" the brain to hear "faster" is a computer-assisted instructional program called Fast ForWord. It is one of the only computer-assisted instructional (CAI) programs that absolutely requires a computer. The way it works is that it slows speech down to 50 percent or less of the normal rate by digitizing the speech and presenting it slowly. It sounds intelligible, but, to the normal ear, quite boring and monotonous. It begins by asking the child do simple things like differentiate between the sounds "ba" and "pa" and later, with slowed speech to "touch the flying cow." If the child clicks on the flying cow, something interesting happens. As the child learns to respond correctly, the computer keeps track and asks the child to do other things. The computer systematically keeps track of the child's errors, noting things such as the words the child has difficulty decoding and whether those words have certain sounds or come early or late in the statement. At the end of every session (and the sessions are sometimes recommended to be one to one and a half hours each), the speech and language therapist who has been trained to use this system uploads the results to the central Fast ForWord computer that returns a customized set of lessons for the next day. Over time, usually 6 to 12 weeks, the child masters all the sound and sound positions within words, and receives drills with increasingly more normally paced speech.

The developers of Fast ForWord believe that actual brain changes occur, and many parents are convinced that the child now seems to "hear" better, and they see corresponding improvements in spoken language. There is not yet enough data, but we lack scientific data on almost all other aspects of autism treatment too. At least this is a treatment with sound theory behind it.

Fast ForWord is costly. There is a similar, less high-tech computer program that aims to accomplish much the same thing as Fast ForWord, and can be used by a speech and language pathologist or teacher in a class or resource room. It is called Earobics. There is even a version that parents can purchase. Both Fast ForWord and Earobics require receptive comprehension (not just for single-word vocabulary) at about the four-year level and the ability to use a mouse. What seems most clear in that these kinds of programs are likely best for children who seem to drop, miss, or slur sounds, words, or parts of sentences—something that is evident if the child speaks. These treatments are not just designed for children with autism, but also for those with a range of problems that might include central auditory processing difficulties. Presently, the developers of Fast ForWord are developing versions for younger children with autism who are either mouse-savvy or can use a touch screen.

BUILDING LANGUAGE THROUGH VISUAL CHANNELS

Children with ASDs who are verbal have many of the same cognitive characteristics as those who do not yet have language. Most notably, "performance" or nonverbal intelligence is almost always significantly higher than verbal intelligence. There are many more finely grained categories that can be used to talk about different kinds of intelligence, but for the purposes of this discussion the main point is that if a child's non-language (nonverbal) abilities are higher than his verbal abilities, looking for ways to use nonlanguage abilities to develop compensatory strategies to develop language abilities is the way to go. If this sounds just like what was said about developing preverbal communication skills in children who are nonverbal, it is. The rationale is similar: The difference is that with the child who has developed some verbal capacity, the tool kit the child has to pull from is larger.

READING AS SOUNDS AND WORDS MADE VISUAL

Reading is big for all children. Reading is particularly big for children with autism. For a number of children with ASDs a big breakthrough in understanding language emerges when they learn to read. Reading means having all the sounds in front of you so even if you miss some of them when someone speaks to you, even if you are not sure where one word ends and the next begins, it is there for you to look at for as long as it takes you to figure the word out. This is powerful for all children, but even more powerful for children who "hear too slow." Many typically developing children and some autistic children, too, will point at words on the page as they make up what that are "reading," even before they can decode the actual words. The power that reading holds is often understood before reading actually begins.

Sight-Reading versus Phonics. Many parents and some teachers notice that children with autism start to sight-read on their own. Even more common are children with autism being drawn to the alphabet and being able to recite its letters and even identify all letters when the rest of expressive vocabulary is still below 10 or 20 words. What does this mean? For one thing, it shows that there is a kind of rote memory operating wherein a short word (like the name of a letter) can be associated with a clear visual image and readily memorized.

If a child who could do this type of sight-reading were Chinese or Japanese, that child would already be really reading! Chinese and some other Asian languages are based on iconographic script (like *kanji*) in which each small figure of several strokes is a unique word. Given that a significant part of the world reads this way, it is clear that the brain can handle recognition and memorization of a very large number of such iconographs. In Western languages, each iconograph represents a sound rather than a complete meaning, so we need many fewer iconographs. However, when a child starts to sight-read, what he is doing is using much the same skill that would be called upon to read in an iconographic language. It is no wonder that some of the words that are reported to be sight-read first are logos on TV, manufacturer names on cars, and the names of favorite fast-food restaurants. Each time these words appear, they are written in exactly the same way.

So what does this mean for the process of learning to read in the child with autism? If he is sight-reading, it is an indication that the child has achieved a partly adaptive self-accommodation to one of his difficulties—decoding and sequencing sounds. The problem is that the English language is not set up to be sight-read, with its prefixes, suffixes, tenses, homonyms, and lots of grammar—like articles that you can't see, or pronouns that change according to who is talking and who is being talked to. How can Mommy be "I" (according to her), "you" (according to Daddy), "me" (some other times), and "Mommy" (when your sister is addressing her)? No wonder autistic children have so much difficulty using pronouns.

There is a long-standing debate in the field of education about reading. Some advocate "phonics first" and point to research that supports teaching children letter sounds before reading words. Others advocate a "whole word" approach and see early and limited sight-reading as a way of consolidating the concept of reading and teaching children habits that they later use in spelling, like "Does this word 'look' right?" Over the years, the pendulum of educational philosophy swings one way and then the other. The truth is that individual differences based on a child's cognitive profile should dictate which method is most sensible for which child. For the very visual child with autism (namely with excellent and early visual memory), sight-reading is the place to begin.

One way to promote sight-reading is to associate word labels with specific visual images consistently. Autistic children who learned to talk using picture-based communication systems are all primed and ready to go with such an approach if their icons included word labels (that may have been attached primarily for the teacher's use).

More formal classroom activities like matching pictures to words, doing worksheets on which the child draws a line between the picture and the word, and using computer programs that have the child drag words to pictures or vice versa are all ways to encourage sight-reading.

There is no reason to ignore phonics while using an initially sight-reading focused approach. Children can practice what each letter says and match individual letters to the letters in words they recognize, sounding out the word as they go. This makes reading a lot like doing puzzles, usually a rewarding activity for children with autism. Getting the child to say each letter's sound as he writes the alphabet, or does an ABC's puzzle places a letter is a good way of associating the intrinsic reward of doing puzzles with learning to read.

Picture and Word Sequencing. Another strategy for using pictures to improve word comprehension is to make captions or copies of the text of a familiar story from a preschool story or kindergarten-level reader and separate them from the illustrations. Then the child can match familiar captions to familiar pictures. If a child is primarily sight-reading, it is more important to use the exact text. After completing the matching activity, the child can verbally tell what each picture is, essentially paraphrasing the caption by linking the words he can say to comprehension of what he has sight-read. Any words that the child uses to describe the picture can be pointed out to the child. As the child begins to read more, the activity can be reversed and pictures can be matched to captions.

Pictures that are quite similar can be a good way of helping the child listen more carefully and appreciate the meaning of grammatical differences. For example, some of the software from Laureate Learning Systems does this using a computer-assisted instructional model, in which the child might have to distinguish past and future tenses by watching to see if the "the boy is about to paint the fence" or whether "the boy just finished painting the fence." An advantage of computer-based software for this type of instruction is that the computer can convey action that is more difficult to perceive in a static picture.

Computer-Assisted Instruction (CAI) to Teach Language. For many children with autism, the non-social contingency of a computer's response to their actions is very reinforcing, and so computer work is intrinsically rewarding. Computer time in the class can be interspersed as a reward activity after participation in more socially based interactive instruction. The computer is a good way to expose a child to reinforcement of emerging concepts for which the child may no longer need direct instruction, but mainly practice. Finally, time on the computer can be a good way for a teacher to deploy staff since a child engaged in a computer-assisted instructional activity might be able to stay meaningfully engaged in his task with less adult supervision, freeing staff for an activity with a child in need of more direct instruction. It is important to remember, though, that using a computer at school is very much like watching videos at home—it needs to be supervised closely enough by an adult so that it does not turn into mental downtime for the child via repetitive use of one mastered segment of the program, or non-functional use of the computer.

The main disadvantage of using computers to teach language is that it largely removes language from a real social context. While this can be appealing to the child with autism, it is important that he not only learn language but learn how to use language socially. This means using the language flexibly—paraphrasing and using related utterances in related situations. One way to help is to provide enough adult supervision during computer-assisted instruction so that peers can take turns at a computer-assisted instructional activity. Using computers in class as the basis of a reverse mainstream activity that involves a child with autism and a peer tutor from a regular education class taking turns at a computer game can be a good way of presenting the child with a natural-language model that elaborates on what the computer says. Left on their own, most autistic children enjoying a computer program will echo it, if they speak at all. A typically developing child is more likely to provide a model for exclamations like those used when scoring or losing points. Similarly, during free time at school (or even at home during play dates, as will be discussed in chapter 8), turn-taking at computer games can help introduce structure and rules of social interaction.

Closed Captioning. Another way to link the written word with the visual and auditory worlds is through television closed captioning. For a reasonable cost, families can order closed captioning with their cable television service. Although closed captioning is primarily designed for hearing-impaired adults and seniors, many programs of interest to higher-functioning children with autism, such as nature and science programs are close captioned, too. Most TVs have a way of turning this feature on and off so it doesn't have to be on when it is not wanted. For younger children, some of the Disney and other "sing-alongs" on videotape have captioned lyrics. Especially when using captions with younger children, pointing out the words, and encouraging the child to touch and follow the words can help him understand the relationship between what he sees and hears, and the activity can help keep the child engaged in a sensory-motor way while watching the action.

UNDERSTANDING NARRATIVE

A very difficult challenge in teaching children with autism to use language in an expressive manner is the issue of developing a sense of narrative. Despite adequate vocabulary, it can be nearly impossible to get a child with autism to recount the plot of a movie that has interested him, or to simply reveal what happened at the school assembly that morning.

Why is this so difficult? One of the big difficulties is rooted in just how visual language is, and how much easier it is for the child to limit his thinking in words to those things that are immediately there to be labeled and described. Also challenging is the difficulty in "seeing" what something in the past tense looks like and how it "looks" different from something in the present tense.

Typically developing children go through a stage in which they have this same difficulty. At two-and-a-half or three, problems with talking in tenses usually takes the form of over-using simple rules of grammar, such as the child's reporting that he "eat-ed" a snack at school today. Modeling of the appropriate grammar—"Oh, you ate snack at school today?"—usually helps. Because the typically developing child readily assimilates a model, this works. But for children with autism who have poor imitation and modeling skills, this transformation is not so easy.

Yesterday, Today, and Tomorrow Books. One way to help children with ASDs develop a sense of narrative and a sense of past, present, and future events is through the construction of "Yesterday," "Today," and "Tomorrow" books. This can be a simple loose-leaf binder, or a blank folio from a photo shop. Teachers and parents compile a series of pictures of key events in the child's day—his backpack by the front door waiting for the bus, the front of the school, the cubby for his backpack at school, chairs or mats ready for circle time, etc. At home, on a weekend, pictures might include the supermarket, mall, park, or lunch spot. To construct a "Today" book, at the end of the day the teacher could pull pictures pertaining to the day's activities and help the child put them in sequence. Numbers (or the words "first," "second," etc.) on each page are very appealing for some children. When the pictures are placed in sequence to construct a narrative of the child's day, the child can verbally or in writing (or both) retell the "story" of the day's events. This is a good way to make adverbs like "next," "after," and "then" comprehensible and useful. (There can be pages with just these words between pages showing activities that the child did.) Alternatively, the teacher could send home a numbered checklist, and the child already familiar with the procedure could be prompted to do this at home, so that he can finally tell his mom what he did in school today. Over time, pictures can be phased out, then the words, until only the verbal narrative remains.

Similarly, the child can learn to speak in the future tense by planning a Saturday's activities on a Friday night or to speak in past tense by retelling a story about an exciting past event like a trip to Sea World, sequencing key pictures in the order events occurred. This activity can be a particularly good fit for the child who likes things to be routine and predictable. Turning the page can also be a good way to keep perseverative talking about past and future events to a minimum.

Treasure Hunting. A slightly more advanced variation on teaching the child to engage in narrative is the "treasure hunt." This activity also takes advantage of strong visual prompts and active involvement on the child's part. In its simplest form, a list of what to do first, second, third, etc., with a reward for completing the list, helps the child follow serial directions. A more complex version is to get directions about the next thing to do from the location of the previous thing to do. For example, the child might start with visual, verbal, and/or written instructions like, "Go to your cubby and find the blue box. Bring Ms. Martina the blue box." Ms. Martina might then tell the child to open the box and read a piece of paper inside that then directed the child to the next box where the activity could be repeated. The last step could be a box with a reward. As children progress, this game can become more complicated, including one-, then two-, then three-step commands. Continuing to link visual cues with written directions helps the child move from a world of only "thinking in pictures" to one in which the pictures have a sound track, and the child begins to think in words.

THE PEDANTIC SPEECH OF ASPERGER'S SYNDROME

The language development patterns of children with Asperger's syndrome (AS) are a bit different from those of other children with autistic spectrum disorders. The description given in the DSM-IV, the psychiatric manual that enumerates the diagnostic criteria, tells only part of the story. One must take a closer look into some of the research that led to AS being designated a new category of ASD—which happened only as recently as 1994—to understand what the salient characteristics of language in children diagnosed with AS really are.

Initially one of two patterns of speech is notable: The child may begin talking at a very young age and have a very good vocabulary, but he may focus language use in an odd way, such as by saying "E is for Elephant" as a first "word" at 11 months. (This is a specific example given to me by a mother whose son with AS scored a 135 on his IQ test at high school age.) He apparently chose this phrase as his first utterance after having been repeatedly read it from his baby quilt. Sometimes the very early speech is not only odd in choice of topic, but uneven, lacking the usual pattern of first words such as names for familiar people and things in the child's life.

Another pattern seen in AS is a delay in speaking that may persist until just before the third birthday, but is followed by sudden development from no words or just a few words into sentence and even paragraph speech within a shorter than expected period (such as six months) especially given the earlier delays. These children often start off with a great deal of delayed echolalia (skipping much of an immediate echolalia stage) and quickly move from non-functional to more functional echolalic use. When these children with AS are young, they may insist on parents' engaging in repetitive verbal routines: "Mom, go to Toys R' Us. Buy blue beach ball?" continuing over and over, irrespective of whether there has been a promise to buy a blue beach ball, or whether the beach ball has already been purchased. Sometimes, these children go so far as to prompt the mother into her (repeated) response: "Say 'We're going to buy blue beach ball after lunch'." This pattern of speech probably works both to assure comprehension as well as to feed the need for predictability, and to enjoy hearing things repeated, something loved by so many children with autism.

One of the reasons that speech and language use is different for children with AS compared to children with other ASDs is that verbal ability is typically not nearly as affected as social abilities. (For this reason, children with AS are often first identified as having a possible ASD in preschool when their patterns of play and socialization are different, rather than when language delays are observed.) Verbal and performance (nonverbal) intelligence levels usually are much more comparable, and unlike autism, verbal ability often exceeds nonverbal abilities. In fact, a subset of children with AS tends to meet criteria for what can be described as "nonverbal learning disabilities" also. While nonverbal learning disabilities are not as well studied a diagnostic classification as Asperger's, they are associated with certain traits such as poor visual-spatial and poor visual-motor abilities—something that is rarely a relative weakness for a child with autism.

As children with Asperger's develop, their language understanding and use tends to be marked with rigidities of use and over-literalness. A ten-year-old with AS and a normal IQ who was in a class for learning-handicapped pupils because of his behavioral difficulties would refer to the other pupils as "stupid"—to their faces. This did not win him friends, and though he was somewhat disturbed by the rejection, he felt it more important to stick to his assertion of their stupidity, since he was the only one who regularly knew all the answers to the questions the teacher would ask. A chapter in the book *Autism and Asperger's Syndrome* provides excellent examples of this type of logic using multiple-choice quizzes on social understanding that can be given to individuals with Asperger's syndrome.

Comprehending of grammar and syntax are typically not difficult for those with AS, though perception and use of vocal affect often is. Not infrequently, prosody is monotone or singsongy and unemotional, and modulated tone of voice is absent, or sounds like it came whole from someone else. Many individuals with Asperger's have unusually monotonous voices, or reflect the emotionality of the topic talked about only by increasing the volume of their speech. (This is consistent with an understanding of Asperger's that is based on the idea that only the social, and not the communicative areas of the brain are affected.) Some individuals with AS may speak too loudly, others too softly. Most of us modulate volume by taking cues from those around us. If you don't take social cues, you probably won't do well modulating your volume to the requirements of the situation.

Many individuals with Asperger's express their autistic-like love of collections and classifications with words. This may take the form of memorizing odd spelling words, dictionary entries, or vocabulary lists in foreign languages (although there is typically no interest in developing conversational fluency, or even a good accent, in the new language).

Some individuals with Asperger's are simply verbose. What most people might use a few words to say can go on for sentences. This may be even more marked when the child feels socially pressured: Quincy, a very smart twelve-year-old with AS (who later was skipped through middle school to avoid social problems there) was asked about his friendships in his sixth-grade class. Squirming in his seat with legs crossed, one hand to his chin and the other to his opposite elbow, he said, "Well, it can be hard to specify exactly who among my classmates I might refer to as friendships . . . " This pattern of speaking is what is sometimes referred to as "pedantic." Teenagers who speak in this manner can seem much better put together than they are, something that is only revealed by understanding factors below the surface, like their patterns of friendships, how they spend their leisure time, and whether odd ideas and interests coexist with their seeming normalcy. Such individuals may be more comfortable talking to adults than to peers, which, for a 15-year-old, is quite abnormal indeed.

CHAPTER CONCLUSIONS

In this chapter, we have explored aspects of how verbal language understanding and use is different for children with ASDs who develop functional and significant verbal capacities. As is the case for nonverbal and preverbal children with ASDs, most verbal children with ASDs benefit from methods of enhancing language understanding by pairing visual cues in the form of pictures, computer games, videos, or other narratives with the words they hear or read. This chapter has focused more on some of the didactic issues of developing expressive language capacity. The use of these language skills is inextricably linked to the development of the social interactional skills that were discussed in chapter 4, as well as to the development of play skills with toys, which serve as the rehearsal studio in which children can work out the meanings of words they have learned. The development of these play skills and their links to moving speech into language will be discussed in the next chapter.

Autistic Learning Disabilities in Relating to the World of Objects: Description and Treatment

How the Child with Autism May See the World Differently. In this chapter, we will begin to explore the third and final area of autistic learning disabilities. These are the learning disabilities that result from how children with autism take in information about the world differently from other children. From the point of view of diagnostic symptoms, these disabilities in learning stem from processing sensory information differently, and apparently extracting and processing meaning differently. Children with autistic spectrum disorders may over- or under-respond to different sorts of sensory stimuli: A child with autism may hear something and ignore it; or he may hear something that is so apparently intense that he covers his ears with his hands or flaps his arms and vocalizes in a frantic perturbed fashion. A child with autism may see something (or someone) and seemingly "look right through" what he sees; or he may seize the object with one hand, hold it to the periphery of his vision with a strong vertical orientation, and stare fixedly at it out of the corners of his eyes, while rotating it slightly back and forth. A child with autism may assiduously ignore strangers, but selectively approach anyone with fluffy hair and grab the hair and smell it.

Yes, these actions are all odd. Yes, these actions all contribute to making a diagnosis of autism. But what else? What do they tell us about how the child with autism is able to make sense of the world around him? What do they tell us about how to go about treatment? Here, we will catalogue how these odd behaviors are our window into how the autistic child's world is differently shaped, and how issues around subsequent exploration, motivation, and play are affected. There are three parts to developing such an understanding: First, there are the sensory abnormalities that "gate" how much information is taken in by the child on each of his sensory "channels." Second, there is the repetitious behavior often associated with autism (like rocking, flapping, humming, spinning, or flicking things) that can serve as a blockade against a fuller range of stimulation being understood or even noticed. Just think about how such misperceptions can alter the base of data the child can refer to when trying to understand new things. Third, there is a typical impoverishment in play in children with autism. Basically, this reflects how a disorganized sensory world can disrupt the expected functions that imagination and play should occupy in coming to understand the social world.

In the first part of this chapter, these sensory and processing abnormalities will be described. In the second part of this chapter, we will use this understanding to discuss ways in which these differences can sometimes be viewed as weaknesses—and sometimes as strengths—and in any case, how teaching can proceed to help a child overcome some of the limitations imposed by these differences.

BEHAVIOR THAT CAN INTERFERE WITH LEARNING
Repetitiousness

In chapter 2, we talked about perseverativeness as a primary, innate defect in information processing for some children with autism. While severe perseverativeness is usually considered a limitation to learning, like other weaknesses in autism, it can be made to work to the child's advantage, minimizing potential negative impact.

Stereotyped Motor Movements. Stereotyped motor movements, especially certain flapping and flicking the hands at the wrist, rocking back and forth or side to side with a certain rhythm, or posturing figures, are considered hallmarks of autism. It is important to note, however, that it is not only children with autistic spectrum disorders who do these things, but also children with other neurologically based conditions, those with mental retardation without autism, and occasionally, the otherwise normal siblings of children with autism.

Depending upon the situation, there are different reasons that parents and teachers try to stop a child engaging in stereotyped motor movements: First, as we were discussing a moment ago, some children with autism may focus in an overly strong manner upon some perceptual feature of an object such as its spinning. Instead of getting bored with a spinning toy after a few moments, as we might expect from a typically developing child, the child with autism not only may fail to grow bored, but may grow more excited. It is not difficult, therefore, to understand why children who are strongly drawn to one perceptual feature, like spinning, engage in repetitious activity—it's exciting in certain ways—rather than boring. Stereotyped motor movements are often a reflection of excitement, too. They are a kind of motor overflow in an immature neurological system that can't seem to regulate arousal in any other way. This implies that stereotyped motor movements result from joint primary, innate deficits involving perseverative tendencies as well as arousal-regulation deficits.

When a child becomes bound up in a repetitive behavior and the rate of stereotypies increases, it can be like a computer that has crashed its application— it appears to be doing the same thing endlessly, but in reality is going nowhere. Nothing progresses until the application is ended or the whole system is re-booted. From an educational point of view one reason that motor stereotypies are undesirable is that they tend to be pretty effective at thwarting the processing of any further information.

A second reason that we don't like children to engage in motor stereotypies is that it simply doesn't look appropriate. Some people refer to stereotyped motor movements as "self-stimulatory" or "stims" for short—meaning that they are hypothesized to exist because they feel good to the child—so he keeps up the behavior.

Because "stims" don't look "right," one treatment is simply to use behavioral methods to reduce or extinguish them. This may be fine, but to simply proceed to do this in the same way for all children ignores a potentially important thing: The preferred sensory modality of the "stim" may shows us things to which the child prefers to attend, and it may indicate which things have an intrinsically reinforcing quality. If carefully titrated, objects or events that engender repetitive motor stereotypies may be useful for teaching purposes as reinforcers.

Some repetitive motor movements, however, are simple overflow, as in a younger typical child. This appears particularly true of hand flapping, hopping, and some vocalizing that occur briefly when something exciting has happened. So when self-stimulatory behavior appears to result from discharge of motor overflow, it is likely to be transitory, and mild redirection of the behavior (such as making flapping hands into "hands together") is likely to be effective and teaching can proceed. The antecedent to that type of motor stereotypy has been some exciting event.

In the case of the most persistent motor stereotypies there is a less transitory, more truly self-perpetuating quality. The real down side of this more intense repetitiveness is the way it can function to exclude subsequent novel stimulation. So, for example, a child with autism who rolls cars down a spiral ramp twenty, thirty, sixty times in a row, may not notice that the toy he is playing with also has a garage for the cars, people to put in the cars, and a gas station at which he might pretend to fuel the cars.

Of course, what looks appropriate, and how much repetition looks appropriate, varies with age. Some repetitious patterns become entrenched and their self-satisfying value is well understood by the child before they begin to look inappropriate to others. A good example of this would be the little guy who lies on the floor watching cars' wheels roll back and forth at eye level. This looks like a fine idea for a 16-month-old, but it looks odd if it is still the predominant form of car play at eight years old. We also saw this type of behavior on one home video that a parent provided as part of a study about early signs of autism prior to diagnosis. Sixteen-month-old Amanda was videotaped "showing off" her "rain dance," prancing in front of a chain-link gutter spout as water dripped from it after a storm, flapping her arms. On a video made a year later, after her diagnosis, Amanda began her dance again, and off camera her mother could be heard, upset, saying, "No, no, turn off the camera now."

Some repetitive behaviors that look odd at an older age would have seemed more typical at an earlier age. In treating some overly repetitive behaviors, the same approach can be taken as with some persisting undesirable behaviors in typically developing children, like a seven-year-old's sucking his thumb, or a four-year-old's still in diapers. The parent can just set things up so it is more rewarding to stop the behavior, and less rewarding to continue the behavior. This is what "redirection," moving a child to a nearby, acceptable, alternative activity is all about. Sometimes parents ask if it will be harmful to make the child stop flapping his arms, staring at postured fingers, or tapping objects held to the eyes. I'm asked, "Does he 'need' to do it?" The answer really seems to be "no." The main reason to stop some stereotypies is that (like thumb sucking) they may have a self-satisfying quality that tends to promote withdrawal from the rest of what is going on around the child.

Other Repetitious Behavior and Obsessive Compulsive Behavior. Children with autism who demonstrate strong perseverative qualities usually not only have stereotyped motor movements, but also tend to use repetitious speech if they are verbal, and may gravitate toward repetitious play, too. The form that the repetitious behavior takes may vary with age and functional capacity.

Many children with high-functioning autism and Asperger's syndrome often have repetitive behaviors and specific repetitive rituals that have many of the qualities of an obsessive compulsive disorder. A few may even meet criteria for obsessive compulsive disorders. One main difference that may distinguish those in the autistic spectrum with repetitious behaviors from those with obsessive compulsive disorders is that those with autistic spectrum disorders are often quite comfortable with their routines and rituals. In many individuals with obsessive compulsive disorders, but *without* other signs of autistic spectrum disorders, the drive for repetition may be very similar and the need to repeat perfectly may be similar, *but* the individual may find it very unself-satisfying, and in fact, aggravating to be compelled to check or repeat his own behavior.

What Repetitiousness Means for Learning. Repetitiousness and the satisfaction it can bring an individual with autism can be a two-edged sword. As already implied, it can limit learning by filling time with repetitions, the need to redo things, and the general inability to move on. However, the desire for repetitiveness can also work to the individual's benefit by using the drive for routine as a prosocial strategy to organize activity in a functional, albeit highly structured and repetitive manner. When repetitiveness is self-satisfying, it is a natural reinforcer for the behavior or routine containing the repetition. Therefore, using some teaching methods that are very high on structure and repetition can be quite naturally reinforcing, even as content is varied. An example of a treatment approach that can be particularly well suited to the highly repetitive or routine-bound child is the TEACCH curriculum, which will be discussed in chapter 11.

PLAY

Why Do Children Play? Play keeps children busy, happy, and one hopes, meaningfully engaged. Children play because it is convenient for their parents.

Parents need time to cook dinner, talk on the phone, and clean up after their children. But why else do children play?

Play is the natural laboratory for children's self-generated experimentation and learning. Children need to be taught, but children also need to "learn to learn" on their own. That's what play is, even—especially—for children with autistic spectrum disorders. Play is a child's forum for conducting "experiments" on the things around him. These experiments need to involve all the senses: How things move, how they look, how they feel, how they sound, and maybe even how they taste. Children with autism have all these senses, but it often seems like their input from certain senses works rather differently from that of typically developing children. In the next section we will examine some possible reasons for this, and what implications these sensory processing "malfunctions" may have for *how* the child explores, understands the world, and is motivated to learn new things.

In His Own Little World. Children with autism are often described as "in their own little world." Indeed it can seem that a child with autism lives inside a big bubble, just like the Good Witch of the East in *The Wizard of Oz*, traveling everywhere in it; there, but not there; isolated from the "real" world. Some autism investigators have suggested that this seeming lack of connection to the larger world may be due to the fact that children with autism overattend to certain kinds of stimuli, especially things that are close by and can be experienced through touch, smell, and movement of their bodies (vestibular stimulation). Some researchers have speculated that these sensory experiences may be overattended to at the expense of things taking place at a greater distance. By this account, information delivered on more "distal" processing channels, like hearing and seeing, may not be attended to nearly as well.

If the child finds certain things quite positive and tends to overattend to them, he may seek them out and may also overattend to them when they are encountered. Sometimes this overattention to certain kinds of stimuli is referred to as "stimulus over-selectivity." This concept also helps us think about what the autistic child experiences as he peers out at the world. Filters that magnify some perceptual information and mask other sorts of perceptions produce a distorted view.

Problems Calibrating Incoming Stimuli. We have already talked (in chapter 2) about "perceptual inconstancy" or "proximal over distal preference" as an innate impairment in which some sensory channels seem to be turned on "louder" than others, with hearing often significantly turned "down," and visual attention to things not in immediate proximity turned "down." An idea related to perceptual inconstancy is the idea that thresholds for perceiving different kinds of stimuli may vary over time, from experience to experience. This can be seen in the child who is seemingly oblivious to certain things, or persistently overfocused on other things. The idea of perceptual inconstancy is more of a heuristic than an established neurological reality, but can help adults understand why the child with autism is doing what he is doing. For example, there is the child who is guaranteed to run to the nearest top and spin it, or try out the "flickiness" of every decently long bit of carpet fiber he encounters. When the child is also a child with strong perseverative tendencies, getting the top away from the child once he's had a chance to immerse himself in its delights is likely to be a struggle. But the child who can become intensely involved in a spinning top for a prolonged period may be one who, apparently, can ignore his name being called until the speaker holds his chin in both hands and turns his face toward her. Why is this?

Sensory Thresholds. We have known for a long time that one of the hallmarks of autism is that many children, especially the youngest children with autism, have disturbances in how thresholds related to these senses function. As we discussed in chapter 2, the innate mechanisms that take in sensory information often seem like volume knobs that are turned up to high or too low or are spinning wildly back and forth sometimes. This concept of "perceptual inconstancy" is a very good way of thinking about the disorganizing influence of abnormal sensory thresholds. We've discussed how it may influence perception. How might it influence the child's activities and interest?

Think about what perceived perceptual inconstancy can do to a child's natural attempts to repeat "experiments" that are a normal part of learning. Things "turned up" too loud might be particularly hard to ignore or pull yourself away from because they so fully captured your attention, like very loud, rhythmic music. Things turned down "too low" might be hard to attend to—it might be as if you were constantly trying to "find Waldo" (a figure in a series of children's books with complex cartoon illustrations of hundreds of tiny figures on each page, only one of whom is "Waldo"). What if sometimes you could readily find Waldo, and other times you could not? Would it make you irritable?

Not all children with autism have these problems processing sensory stimuli, and most have such problems mainly with respect to one or two sensory "channels," like hyperacussis (auditory hypersensitivity) or lack of a notable pain response, especially when younger. Nevertheless, a child constructs his understanding of the world and the way things in it work by making sense of the results of his own actions. If these experiments are very limited in scope, because, for example, the most salient experiments always involve seeing how something spins (moves), learning can quickly become limited to acquiring knowledge about "spinability." Therefore, exploring a diversity of objects and learning how to conduct many different "experiments" on each object become key to teaching the child with autism to open himself to knowledge that all other children accrue through these diverse "experiments." Viewed in this way, teaching a child with autism how to "play" is tantamount to teaching the child with autism how to learn.

These sensory-regulation and threshold problems can be thought of as calibration problems: If you were conversing with someone as you walked down a sidewalk approaching a construction site, your ability to hear and attend to your conversational partner would likely be unaffected by the construction sounds—at first. As you approached the sounds, it might be hard to shut them out and concentrate on what was being said and, at some point, it might become physically impossible to hear speech over the sound of a jackhammer. It has been suggested that the child with autism may reach such thresholds more easily, perhaps especially with certain sounds—low rumbling noises like a hand dryer in a restroom, a garbage disposal, or a vacuum cleaner. Visually, there may be miscalibration of thresholds of the opposite sort: Instead of avoiding certain sights, the child might overly attend to them, as with spinning or rolling things, or flickering lights.

In those children in which there does seem to be a preference for taking in information sent on certain sensory channels, but ignoring information received on other sensory channels, the child's learning experience is going to be distorted by what he misses and by what he attends to too much. Since "overattention" includes the capacity for close and prolonged attention, overattended materials and all things with related sensory properties can and should be used as teaching materials. Strong sensory preferences show us that these stimuli have a high reward salience for the child. Therefore, in planning interventions for a child with autism, it is important to get ideas about what materials to teach with, how long teaching sessions with preferred materials can be (longer), and the ways the materials themselves become instrinsic reinforcers. The Autism Learning Disabilities Inventory in Appendix A was designed to help organize such observations systematically.

MOTIVATION, CURIOSITY, EXPLORATION, AND IMITATION

There are two main reasons that play is a critical domain of learning for children with autistic spectrum disorders. Correspondingly, there are at least two types of autistic learning disabilities present when an autistic child has deficits in spontaneous play.

Motivation in Play. There is a strong link between motivation and self-determination. Most parents of autistic children are well aware of this. When the child really wants something, he can always figure out many straightforward as well as surreptitious ways to try to get what he wants. A child who seems completely uncomprehending and incompetent when asked to assist in putting on his own shoe (and who lacks interest in having shoes on), may be able to engage in seemingly much more complex problem solving: pulling a chair across a kitchen, climbing across a counter and opening a cabinet containing a bag of Cheetos, getting the snack down, and opening the bag. The latter is clearly a multistep activity requiring more coordination and planned execution than what is needed for pulling on a shoe. What differs is the child's motivation. We can assume that it was someone else's idea that he get his shoes on; it was his own idea to fetch the Cheetos.

Deception Deficits. Interestingly, the surreptitious part of self-determined behavior can be a little differently organized in a child with autism than in a more typically developing child. Being deceptive is closely related to having a theory of mind. To be really good at being deceptive, it helps to know whether someone else (say, your mom) has any way of knowing what's on your mind. So, if you want Cheetos and you have just asked for them and been told "No," then it is probably not a good time to go in the kitchen and start pushing a chair around so you can climb to the Cheetos. It will be a no-brainer for Mom to guess what you intend to do. Autistic children who carry out prohibited behaviors in plain sight of whoever just did the prohibiting are wearing their "mindblindness" on their sleeves. On the other hand, if you have learned through cause-and-effect experience that climbing on the counter in front of Mom results in a smack on the bum and a loud "No!" (and no Cheetos), you might not try that escapade in full view. You may succeed at being deceptive simply by working out the probabilities and planning so that things go in your favor. This does not necessarily mean, though, that you have the ability to guess what others might know (that is, "mind read" or have theory of mind skill). This distinction is important because your ability to comprehend the intentions of others plays a pivotal role in a whole range of rule-oriented activities you may or may not be able to engage in, ranging from hide-and-go-seek to soccer. In fact, many things that children play at *are* their way of practicing their "mind-reading" skills. Understanding the activities and interests of children with autism provides a short course in understanding how motivation and imitation fuel social interaction.

Motivation and Choice. When you choose an activity for yourself, chances are that you will more likely be motivated to finish your activity and to do the activity well, compared to when someone else chooses an activity for you. All other things being equal, would you be more enthusiastic about reading a book you chose, or one that someone decided would be "good for you" to read? The power of self-choice also operates in the motivational system of children with autistic spectrum disorders.

Many children with autism seem to have motivation problems. These motivation problems can be broken down into two areas: First, there is the problem when the child does not find rewarding those things we think, hope, or expect him to find rewarding. (We have already discussed this aspect of reinforcer saliency with respect to lack of response to social praise in chapter 4.) The second motivational problem for children with autism, therefore, is that the things that motivate them can have very low educational value because they are repetitive, unvarying, and consisting of a limited number of things.

"Educational" Toys. Typical children are motivated to play because they are curious about almost everything. They are often curious about how an object functions; when they are older, they want to discover what the object may represent or how it may be used to represent actual things in the world around them. Play comes to equal imagination—representing things as they have seemed, or might be. One aspect of this is that children can play with anything, not just a specially designed "toy." Toys as we know them are a rather modern concept.

Autistic children often reject toys and, as a result, their parents buy them more toys! Alternatively, because formal learning is often slow and toys that foster imagination are seldom sought-after objects, some parents of autistic children eschew such toys for their children and instead, understandably, focus on only those things seen as "educational" toys—puzzles, flashcards, electronic toys that teach letters, and so on. This actually further limits what the child has to explore, as most toys designed with an educational focus have a limited number of functions. However, if the child is mostly interested in such toys on his own (without someone "helping"), they may be a better place to start building "self-interest" in objects than anywhere else.

Curiosity. Autistic children tend to have limited, or rather narrowly channeled curiosity. Curiosity can be defined as the self-generated tendency to explore things in multiple ways. The lack of curiosity seen in autism seems to have two sources: one is the degree of mental retardation the child may have, with more mentally retarded children tending, on average, to be less curious or less "sparky." Second, curiosity is sometimes quashed in children with autism by the countervailing tendency to be perseverative and to enjoy sticking with old things rather than checking out new things. The odd exception to this is that many autistic children limit their "curiosity" to the domain of a perseverative interest: A child with autism who likes to flick long stringy things may seem *compelled* (and this is the more operative word here than curious) to explore every belt, necklace, fern frond, and rubber boa constrictor encountered in a new setting with respect to its "flickability."

Self-Initiated Learning. One challenge of teaching children with autism to play is finding activities that promote self-learning and that also have some reward saliency to the child and thereby become motivating to pursue. (In chapter 4, we discussed many such approaches.) Creating a self-generative learner through play holds the potential for subsequent self-learning of many formal educational skills and adaptive behaviors as well. In the longer term, it is critical that children with autism become self-learners and perpetuate their own learning experiences. One-to-one teaching is great before functional self-learning skills arise. As children begin to learn from self-initiated experiences, they need opportunities to do so. This is why full-time adult-initiated and directed one-to-one teaching can sometimes be disadvantageous.

Exploring versus Imitating As Self-Guided Learning. Yes, children with autism can learn some of the same things as typical children on their own. Initially, however, this may occur by watching or participating in "experiments" that someone sets up for them and steps them through. In fact, for those autistic children who are the least exploratory, or the most repetitive, this is critically important. The ability to problem-solve using self-generated activity is part of successful mastery in any situation. The goal of play "instruction" therefore should be twofold: to teach the task, and to help the child learn to do this "experiment" more independently next time.

As was said earlier, children learn new things through exploring and experimenting. They also learn through imitating others. A child with autism who neither explores nor imitates is cut off from the two most important tools that young children have for learning new things. Imitation, more than exploration, interfaces with the various social autistic learning disabilities that may be present. So, for many children with autism, increasing spontaneous exploration of things in the environment may be an important way of taking in new information, but in a non-social (not socially dependent) way—a possibly valuable compensatory strategy.

Imitation in play is essentially a social act (as we discussed in chapter 4). Imitation arises from wanting to "be like," or "do like" someone else. If the social drive is missing and social motivation has not yet been developed, social imitation will likely be low. Teaching a child to respond to social reinforcers and teaching formal imitation skills must go hand in hand for spontaneous social imitation to begin. Play, games, or group activities in which the child with autism may initially play along out of a drive to explore the mechanistic aspects of the activity (like "Simon says: Touch your toes! Touch your head!") can be guided into an activity that includes more mutuality and imitation, because watching others can help the child engage in the activity more effectively.

Private Speech. The part of play that is often most difficult for children with autism, is the representation of things as they might be or as they may have been in the past. Imagination, described earlier as the "script" for so much children's play, is lacking in much of the child with autism's interactions with objects. One reason for this is that there's simply no "script." In the simplest and earliest forms of play in typically developing children, toddlers reenact things that have happened. For example, a 32-month-old who is just starting to use sentences and who knocked an open cup of juice off the table might be seen throwing a pretend tea cup to the ground, saying, "What a mess!" and then retrieving the cup and throwing it again. In this type of reenactment play, the 32-month-old has an opportunity to review what was said to her, what the words meant, and how the whole thing felt. A psychoanalyst might say that the 32-month-old was working through the Eriksonian stage of Autonomy versus Shame and Doubt, but a developmental psycholinguist would say that the child's play and language were ways of increasing her understanding of an abstract, but seemingly important-to-Mom, concept—"messy." Key to this episode is the fact that the 32-month-old was using her own language to narrate her behavior, something that can be referred to as "private speech."

Children make a major mental transition when the language they are learning starts to guide their behavior. It is only after this occurs that the child can begin to think in words and verbal "scripts." Many parents and teachers who have enumerated long lists of words that a child with autism "knows" will acknowledge that they seldom hear the child utter the word when he interacts with the "known" object. There is no "private speech." In these cases, the child's interaction with the toys is usually either sensory (squeezing, rubbing), motor (moving), or consisting of a simple functional use of the toy (like going through a bin of rubber animals and piling all the mammals in one place and the birds in another). Such play is seldom representative or imaginary in theme. Words are not used to narrate activity. The reason for this is that the way a child plays with the object does not include a verbal script specifying a plan of action. "Private speech," as it was just described, begins when the child's play becomes more representational of events. It is logical therefore that the child with autism is not likely to "need" to script his play verbally until he begins to engage in more elaborate and sequenced actions with objects, like sequences that represent observed activities. For children with autism, there is often, to use Piaget's term, a "decalage" in this regard. This means that while language may be at one level (like single words), play is at another (lower) level. The car carrying the child's imagination is stuck in neutral with the engine revving.

Bringing Words and Play Together. The time of this "decalage" is an ideal time, developmentally, to show the child how to link simple actions with toys in a way that the play actions can be fitted to "scripts" of the activity. In this way actions in play come to foster language. This means that children with a good repertoire of single-word labels and the ability to use those labels for objects are ready to learn to play representationally, making the objects "do things." This "doing things" can be scripted action accompanied by prompted, scripted, illustrative language at first, but should be prompt-faded so that the child is encouraged to begin to verbally script his own play spontaneously.

Typically developing children start simple: An 18-month-old will drop scrambled eggs off his high chair and say "Ut-oh!" Then the spoon may go, accompanied by another "Ut-oh!" Adults tend to be a bit annoyed by these repetitive (and not always fruitful) activities, but they are early language experiments with verbal scripts for actions. The "play" (representational) version of this verbal script is the same toddler, a few months older, squatting over a bin of plastic food, picking up each item, labeling it and then throwing it, uttering "Ut-oh!" after each toss.

Usually, the things the child with autism will do with objects is a repeat of things he has been shown—without elaboration or linking to further novel actions he has not been shown. When the child with autism can be helped to have his words guide his play and his play illustrate language, a link tied to language meaning is forged. This becomes the means for further developing abilities in both of these domains. It may be that some children with autism need the opportunity to step back to the "Uh-oh" stage of verbal scripting to develop a concept of how verbal scripts can make play more interesting.

Laying Down a Soundtrack with Play. A main goal of teaching play to children with autism is to create a "sound track." The way children with autism initially come to understand complex sequences of activities, and come to expect routines, is by having hundreds of short "videotapes" that illustrate a sequence of activities that must be carried out to achieve a desired goal (like the story of the child who pushes the chair to the counter in order to climb up and get the Cheetos). But, initially, the "videotape," initially has no "sound track." This is the same metaphor that was used in the earlier chapters on language development. The child needs to have a soundtrack for play, even more than for functional routines, if language is to become self-generative. This occurs by demonstrating the links between objects and their noun labels, actions and their verbs, and sequences of actions. Social reasoning is carried out using language and language concepts, and so building language is an important prerequisite to building social skills. Similarly, in the case of play, adding a sound track is prerequisite to the capacity to make new videotapes of new experiences that can then be added to the play repertoire.

Play and the ALD Profile. Another consideration in teaching play to children with autism is the rest of their autistic learning disability profile. How can play and representation be motivated? This is where looking at the Learning Disability Inventory in Appendix A can be helpful for brainstorming treatment strategies: If the child is one who loves repetition, early representation through play that is taught should be repetitious. If the child is one who loves repetition, and also loves things that are flicky, early representation through play should be both flicky and repetitious—maybe using a rubber snake that eats all the play food one piece at a time and says the same thing as he finishes each piece.

TEACHING PLAY

Who Needs to Play? Sometime I hear that a particular child is "in program" and at therapies so much, that there is no "time" for "play" left in the day. Well, play is child's work. If a child with an autistic spectrum disorder is very involved in a structured program with one-to-one teaching for most of his working hours, does he still need to play? Yes, but it's not just so that his teacher can "take data." Even if the child has a two-to-one instruction program so that one teacher can teach while the other takes data, does the child still need time to play? The answer is still definitely yes, but why?

Life, and the things that can happen in it, are open-ended. We need to prepare for things that have never happened. This might be someone new talking to you, seeing a new and interesting-looking object, or seeing something happen that is unusual and unexpected. Through play, children learn to step up to the plate and swing at what comes at them, using whatever strategy they think might work. Normally, play is open-ended, usually not exactly the same twice, and it is self-initiated by the child. The child decides what to play with and what he will do with the things he has taken up. This is an early simulation of the adult world. In some structured teaching, especially one-to-one teaching, the child more or less remains under the adult's control. Being able to be under instructional control *is* a critical learning skill. However, being able to self-initiate activity in novel ways with novel objects is also a critical learning skill—and adults can help the child develop it by supporting the child's activities, not by always telling him what to do, step-by-step. If the child is told what to do step by step, then it isn't play, and it's not self-initiated exploration and problem solving.

The conundrum here is that the child with autism both needs to be shown how to play and also needs to initiate his own play (without being repetitive, narrow of interest, or overly focused on one sensory "channel"). How can this be accomplished?

REDUCING STEREOTYPED BEHAVIOR, INCREASING PLAY

As stereotyped behaviors such as repetitive motor movements and repetitive play are reduced, it can create a bit of a void. These behaviors, after all, had a function and took up time. Replacing stereotyped behaviors with more functional, typical activities is key to developing play and the ability to learn through self-initiated activity. In this section, we will discuss enhancing both toy play and peer play with the overall aim of increasing both cognitive and social capacities.

LEVELS OF PLAY

When we talk about play, we need a vocabulary and a sense of what kinds of activities occupy a child's play at different stages of development. These stages have a great deal to do with the exigency that one stage necessarily follows the other, and the fact that stages of play logically cannot be skipped, but coherently build upon one another.

Sensory Motor Learning and Play. The youngest children simply explore the sensory properties of toys, and this is called sensory motor play or the stage of sensory motor development. How things look, sound, feel, taste, and move are not only the main topics of interest, they are the *only* topics of interest at first. As we've discussed, because children with autism can be over or under-selective in their responses to sensory stimuli, this sensory motor stage is, for them, typically, quite a prominent and pervasive part of early play, and vestiges of it may persist throughout development. Part of intervention is getting the child with autism to tolerate more stimulation on sensory channels that he does *not* prefer as sensory-motor learning in any modality will tend to develop before more concrete, representational, or imaginary play using that modality. (This can mean something as simple as starting a child who does not explore things tactilely to first recognize things by touch—which is sensory-motor; classify things by touch—hard, soft, and so on—which is functional; use representation with touch—like hugging various things that are soft, bouncing things that are rubbery; and finally, using imagination—like pretending a pillow is a baby because it is soft.) The goal is to increase the range of perceptual experiences the child can apprehend and from which, over time, the child can extract information and build new experiences.

Learning via sensory modalities is what does happen first, developmentally, to all children. Giving the child a range of things to explore that are heavy in the sensory modality he prefers can expand self-initiated, self-sustained play. Additionally, by introducing toys that embrace both a preferred sensory quality as well as a non-preferred one (for example, a spinning top that also makes music as it goes round) would be a good way of developing tolerance and calling attention to the world of sounds. As the child becomes aware of a wider range of sensory information and develops mastery at regulating how he gets and stops different kinds of information, this consolidation leaves him better prepared to play with things that can be experimented with in many different sensory ways. After young children learn through their sensory and motor activities about the characteristics of objects, they can transition into the next stage—functional play.

Linking Sensory Motor and Functional Play. With each qualitatively different stage of development, there are new tasks. After children get to know the "identities" of things—how they look, how they feel, how heavy or light they are, and what sounds they can be made to produce—they are ready to begin to assimilate other information. This includes concrete information, like what the thing is called, whether it is considered big or little, how many of them there might be, and how the object functions. This normally begins when young children are interested in *One Fish, Two Fish, Red Fish, Blue Fish*, and thematically related literature. This is a particularly important point to think about in devising a teaching plan for a young child with autism, because he should not be expected to master concrete information until he has a sensory-motor knowledge base for an object. This means that when a child is taught a new label for something, let's say a frog, he also needs to be able to have a frog to touch, hold, move, and hear croak to know what its "frogginess" is. This is how children consolidate sensory motor information with concrete information. This is developmental. The initial sensory motor knowledge base becomes the foundation for concrete, functional understanding about an object. If the child has no sensory motor information about an object (say a flashcard of a frog), there is no "frogginess" to which to relate this word. (This does not mean that the child cannot memorize that he should touch or say "frog" when presented with the card, just that it is not information he really understands and can use whenever something that seems "froggy" occurs again.) Play is a way of linking the sensory motor knowledge base to a concrete database of functional meanings that represent *why* things have the sensory properties that they do.

Sensory motor play predominates in the first two years, and more concrete and functional use of toys characterizes play in the third and fourth years of life, especially after language begins. Much of what preschoolers are doing is linking up these sensory and functional databases of information; play is how they do it. This is another reason that the development of play is essentially the development of the capacity to think. Words bind together the sensory-motor perceptions with the related functional knowledge of objects, supporting reasoning about parallels and differences, and forming the basis for language as a rationale tool.

Functional, Concrete Play. Functional play, as the name implies, is using objects according to their functions—rolling cars, zooming planes, hopping dinosaurs, and feeding babies. It represents actions as the child sees them live, on TV, or in the actions of others with those objects. At first, the capacity for reenactment is fairly limited, and so play starts out disjointed—feeding the dolly, putting it down, playing with something else, coming back, and putting the dolly to bed. At this stage, there is no link between feeding the dolly and putting her to bed. Feeding and going to sleep are just two out of many things the child has seen done with dollies (or babies). For typically developing children, it is as if they start out with a catalogue of photos of interesting things they have seen, and they create little tableaux representing each photo, one at time. Later, the "photos" become "videos," which is where thematic play comes from.

We know that children with autism are probably at least as visual as typically developing children of the same age and also build photographic catalogues. Therefore, it is a reasonable strategy to think of ways of using their catalogues to develop videos with scripts that can narrate thematic play for them. However, children with autism are not likely as interested in building and organizing these tableaux quite so spontaneously as typically developing children. With autistic children, their photographic catalogues tend to contain single-object stills rather than objects in action relationships with one another. Behavioral methods may be needed to provide structure and incentive to carry out the activities required to animate these simple photos to form more complex tableaux. At first, teaching play in this way can seem Sisyphean, but the goal is to achieve a momentum for what later can be more self-generative play and learning. Examples of teaching play this way include taking "stills," like Barney riding in his car and Barney sitting in his playhouse, and animating the scene with prompting and prompt fading of Barney getting in his car, driving over to his playhouse, getting out of the car, and going inside—a theme that can be elaborated with the inclusion of Baby Bop, BJ, and even Winnie the Pooh.

Stimulating Symbolic-Thematic Play. Symbolic play has two key dimensions not yet present when play is primarily functional and concrete. As children develop the capacity for symbolic and thematic play, at ages three and four, two new things happen: First, the catalogue of photos used in the earlier phase of concrete play becomes a moving picture, or as it has been referred to earlier, a "video." Second, there is a leap at which point there is an integration of sensory as well as functional characteristics of things, and narrative, flexible sequences of actions become coherently joined. From this flexibility, the ability to deal in symbols arises. If data from the sensory database tells you that cars are roughly rectangular and move mostly forward, that means you can pick up anything that is roughly rectangular and move it forward and say, "It is a car!"—the label in your functional database for things that are roughly rectangular and move forward. A friend might argue and say, "No, it's a bus!" and another might insist, "No, It's Thomas the Tank Engine,"—but each is basically addressing the same issue. When three rectangular blocks become a car, a bus, and a train for three different boys, and then race and crash, it's symbolic, imaginative play.

The foregoing example should make clear why it is not helpful to try to teach children with autism play in a way that is primarily designed to be chronologically age-appropriate rather than developmentally "age-appropriate": If the child has not yet had an opportunity to develop earlier stages of play, he does not yet have the prerequisite skills to understand the meaning of more sophisticated play activity. To simply "shape" a play action that *could* be symbolic (like Thomas's flying and crashing) would not be a symbolic action if the child had no functional database that told him whether or not trains fly (so that it would be funny when one did) nor sensory knowledge that trains say "choo-choo" so that might be why Thomas was saying "choo-choo" as he flew. Putting flying trains into a narrative will not promote future variations on the theme if the child does not yet recognize the components. Instead, the teaching (shaping) will result in a learned behavior, not an understanding that can serve the child in a generalizable way. No wonder pure behaviorists who teach such actions through shaping often point to the child's failure to pretend that a block is a car and can fly as evidence that the skill has not "generalized." The real problem is that the prerequisites have not been taught. Teaching play developmentally is how we must prepare children to "generalize" the knowledge they acquire.

ASSESSING CURRENT STAGE OF EXPLORATION AND PLAY

The first step in developing a plan to enhance play skills is to conduct an assessment of the autistic child's strengths and weakness with respect to play. By considering the child's autistic learning disability profile, one can organize observations relevant to this goal: How do the specific autistic learning disabilities we have discussed, like those around interest in peers, awareness of peer interests and norms, formal imitation (ability to copy explicitly on request), incidental imitation (like copying the way someone else moves his hands, throws a ball, or dresses), and use of receptive and expressive nonverbal communication limit the tools that a child has to engage in activity with others? The answers to many specific questions about an individual child's strengths and weaknesses in these areas should form the basis for selecting which of the various methods described in this section may work for a particular child.

WHERE TO START?

Interest in Objects. Is the child interested in conventional toys? What kinds of things does he prefer? Does he play with just one aspect of a toy (like getting it to make a sound), or does he play with the "whole" toy? Does he pick toys based on one sensory property (like its being "flicky"), or are his tastes more eclectic? Does he ignore or actively reject dolls, stuffed animals, action figures, and other proxies for animate beings? What about dinosaurs, or our modern day half-man/half-beast Minatare—Thomas the Tank Engine?

Some children with autism gravitate toward actions and activities that are high on vestibular (movement) stimulation. Other children show very age-appropriate climbing, running, and other gross motor skills, but have much less interest or aptitude for fine motor activity such as using crayons, pencils, and Play-doh. Any of these things that a particular child likes can be put on a list of things or contexts that can be used for teaching other less well-liked or well-mastered abilities.

To begin to teach a child to expand play interests, it is important to start with where he is. This means inventorying what he will play with, how he'll play with it, and under what conditions. From there, the ways in which the child plays with a preferred toy can be broadened, the contexts in which it is used can be increased, and related objects can be introduced. One interesting controversy that comes up in this respect is that some will argue that a child with autism should never be taught with the object that interests him most, if that object has the possibility of being used in a repetitive or stereotyped manner. As we discussed in chapter 4, this can create a real "cutting-off-your-nose-to-spite-your-face" situation when it comes to building intrinsic motivation into play. If a child is in love with Thomas the Tank Engine, he may not want others to "take turns," but if taking turns or not playing with Thomas are made to be the only two alternatives, just getting any contact with Thomas can be a powerful motivator. This example stands in contrast to motivating play in which the child rolls a ball back and forth and has half a Gummy Bear popped into his mouth from behind after the ball is rolled forward. Rewards that are topical and contextually relevant, as we have discussed in chapter 4, are more likely to be associated with self-initiated and self-sustained learning and exploration in related situations. This is especially true with play.

SENSORY INTEGRATION: IS IT A VALID IDEA?

Sensory Integration. Why do children with autism prefer some sensory activities over others? It has been suggested that some sensory or perceptual "channels" may be too "loud," others too "low." Information (such as sounds) on a channel that is tuned too low may result in things like the child seeming not to hear, even though hearing has tested out fine.

The other interesting idea that has been around for a while is whether certain preferred activities should be considered "nutrition," in the sense that if the child is "fed" what he craves (sensory input on a preferred channel), apparent sensory disregulation will equilibrate. I refer specifically to what is frequently termed the "sensory diet," the treatment method prescribed to accomplish "sensory integration." The term "sensory integration" originated with the work of an occupational therapist, Jean Ayres in her first, 1973 book. In 1979 a second, less technical book for parents of children with various problems called *Sensory Integration and the Child* was published. The books, written before we knew as much as we know today about the complexities of brain function, offer the hypothesis that many of the smaller and more subtle developmental problems in coordination—hearing and movement, vision and movement, and seeing and knowing—are the result of the brain's not receiving the "nourishment" it needs from the senses. A sensory "diet" is a ramped-up level of stimulation on some sensory channel, designed to fuel the brain, which when capable of being more active, is supposed to be better able to integrate incoming stimuli. Over the last ten years, particularly, this has become a very popular approach with occupational therapists and opened them to work with children with autism. In fact, "sensory integration" has, in some places, become so popular that the cart often drives the horse, with occupational therapy being recommended *because* the child has autism, not because of some specific developmental aberration in sensory information processing.

Sensory Integration Therapy. The sensory integration therapy approach (often referred to as "SI") has proliferated, though it is completely without data demonstrating efficacy. Given what we now know about brain function, the theory upon which SI is based makes a whole lot less sense than it did in the early 1970s. I personally think that spending precious special-education dollars on an unproven theory like sensory integration is an exploitation of parents who seek anything that might help.

It does not mean, however, that children with autism don't love receiving sensory integration therapy. (I like receiving a massage, but I won't try to tell my insurance company I need it to nourish my brain and integrate my senses. That would be too New Age, even for San Francisco!) Because so many children with autism enjoy SI sessions, let's not throw out the baby with the bathwater.

A closer examination of sensory integration approaches is warranted because it can often be included on the list of activities that a child with autism prefers. Sensory integration therapy activities can be many of the things on an autistic child's "most wanted" rewards list: These might include being squeezed between cushions or thick mats; being rubbed; being brushed with a brush designed for baby hair, corn, or mushrooms being pushed into a big beanbag chair; being spun around on a merry-go-round; and being swung on various devices—swings, hammocks, even carpeted logs suspended by ropes from the ceiling.

If these activities sound like fun—it's because they often are. Many parents talk about how their children run willingly from the car to the occupational therapist's office on therapy days—a sure sign he likes it. But does liking your sensory integration therapy mean it's integrating input into the brain? There's no evidence for that. But if the child likes it, it may be a way to get a child to use language to ask for more, to interact with peers in a reciprocal activity like jumping on a bed or trampoline, or to make eye contact to request that an activity be continued. These would all be fine examples of intrinsically rewarding situations that might reinforce language development, peer interaction, or nonverbal communication—likely all areas of deficit for any child prescribed "sensory integration."

It is not clear, however, that an occupational therapist is needed to do these kinds of activities, or that particularly special equipment is needed. In fact, most of the skill development is more in the domain of a speech and language therapist rather than an occupational therapist. There are some programs in which children with autism receive combined speech and language therapy and occupational therapy sessions, with the occupational therapist's structuring the activity around the equipment used, and the speech and language therapist structuring the content of the communication that is encouraged—a much more sensible model.

Where Good Intentions of Sensory Integration Go Bad. Another reason to be skeptical about sensory integration is that it can stand in opposition to solid, much more scientifically established behavioral principles. For example, I visited a class for children with autism and other severe handicaps in which sensory integration is widely used. One boy became increasingly disruptive during morning circle time, as another pupil took quite a while to complete his turn at circle. After a few minutes, his loud vocalizing, jumping up from his seat, and hopping up and down had begun to have quite a disruptive effect on other pupils—one rocked in his seat covering his ears, and another bounced in his chair moaning. The autism program specialist who had helped the teachers implement their sensory integration program removed the child to the back of the room, settled him in a beanbag, and rubbed his shoulders, and after he began to settle a bit, went off to get a brush. After being left alone, the boy settled further and readily accepted the brushing when it began. According to sensory integration theory, the boy had become sensorily "dis-integrated," and craved the sensory stimulation that would enable him to reorganize. The autism specialist thought that once this young man received some strong sensory input he would calm down, which he did. A behaviorist would say that since the boy preferred not having to remain with the circle, found the beanbag more comfy than his little wooden chair at circle, and certainly enjoyed a back rub, the autism program specialist was reinforcing the presence of inappropriate circle time behavior, and was in fact reinforcing his efforts to escape from circle time. The behaviorist would predict that this pattern of adult responding would result in more disruptive behavior in the class, and indeed the class was observed to have a very high rate of ongoing disruptive, inappropriate vocal and motor behaviors. The bottom line is that sensory integration activities may be fine reinforcers and may provide fine teaching contexts, but they may be absolutely counterproductive if the sensory integration hypothesis is applied in circumstances that call for widely accepted behavior management principles. If the preferred sensory integration activity can be obtained by being disruptive during a less preferred, harder, or disliked activity, the child who can get SI for being disruptive will become more and more disruptive whenever he is asked to do something not quite to his liking.

WHERE DO CHILDREN PLAY?

Other Play Contexts. Using the activities of sensory integration therapy may be a constructive, reinforcing context for structuring new play activities. What other variables are likely to influence successful play environments? For children sensitive to new places, facilitating play in a home-like environment may work better than doing it in a more formal "therapy" setting. Some children may prefer to play with only one or two peers; others may not mind being in a group setting such as a school, an after-school program, or a preschool. Some children are much more amenable to contact outdoors than inside; some are the other way around. Sometimes a small confined space in which play with the playmate (adult or child) who is the main alternative to doing nothing works best. In developing more varied and imaginative solitary play, a confined space may promote innovation because following suggestions as to what else can be done with what the child has becomes relatively more interesting.

Interactive Play Activities. In chapter 4, we talked about the roles that adults can take in interacting with children with autistic spectrum disorders to facilitate social interaction and play. Now we will talk about the play content, the things that are likely to work better than others in developing increased interest and the ability to participate in group settings. Depending on the age of the child, the type of play that children of his developmental and chronological ages usually engage in, and the child's interests, the activities selected for a particular child should vary. The central principle is to play (pun intended) to the child's strengths.

There needs to be an awareness of specific autistic learning disabilities that may affect participation in certain types of play activities. These may include whether the child can quickly process verbal directions, whether the activity includes compensatory visual models, whether the child must be able to imitate, and whether the child must be able to "read" other children's responses to his actions. Choosing initial social play activities that are geared to developmental level, complement autistic learning style, and circumvent these autistic learning disabilities should all be elements in designing and choosing play activities.

Starting Interactions. In typically developing young children, mutual play skills develop almost like the early scenes in a ballet in which the dancers first think each is alone on the stage, then discover one another, then, dance alongside one another, and finally dance together. In earliest play, the child first has a desire just to play near another, rather than to play elsewhere. Many children with autism are fairly comfortable with this stage—though not all. Next, an awareness that the other is playing with similar things, or other interesting things begins to develop. The children glance at one another's activities and occasionally catch one another's eye, perhaps smiling, perhaps (accurately) expressing concern that the other child might want his toy. Next, mutual play with the same or related items begins, or, alternatively, the child plays in deferred imitation of what another child has been seen earlier to do with the toy. Finally, children begin to play with toys jointly.

As has already been said, in teaching children with autism to play together, one must follow these rather invariant stages in the development of play. No typically developing children "skip" stages and go straight from tolerating the presence of another to turn-taking in a mutual activity with a toy. We want to take care that, with the goal of helping the autistic child behave "age appropriately," we do not prompt play that skips stages. Such play will be non-spontaneous and will not be self-generative, as is play that has been developed in stages, consolidating the gains and new skills of each stage as activity becomes more complex.

Solitary Sequential Play. When children initially show mutuality in play, the mutuality is usually manifest as both children doing the same or similar things with the same or similar toys. If one guy wants to dump pebbles into the super-sized Tonka dump truck, other dump truck fans in the vicinity will soon want to as well. With children with autism, the easiest way to spark this type of play is to put them near others who play with the same kinds of things they do. If the child doesn't have any functional toy schema, teach him some first. A Thomas-the-Tank Engine fan who just carries Thomas, looks at him, and sometimes brings him close to his eyes may best learn about dump truck exploits by learning about dumping with Thomas's coal-carrier friend. If that gets to be OK, it means the dumping schema is emerging. Tonkas can be next. Then if the new dump truck fan meets an existing dump truck fan on the playground—well, they now have something in common. The chances that some imitative play will develop increases. Paired with this, such play forays should be supported by all of the strategies discussed in chapter 4 about shadowing and teen play experts.

There are times when a child with autism will play alongside another child with similar toys, but there is no mutuality—no glancing at one another, no commenting on the others comments, no grabbing at what the other has. When the mutuality is missing, the first task is to build it into such simple play. Don't assume that the child with autism must somehow be covertly taking in what the other child is doing. He is probably happily ensconced in his own little world with the most marginal awareness of other children. A systematic effort must be undertaken to move him off this position. Often this type of side-by-side play is erroneously referred to as "parallel play." It's not parallel until there's some interchange of awareness and ideas. But true parallel play schemes need to be established before true interactive play in which one child's actions or words build on another's can take place.

To begin to move from solitary to parallel play, mutuality can be built up through participation in after-school or other recreational programs in which everyone does the same thing—though not necessarily at the same time. These solitary sequential activities can be seen as the bridge between solitary and parallel play. Lets enumerate examples:

For younger elementary school-aged pupils, solitary sequential activities include things like gymnastics, tee-ball, and karate—any game in which kids follow an adult in unison or turn by turn. For older elementary school children, these activities tend to be better liked and work out more successfully than activities like team sports, that require a capacity to understand strategy and what others may be thinking and planning. We will talk more about this later in this chapter as we consider developing skills for more rule-oriented play. As imitation skills improve, these "solitary sequential" activities include sports such as junior bowling or competitive swimming in which people take turns, with each serving partly as a model for the next person, and in which some strategy is needed. One's own competitive savvy (or lack thereof), though, does not penalize teammates. For the child with autism, this protects social acceptability.

For high school-aged pupils, a sport like track or the swim team may offer similar additional advantages. In between turns, the child can watch or talk with others, but there is no need to talk with others if you choose not to. There are also group activities like karate, judo, or band, in which conversational pressure is less, but the activity is age-appropriate. Gaining expertise not only gives a child or teen with autism some confidence, as it would anyone the same age, it also gives peers a circumstance for positive valuation of a classmate with autism who may seem less able at other school activities.

These somewhat solitary, somewhat group, activities sometimes work more easily if the child with autism can attend with a peer he already knows and with whom he has some degree of comfort, and who he is perhaps more likely to imitate, such as a sibling or cousin. Having a ready repertoire of activities with at least one other peer can make fitting into a new group, class, or team less trying and more transparent for the child with an ASD.

PARALLEL GROUP ACTIVITIES

For many children with autism, a good way to begin to participate with groups is through parallel group activities. At the preschool level, this includes singing and action-song games (like the hokey-pokey) that everyone does in unison. Prior to entry into a group, the child with autism can be pre-taught these activities so that his ability to participate does not fully hinge on his imitation skills (which are likely not his strength), but rather on his memory (which is likely notably better). When memory passes for imitation in the peer group, it lays the groundwork for the child's acceptance into the group by allowing him to be more like others.

Guided Turn-Taking as a Bridge to Interactive Play. Just as solitary sequential play activities can serve as a bridge between solitary and parallel play, guided turn-taking can serve as a bridge between parallel play and more interactive play. One thing that can be difficult for children with autism when it comes to group participation is the waiting and doing nothing before the activity starts. Many times in pre-K and kindergarten classes, children sit, fidget, and wait while their peers finish a previous activity and all are ready to transition to the group activity. At times like these, typically developing children will whisper sweet nothings to one another and giggle; little girls will explore the poodle pocket on their sweatshirts. The child with autism is more likely to frame this experience as "What's in this for me?" so that if waiting seems a bore, and something else in the classroom is more interesting, he will be off.

One class I visited handled this issue of getting autistic children engaged in parallel activity particularly well: the teacher began circle time (the big time for parallel activity) as soon as two children had arrived at the circle from their previous activity. As the first song began, the other children still dawdling over the end of snack (the previous activity) heard the music coming from the circle area and got on the ball. The circle grew and participation increased; no one had time to get bored and run off. One classroom staff remained behind at the snack table to oversee the finishing of that activity while another made sure that each child finishing snack headed in the right direction.

Guided turn taking during a familiar parallel play activity can serve to form the basis of more truly interactive play. Some toys lend themselves particularly well to these types of activities: sending cars down a ramp, dropping a ball through a chute, finding a letter of the alphabet electronically on a desktop toy.

An adult can introduce the concept of taking turns, for example, by holding all the cars, and giving them one at a time to whoever's turn is next. Outdoors, throwing a beanbag or a basketball or taking turns on the front and back of the tricycle can be examples of this too.

JUMP-STARTING IMAGINATION

Scripting Play from Video Models. In chapter 4, we talked about the great difficulties that most children with autism have with imitating, and in particular, the difficulties they have modeling others. This lack of a native drive to "do like" and "be like" others is fundamental to the core of autistic spectrum disorders. Overcoming and compensating for imitation deficits is central to developing a capacity to engage in play with peers. For a typically developing child, coming into a room with twenty peers who are all standing with hands joined in a circle singing, makes most newcomers want to join in too. Some are shy, might need a minute, or might need adult encouragement. The child with autism, though, would be the one most likely to run away from such a scene. How then do you harness the power of this type of imitative learning and get the autistic child to participate?

A nice body of research exists on the use of video models to teach adaptive, social, and play skills to children with autism. Intuitively, this teaching strategy makes sense. Many parents of small children with autism can describe how their child is drawn to the Barney theme music and will bop along with Barney and even copy some of the things Barney and his friends are doing. Some prefer Teletubbies, perhaps because they present a simpler model for the (limited) things they do. One hypothesis is that the attraction to video models over live models for children with autism is that the scary feeling of being with so many unpredictable "others" is completely factored out of the equation. Some educational videos have been developed that take advantage of the observation that children with autism seem to learn more readily from a video model than a live model and have been successful at teaching skills like pulling up pants, brushing teeth, and so on. If specific adaptive skills like these can be taught from video models, can videos be used to "jump start" play?

MOVING FROM MODELING TO IMAGINATION

Getting true interactive, imaginative play going between children when one of the children is autistic is hard work. Learning to model actions after the actions are seen on videos is just one step. It gives the child a tool for taking in information and creating a schema, a kind of mental representation of what has been vicariously experienced. Turning those modeled actions into play is a trickier step. It requires a lot of creativity because it may be the first type of play that relies both on the child's self-generative speech as well as a capacity for representation.

Enter the Disney Corporation! Teaching these skills to children with autism today is much easier than it once was because all the Disney animated cartoons (except the one that's in the theatre at the moment) are available on video, and a host of corresponding action figures, ready for purchase at the time of the video's release, are at your nearest toy store (if not free at McDonald's). Many children with autism initially prefer videos with cartoon characters rather than people. (This may be due to the fact that animate characters emit less "noise" from their facial expressions and body language than do real characters and are therefore a little easier to recognize and "read.") Cartoon characters also tend to be heavier on easily memorized, fun to replicate sight gags—like Buzz Light Year flying to "Infinity and Beyond." It is easier for a child with autism, who is very visual, to recognize and copy Buzz than some animate character who mainly stands around and flaps her mouth, like Cruella deVille.

How Echolalia and Echopraxia Can Help. For the child who has established some one-to-one mutuality in play with others and can participate in parallel group activities, video scripts can be a really good "primer" of play schema. Many children with autism have a tendency to engage in echolalia (repeated speech), and echopraxia is its motor "cousin."

Echopraxia is a tendency to repeat particularly interesting motor schema—unsurprisingly, often from those videos that have been watched numerous times. A close "cousin" of echopraxia is what is sometimes referred to as "playlalia." Playlalia is echopraxia that is rote repetition from an interesting model (essentially the same activity that a typically developing child might show), but coordinated with accompanying language from the video. A typical six-year-old might grab his Buzz shouting "To infinity and beyond!" while leaping off the sofa, rolling on the floor, and pretending to be attacked by the "bad" Buzz. If the autistic six-year-old can be helped to the playlalia stage of this scenario, the two six-year-olds will have something in common.

When Can Videos Be Good for Kids? We've already discussed some aspects of TV viewing. But how can it influence development of play skills? Obviously, too much repeated watching of anything on TV is bad. It's mental downtime. But, if the child is given access to all the action figures that go with his video, however, and someone (like a teen expert player) can watch with him, together they can do what the TV does while the TV does it. Later, with the TV off, they can do the same things. Later still, they can "go off road" and innovate from the script. In this way, the child learns by example how to move from echolalia, echopraxia, and playlalia to incorporating innovation in his play. In moving beyond what is seen on TV, the child is being primed to develop a repertoire of play schema that then can be used in more interactive, imaginative play with peers.

Innovation from Scripts. Not too long ago, I visited a wonderful class for children with autism in which the teacher was doing some of the best work I'd ever seen with respect to developing imagination. Three five- and six-year-old boys with autism, Scott, Aidan, and Miguel, participated in this "adventure." (The teacher later told me that each day there are repetitions of the adventure I saw, with some of the same and some new pages to their "script.") The guided imaginative play started with the boys and the teacher seated in four chairs that had been placed in two rows, with the teacher sitting in the back row. The teacher called out, "Anchors away! Where we headed today Captain Scott?" Captain Scott thought for a minute and said, "To get pirate treasure!" The teacher said, "Navigator Miguel, do you spy land?" (Miguel put a pretend spyglass to his eye and said he saw an island.) Next the teacher asked First Mate Aidan whether they were ready to trim the sails, and when he said, "Yes," the teacher said, "All hands trim sails." All the boys stood up and made motions like they were pulling on vertical ropes. "What next Captain Scott?" Captain Scott told the crew to go ashore. "What's on this island?" the teacher asked. "Buried treasure," First Mate Aidan replied. This whole scene went on for several minutes. Later in the morning, the teacher explained that each day their adventure took place on either a spaceship or a pirate ship—it was up to the captain of the day to tell the other crew on the spur of the moment. Sometimes they landed on an island, sometimes a planet, sometimes the moon. Once landed, they might look for treasure, bad guys, or wild animals. At each step of the way, a child was prompted according to his role and made a choice which the others might add to or comment upon.

While the play was contrived compared to what boys that age might typically do on their own, it was easy to imagine integrating typical peers into this game or taking the game with one of these kids to his after-school program where peers could be recruited to play along, too.

Rule-Oriented Games of Probabilities. As kids mature, they outgrow the more imaginative activities that are so common to children under six or seven. Integrating children with autism with typical peers after age six or seven means preparing them to engage in the types of interaction common to that age group. Between the ages of six or seven and the ages of ten or eleven, children reach a stage sometimes referred to as "latency." At this stage, they are very interested in rules, absolute rights and wrongs, collections, how things work—all things concrete and rule-oriented. It is at this age that children become involved in team sports and a formal sense of competition develops; by the end of this period peer relationships may be both hierarchical and cliquish. There is less boy-girl socializing during latency than at any other time in development, and activities that preoccupy the children are more gender-specific.

In many ways, the preoccupations of latency are favorable for the child with autism: Autistic children with stores of knowledge of a particular topic can get some respect for it from peers. Billy, who was ten and had Asperger's, was a whiz at sports statistics, especially baseball. He started at a new school for learning-handicapped children. One classmate commented in an admiring tone of voice, "That Billy's a little weird, but he sure knows a lot about baseball!" This is a real compliment coming from another 10-year-old. It protected Billy from being as isolated as he might have been had he been judged on social skills alone. An aspect of autistic learning style—amassing rote facts—in Billy's case, counterbalanced a lack of affiliative drive with peers, an autistic learning disability.

In addition, latency-aged child care a great deal about rules—who's fair, who is a cheater. Children with autism care about rules. On top of that, children with autism aren't sneaky and don't cheat because they have such difficulty with the theory of another's mind, a skill needed to be successfully deceptive. For many latency-aged kids with autism, you either follow the rules or you're wrong. In fact, this black-and-white way of seeing the world tends to persist throughout life. But when typical latency-aged kids and autistic latency-aged kids all know the rules—and can agree upon them—they can play together.

A speech and language therapist for fifth graders took advantage of this rule-oriented mentality in a group language pragmatics/social skills development session I observed: Six children, including one high-functioning autistic boy, were playing "Go Fish." They all knew the rules. The therapist structured the interaction, reminding them to look at the player from whom each was requesting a queen, a six, or an ace. She reminded them that others could see the cards of a child not holding them properly and might therefore cheat. Soon they were all reminding each other to hold their cards better. "Go Fish" tested their memories of who held each card. They also had to remember to use each other's names as they made their requests. When a pupil erred by asking for a queen from someone other than a player obviously already holding a queen, the other kids would reprimand him, and he had to learn to say something like "we all make mistakes sometimes," or "I forgot; but it's OK, it's just a game." In the safe, structured, completely rule-governed context of a simple card game, all the children were learning skills for more effective social interaction.

"Go Fish" and rule-oriented board games of chance or probability, like Candyland, Chutes and Ladders, and Hungry Hippos, are great places to start social interaction. They allow for participation that involves taking turns, without having to add extra, spontaneous commentary to be a player. While you play, though, you are exposed to models of peers using exclamations of delight and disappointment and get to participate in discussions of rules ("Whose turn is it?"). These are things the child with autism can do quite well if he has been pre-taught the activity in play with an older child or sibling.

Strategy and Theory of Mind versus Probability. For older and higher-functioning people with autistic spectrum disorders, the capacity to memorize and follow rules, and understand mathematical probabilities can transform into higher-level game playing. A number of people with high-functioning autism are great chess players. They can focus concentration, are not easily distracted by extraneous (or even intentional) social signals, and can deal with the math while drawing on a vast memory of previously played games. Monopoly, card games, and even word games like Scrabble can be viewed as meeting these criteria, too. While most of us probably use higher-level theory-of-mind skills to form strategy ("If I move here, he'll think that I think that he'll move there . . . "), individuals with autism rely more heavily, and probably more reliably, on math, memory, and concentration.

RULE-ORIENTED GAMES USING THEORY OF MIND

The one area of peer play that tends to remain off-limits for most kids with autism consists of those activities requiring theory of mind—the ability to "mind read" what someone else must be planning to do. Problems with theory of mind are core to autistic deficits. Quickly reacting to social signals is not an area of strength. In a ball game, the direction in which an opponent gazes, the times in a game when the opponent seems nervous or confident, and discerning why the other player might be moving in a particular direction are key to strategy. Situations that call for reading nonverbal cues and gestures and thinking quickly about strategy are not playing to the strengths of an individual with autism. This means that team sports like baseball, basketball, soccer, football, and, to a lesser extent, individual sports like tennis are very unlikely to be successful social experiences.

Sometimes parents will want to try one of these sports anyway because there is a Challenger or Special Olympics league, or the child seems to like the activity. These are good reasons. Certainly, special teams afford a great opportunity for the child with autism to excel.

For five- or six-year-old children with autism, playing team sports can be good for socialization and less limited by their theory-of-mind problems than when they are older: This is because, among typically developing children under six, the percentage of six-year-olds who are really sure in which direction to kick the soccer ball and who know who's on which team, and which goal is theirs— can still be a bit murky. When this straightens out at around seven or eight, typical latency-aged kids get very insistent on doing things "right" and can be very punishing to the kid who seems oblivious to the rules. It is always important not to set a child with autism up for more of an uphill struggle than necessary.

SOCIALIZATION FOR THE HIGHER-FUNCTIONING ADOLESCENT

As children grow, the activities that define how time is spent change. Adolescents don't see themselves as "playing" so much as "hanging out," spending time together in increasingly informal ways with less of a planned agenda or engaged in rule-oriented activity. Part of being "cool" is *not* following rules. This can mean knowing which rules can be ignored and when. It means knowing which rules can be violated a bit, and where and with whom such violations are likely to add to your coolness (your positive peer valuation). Part of being socially acceptable as a teen is perceiving and following an ever-shifting set of principles that guides such adolescent behavior. The higher-functioning child with autism or Asperger's syndrome who has done well through the elementary-school years by memorizing and adhering to lots of social conventions that have been memorized as concrete rules (like not sharing items of personal hygiene) can be flummoxed when girls in high school brush, comb, and rearrange one another's hair. Protesting the inappropriateness of such behavior will only serve to delineate how uncool (and not worthy of affiliation) you are.

This set of social norms presents a whole new level of challenge for higher-functioning adolescents and young adults with autism or Asperger's syndrome who may find a niche in the more latency-aged rule-oriented world, but can't begin to understand a world in which exactly how you dress, stand, or walk, and what you smile or laugh at—makes all the difference in social acceptability.

Perhaps the cruelest time for young people with Asperger's or high-functioning autism is middle school. They are smart enough to know that things are not going well as this transition to adolescent values begins, but are quite vulnerable to anxiety, clueless as to what is wrong or how to fix it. A typical defensive strategy is to become increasingly isolated from peers. Since such individuals may have had one or two friends at best, this can be made worse by the likelihood that these friends will reject them too. Affiliating with a kid perceived by the adolescent peer group as being weird in any way puts you in the isolated world of the weird group too. Many parents report that at middle school, their child's one or two friends from elementary school will now only be seen with them when no one else from school is around.

There are no real good answers here, but there are some strategies that, on an individual basis, may help, depending on the social ecology in which the young person lives. One of the most protective things is a few good friends. Sometimes these friends are situation specific (from home, church, or computer club) or are siblings. For one young man with Asperger's, Chris, his protection was his learning-disabled, but jock, twin brother, who brought him along with the other guys on the football team. They called Chris their mascot and importuned him to carry equipment, but it was OK with him because he felt safe having his brother there. For others, this safety net it is a special school for Asperger's or learning disabilities, a protective environment in which all students have some vulnerabilities—though maybe not all have social deficits—and in which the autistic spectrum pupil, especially, can be segregated from the more conduct-disordered young person.

Young incipient sociopaths of various sorts seem to have radar for picking up higher-functioning autistic spectrum kids and just bear down. These are the kids with uninviting diagnoses like "conduct disorder," "oppositional defiant disorder," or sometimes "severely emotionally disturbed." The young sociopaths need the same sort of highly structured, behaviorally regulated environments that many young people with Asperger's and high-functioning autism do, and, in school settings particularly, there is always a risk that these two groups will be placed together. It is not a good idea for pupils in either group that they be integrated. It's like throwing the lambs to the lions.

On the other hand, kids with other kinds of neurodevelopmental disorders, like those with some forms of attention deficit disorder (ADD), can be good buddies for higher-functioning kids with ASDs. If anything, the child with ADD tends to be socially *too* initiating. The ADD-type social initiative sometimes provides the additional level of intrusion and persistence that a young person with Asperger's or high-functioning autism needs to form a bond.

Another approach is to identify a peer buddy who will sit next to the kid with Asperger's in a class and be responsible for walking to the next class with him. Individual teachers can be recruited to identify peers who share class schedules. Using different peers for each class change provides an opportunity for the child with Asperger's or high-functioning autism to get to know more students and also makes the activity more of a responsibility than a chore for the peer buddy. The peer buddy is more likely to be seen as altruistic by his peers if his help is limited than if he is expected to do more open-ended "hanging out."

The high school socialization of lunch and PE is usually the hardest on students with high-functioning autism and Asperger's. Solutions include taking lunch in the library or a resource room, or having a quick lunch in a resource room and then getting some one-to-one instruction or computer time. Adaptive PE, which is often needed anyway, or an individual sport like track that can be done during lunchtime can help cover for what will otherwise be very stressful open-ended social time. Large group, free-form socialization is not likely to help the pupil with Asperger's or high-functioning autism, and can make the student so anxious and avoidant that the two or three periods of the day before lunch and couple periods after it become danger zones for inappropriate acting-out behaviors. Be practical. Ask the student which solution he prefers rather than imposing one. If he's bought into the plan it has a better chance of working. Adolescents with Asperger's or high-functioning autism don't appreciate having adults running their lives any more than any other adolescent. Simply giving two or three socially acceptable ways to spend a lunch hour can be fine. Including the young person in decision making about how his time will be spent doesn't have to mean bringing the pupil to his IEP meeting—I am not a big fan of that, as I think it precludes necessary and honest discussion of a pupil's weaknesses as well as strengths.

One place that extracurricular socialization can work relatively well is in the context of religious organizations. One of my colleagues maintains that the monks of the Middle Ages who took vows of silence and poverty and produced beautiful, labor-intensive calligraphic religious manuscripts must all have had Asperger's syndrome. A more contemporary example is one of my patients, Roger, who converted from Judaism to Mormonism. He was a social isolate with no real friends. Somehow, Roger was evangelized by Mormon missionaries and suddenly found himself with friends who called a few evenings each week asking him to join a bowling party, go out for pizza, or join a hiking trip. Roger was accepted for who he was and for the first time felt he belonged to a group that didn't tease him and did not say things about him behind his back. As a 25-year-old faced with whether he wanted to move with his parents to Scotland or stay where he was, Roger was undecided. His parents persuaded him to accompany them on a look-and-see visit to Scotland. Soon after they arrived, he was contacted by members of the Glasgow Mormon Church who welcomed him and talked to him about living there. Roger moved.

PEER COMPANIONSHIP

Out-of-school contexts may present better opportunities for socialization. For high school-aged students with Asperger's or high-functioning autism, hiring a peer buddy can be a good way to provide a model to foster age-appropriate language, dress, and interests. A community college employment opportunities office may be a good place to find a 20- to 24-year-old who is interested in a part-time job as a leisure-time companion for a person with Asperger's or high-functioning autism. Sometimes this arrangement can be presented to the young person with Asperger's or high-functioning autism as another student who can drive, and who can take him to the mall to buy a desired video game, have lunch, etc., so he does not have to go with his mom. (Remember this is age-appropriate; even if he would rather go with his mom, it can be a positive step toward independence to learn to go with an age mate.) Sometimes, when I suggest arrangements like this, the parent worries about what might happen if there were a car accident or if they didn't return at the appointed time. Well, that's a concern with any teenager. Nowhere is it written that parents of kids with AS or HFA are exempt from the concerns they would have as parents of a child without AS or HFA.

Sometimes after-school activities that play on a student's strength, like a chess club or astronomy club, band or a computer lab, can be a good setting because there is a much smaller number of pupils and one teacher is pretty much keeping things structured, but there are some opportunities for more informal interactions during chess games, science labs, and other small-group cooperative activities. If the person with AS or HFA is one of the more competent members in the activity group, his differences may not result in any negative valuation in such a setting.

Autistic Learning Disabilities and Socializing. The truth of the matter is that by high school, most young people with high-functioning autism or Asperger's are pretty clear about their own attitudes toward peer relationships. Some may characterize one or two people as "good," "best," or "close" friends. Usually, their contacts with these people are not as intense and frequent as those of others their age. Others may allude to having friends, but seem unable or unwilling to specify who these friends are or what they do together. Still others simply say they don't really want friends, don't have time for friends, or are happy having "friends" they meet in Internet chat rooms. What they all have in common is a limited ability to define the qualities of a true friend. This means that being a true friend has got to be just as hard.

Like the rest of us, those we describe as having Asperger's syndrome or high-functioning autism vary in how much effort and attention they want to give to maintaining social appearances and a network of close friends. The social qualities that cause us to categorize early-arising aloofness and absence of preschool-aged affiliative drive as part of autistic learning disabilities are precisely what remain as a personality variant in adulthood. This can range from an appearance of extreme shyness to aloof disregard for others to seemingly clueless insensitivity.

If you ask your "typical" adolescent with Asperger's whether he'd like to meet the guy he talks with all the time in the Star Trek chat room, he's likely to say, "Not really!" Sometimes dealing with this type of response is more an issue for those around the person with Asperger's than it is for him.

CHAPTER CONCLUSIONS

In this chapter we talked about how children with autistic spectrum disorders can have difficulty in relating to the world around them. When we think about children relating to things outside themselves, we usually think of the world of other people—the social world, and the world of objects—the play activities that especially occupy the youngest children. These worlds are, of course, overlapping. In this chapter, we focused on how the child with autism may, because of sensory difficulties, weigh and perceive incoming information differently, creating a whole new weltanschauung—filtered through these sensory alterations. This makes the information available through play with toys different, and makes social interaction very different, a related topic discussed in chapter 4. In chapter 9, we will use the conceptualization of autistic learning disabilities and autistic learning styles to see how these differences affect ability to adapt to everyday life. Parallel to issues of learning to communicate and becoming socialized are issues about how children with autistic spectrum disorders encounter difficulties in the adaptive challenges of everyday living. These are the skills that other children naturally pick up along the way, like staying safe, eating a variety of foods, getting potty trained, and learning how to get dressed. In the domain of adaptive functioning, just as in the development of social and communicative skills, principles of how autistic children learn can be applied to consolidating meaningful functional accomplishments.

CHAPTER NINE

Autistic Learning Disabilities and the Skills of Daily Living

DAILY LIVING SKILLS

In the preceding chapters, we have seen how the symptoms of autism affect main aspects of life such as communicating and relating to others and taking in information from the things in one's surroundings. An important question that is raised by the presence of these autistic learning disabilities is how does the child with autism compensate for his disabilities in a way that ensures that his basic needs are met? An evolutionary psychologist hearing about all these deficits in social development and communication would have to wonder how children with autism ensure their survival, as it seems that the usual social interdependence doesn't work very well.

The answer, of course is that children with autism manage to elicit caregiving from their parents—and manage to elicit a lot of it, just the way infants do. The problem is that this stage of dependency can become prolonged. It often results in all sorts of family problems when the child with autism won't eat what others are eating, won't sleep when others do, has no apparent concept of his own safety or that of others, and generally, as Thoreau said "marches to the beat of his own drummer."

In this chapter, we will examine how autistic learning disabilities affect skills needed in daily life. Keeping in mind the particular motivational and learning style of children with autism that we have already discussed, I will suggest modifications to mainstream behavioral practices. Skills discussed in this chapter, unlike in earlier chapters, are those that most children first develop at home as part of the routines of daily living, rather than in a classroom as something explicitly taught. These skills can, however, be taught in classrooms and in fact constitute important curricula for the more affected children in the autistic spectrum, those who do not acquire spontaneous communicative use of spoken language by age six or seven. These children typically have protracted difficulties in multiple areas of daily living skills. The term daily living skills is sometimes used interchangeably with "adaptive behavior skills," though discussions of adaptive behaviors can have more the implication of concerns about behavior that interferes with daily living, like problems in transitioning between settings or activities, or tolerating new people and places. In this chapter the terms are used interchangeably, as is the term "functional skills."

Picking Your Battles. In developing a child's adaptive behaviors and implementing behavior changes, it is always important to pick your battles carefully. If a child does things that endanger himself or others, such as running away in open public places, or being aggressive toward younger children, this is likely a high-priority item, a battle worth fighting. However, if a child eats only small quantities of a limited number of foods, but is still where he should be on his growth curve, expanding food choice is a battle you may choose not to fight immediately, especially if the child is just starting school or therapy.

Sometimes I'll meet an eight-year-old child with autism who can read on a second-grade level and do math on a third-grade level, but still isn't potty trained. The parents have brought the child in for help with potty training, because the full-inclusion second-grade teacher, the child's one-to-one aide, and the school nurse are unwilling to change his pull-ups on the days he has an accident. Such parents may have worked hard to develop the child's academic skills, but did not take time to focus on the skills of daily living we expect a second grader to have mastered. The chain is as strong as its weakest link. When we apply educational and behavioral methods to the training of children with autism, we must also keep a developmental perspective. If a child who is bright enough to go to second grade, but is restricted by the fact that some of his skills (like being potty trained) are not yet at the 30-month-old level then, it can be argued that someone has failed this child. Any child bright enough to read and to subtract with borrowing is bright enough to use the toilet.

Skill development is a matter of setting priorities. This chapter is intended to round out the picture of how to help the whole child fulfill as much of his potential as possible. Reading while still wearing diapers makes reading look like a rather cosmetic improvement. Our ability to teach and train children with autism has benefited enormously from access to behavioral technology. If such technology can be wrapped around the symptoms of autism to teach academic skills, it can certainly be used just as effectively to allow the child to develop adaptive behaviors commensurate with cognitive functioning.

DAILY LIVING AND AUTISTIC LEARNING DISABILITIES

Much of what we have learned, we have learned incidentally. There are many things all of us do hundreds of times a day, such as in eating, dressing, going to the toilet, using a telephone, or taking a walk, that required relatively little direct instruction to master and even less instruction to refine. Chances are that little or no formal teaching was involved in learning to do some of these things, rather, our skills in these areas are the result of a gradual accretion of knowledge through everyday experiences. The way we carry out these behaviors is very much predicated on the culture in which we live; in other words, our daily living skills are a result of learning the conventional ways of doing these things. Individuals with autism, however, have little to no interest in doing something just because other people do it. The challenge in teaching adaptive behaviors is motivating the child with autism to want to master what we consider necessary adaptive behaviors, like eating the right foods, sleeping at night, and not darting into traffic.

SPECIAL CONSIDERATIONS IN APPLYING
BEHAVIORAL THEORY TO AUTISM

Motivation is key to organizing any kind of learning, as we've discussed in the context of teaching social, play, and language skills. Motivation for the child with autism always goes back to that thought bubble over the child's head: "Why should I care?" The answer can't be "because mommy wants me to" or "'cause everyone else is doing it," but rather must include personal benefit in terms of something the child wants. Alternatively, all of us, including children with autism, can be induced to do things in order to avoid undesirable consequences. Most of us prefer to be rewarded rather than punished; the same is true of children with autism. Just as rewards are different for children with autism, so are deterrents, and this is what we will discuss in this section. The principles of behavioral analysis, unsurprisingly, broadly apply to developing adaptive behaviors in children with autism, but require modification to accommodate what a child with autism is likely to view as rewarding and what he is likely to perceive as deterring. I prefer the term "deterrent" to "aversive" for a critical reason. "Aversive" implies something that anyone would want to avoid and would consider negative. Loud yelling, pinching, spanking, and mild electrical shock are all aversives that have a mostly distant history in behavior therapy. By contrast, a "deterrent" is also something that should decrease the likelihood of an undesirable behavior's recurring, but is something that mainly a person with autism would avoid, such as restriction of personal movement, close presence of another person when not desired, holding hands, or inescapable direct eye gaze.

DEVELOPING A REINFORCER HIERARCHY

A reinforcer hierarchy is simply a list of what the child loves most in life. This was discussed at length in chapter 4. In the simplest case of "external" or "extrinsic" reinforcement, the child gets a desired food for a desirable performance. In the simplest case of "internal" or "intrinsic" reinforcement, the child engages repetitively in a spontaneous activity (like watching something spin) because it feels good. All things being equal, internal reinforcers are preferable if they can be part of the desired activity, and thereby self-perpetuate the drive to engage in that activity. However, the desired activity must be incorporated into a larger activity that leads to a desired performance—if it is an internal reinforcer worth listing in the reinforcer hierarchy. An example in a moment.

Some reinforcers are external or extrinsic, some internal or intrinsic. Some reinforcers are primary, like foods or sensory stimulation; some are secondary, like money or any token that can exchanged specifically for something we want. Some reinforcers have a higher value than others, either because of their excitatory value, or because of their relative scarcity. Most reinforcers can be titrated—broken into smaller allotments (like five minutes at a time of a video); but some can only remain whole (like getting to go buy an ice cream). Some reinforcers can be earned immediately after the desirable behavior has occurred; and some can be deferred using tokens.

The whole idea behind a reinforcer hierarchy is that you get more when you do more. You get the best rewards for accomplishing the hardest things to accomplish. Sometime, "hardest" can be equated with demonstrating a new skill (like pulling up your pants) or achieving a new milestone (like staying in your bedroom all night).

DETERRENCE: NEGATIVE REINFORCEMENT, PUNISHMENT, AND PAIN

The flip side of reinforcement is deterrence. (In the bad old days, we used to say that the flip side of reinforcement was punishment, but that was too often equated with corporal or physical punishment.) Deterrence typically involves altering circumstances so that repeating an undesirable behavior now seems less worthwhile. For example, if six-year-old Amalia lays on the floor, screams, and kicks the refrigerator with her hard little shoes until Dad opens it and successfully guesses what she wants to eat, you can be sure that Amalia will remember and use that strategy the next time she's hungry or has been offered something to eat that she has found to be unacceptable. Walking out of the kitchen and ignoring the screams would be negative reinforcement (an absence of positive reinforcement). Children who are the real pros at modifying the behavior of parents counter this type of adult maneuver by getting up, following, and flopping on the floor in front of the parent while screaming and commencing to kick the parent.

Ignoring. The most common method of negative reinforcement used with children with autism is to ignore the child. Ignoring is the act of turning your back on a manipulative behavior that was previously successful at obtaining a desired end. The idea is that if the undesirable behavior is no longer successful because no one sticks around to respond to it, then it becomes ineffective. For children with autism, this only works sometimes. Attention to the exceptions of when ignoring is not likely to work takes into account some of the autistic learning disabilities we've discussed. There are two instances in which ignoring is not likely to work with a child with autism.

Ignoring Endangering Behaviors. When the negative behavior is dangerous either to the child, to someone else, or to property, it is natural to not want to ignore the negative behavior. If Amalia had kicked her baby sister's high chair while her baby sister was in the high chair, Dad, who had been instructed to ignore tantrumming, would have had a much harder time doing so. Probably, he would have taken Amalia out of the kitchen and tried to distract her in some way. This would have in essence said that "if you tantrum, someone will intervene and offer you something that will make you happier than you are at this moment." That will have essentially provided a low-level reinforcer. If Dad had taken baby sister out of the kitchen with him, Amalia might have "ruined" the ignoring by accelerating to the point of trashing the high chair. Once the undesirable behaviors have risen to the level that the child realizes won't be ignored, like hurting others or property, it is too late to use ignoring to eliminate the behavior, and more powerful deterrents are needed.

Ignoring and SIBS. A good example of a behavior you don't want to ignore is a self-injurious behavior (SIB). Some SIBs are designed to manipulate parental behavior, as with the child who bangs his head and then looks to see if he is about to get the gum he wants from his mother's purse. This rapidly becomes a complex situation as the parent finds herself torn between setting firm limits and preventing real harm. The teacher is in this position when she is caught between setting firm limits and possibly having to file an incident report.

Most SIBs probably start as an "overflow" response when the child is agitated. Universally, there is great similarity in SIBs among children with autism, with characteristic biting of the palm, the top of the hand between the index finger and thumb, or the wrist, or banging the forehead. (This does not mean the child learned a particular SIB from another child, but rather it's hard-wired—like thumb sucking.) However, if at this moment of intense frustration and SIB, the parent responds to her own distress at the appearance of a SIB by giving the child whatever he is frustrated about so as to soothe him and deter the SIB, the parent is probably inadvertently reinforcing the SIB as an effective method of manipulating parent behavior. From that point forward the SIB may appear whenever the child is really frustrated. Over time, the threshold for appearance of a SIB will probably get lower as it becomes more likely that the SIB will produce the desired effect. The child may understand the relationship between showing anger and getting his way and may get worked up to the point of self-injury with the knowledge that it may bring an end to his frustration. A case in point: Ten-year-old, 130-lb. Rashid was in the clinic for a range of behavioral problems including banging his head when he was really aggravated. Another behavioral problem was overeating. Rashid was an obese child, and one of the things he really liked was corn chips. His parents had brought along a huge bag, hoping this would keep him calm during our testing. Rashid knew the corn chips were in his mom's backpack and made many attempts to extract them, but after we had discussed overeating and overdependence on corn chips as a behavior control tool, his mother would not give them to him. Rashid began banging his head. His parents became quite distressed, and his mother quickly reached for the corn chips. To test the hypothesis that this head banging was not pure aggravation but also manipulation, I sat on the floor next to Rashid, ignoring him but playing with a brassy, loud electronic train he'd been showing great interest in all morning. As I played, the head banging became intermittent, and Rashid surreptitiously crept on his belly toward me, whining but stopping for a bang or two along the way. Finally, he grabbed the train from me and began playing with it himself. The train was more interesting than the tantrumming that was being ignored. More importantly, the differential value between the train and the corn chips was not so great that a train in the hand was worth more than corn chips in the backpack.

"I Want to Be Alone." For Greta Garbo it was an expression of a preference. Sometimes the child with autism wants to be alone too. We consider it quite OK for an adult to be alone, but most typically developing children hate being alone. Most autistic children do not. When a child doesn't mind being alone, maybe even prefers to be alone, being ignored will be no deterrent. Ignoring only works for those children with autism who do in fact get upset when they are isolated. If you are agitated because you cannot get what you want, and you are ignored, the social "volume" around you goes down. There is no one talking at you, pulling at you to sit up, or otherwise making you feel worse. This makes the act of being ignored slightly positive. Ignoring may, in fact, be helpful to getting back to a state of equilibrium. As the child calms, he may no longer want what he was tantrumming for as much as his newfound state of left-aloneness and increased calmness, especially if calming is promptly responded to with something the child finds desirable (but not the source of the tantrum). This is fine. This is how ignoring benefits many behaviorally overwrought children.

However, sometimes what the child wants is so important to that child that the possibly beneficial effects of ignoring are not calming. In this case the tantrumming may continue until the child exhausts himself and falls asleep. If the tantrum has gone on that long without ignoring's having a deterring effect, there is probably something more effective than ignoring that can be done.

WHY TIME-OUTS SOMETIMES DON'T WORK

When ignoring a behavior is ineffective because the child is too persistent, or what he wants and can't have is very important to him, the next level of deterrence that can be used is a time-out. Parents can read about time-outs in every parenting book. I am amazed and, honestly, often horrified by how often I see parents of typically developing children threatening them with a time-out for everything from looking at Mom cross-eyed in the market to giggling loudly at a cartoon while Mom tries to read a magazine. Time-outs are not for whenever the child is annoying. It will only make the child more annoying. For the typically developing child, the time-out is supposed to be a "time-out," time away from what he is doing so that he can reflect on his action plan, or lack thereof, and, one hopes, self-correct behavior. Time out also derives punishment power from isolating the child from a desirable setting and placing him in a less desirable one.

This set of assumptions may be only partly true for the child with autism: The part where the time-out is an opportunity to take time out and reflect on what you have done and reorganize yourself is fine, as long as you understand enough language to comprehend what behaviors are expected to change. If you do not understand exactly what behavior needs to be deterred, this approach is more problematic. Unless the temporal association is immediate, there is no power to the time-out at all.

The aspect of the time out that provides an opportunity to calm down by interfering with the child's cycle of misdirected activity can work, even for a preverbal child who may not understand the words designating the reason for the time-out. However, for the child with autism, the aspect of time out that is often the deal breaker is the isolation. If the child's behaviors are undesirable because he is socially over-stimulated or being pressured to engage in a non-preferred activity, a conventional time out is just what the child should *not* have.

If a child comes to feel that the best way to get out of class work is to vocalize in a loud disruptive way, hit another pupil, or trash a desk, he can be expected to do those things with increasing frequency. Yet many teachers take autistic children who have engaged in just such activities and sit them outside the classroom or on a chair in the back, or direct the pupil to fold his arms on his desk and put his head in his arms for a "time-out." As isolation is increased, the positive value (rather than the deterrent value) of the intervention is increased for most children with autism. They often do not mind being alone. Absent a drive for peer affiliation and approval, a child with autism will not find a time out stigmatizing in the context of his class the way another child might. At home, a time-out alone in his bedroom is just fine for many children with autism as it affords the perfect escape from pressures to do as others wish.

Accompanied Time-Outs. An alternative method is the accompanied time out. The idea is to obtain the achievable benefits of time-out, such as a calm-down break and a chance to reflect, but not to add the "positive" of isolation. An adult who sits behind the child without speaking or looking at the child, perhaps resting her hands on his shoulders to deter exit, ruins the positive experience of being alone. The child should be isolated way from classroom noise and activity as much as possible, or from TV. If the child struggles to leave time out, a gentle but firm "human seat belt" restraint from behind is fine. The accompanied time out should be as immediate to the negative behavior as possible, and should be short. (Some parents complain to me that they place their child with autism in his room for a 15-minute time-out and come back to find him playing contentedly. Some punishment.) A short time out means a slow count to 15 or 30 for a toddler, or a couple of minutes for a school-aged child. The adult, however, needs to stay with the child, needs to stay in restraining physical contact if needed, and should be prepared to end the time out when it is clear that the undesirable behavior is gone or significantly decelerated. The point is for the child to see a strong relationship between getting calm and getting free. After an accompanied time out the child should be redirected to another activity that is, if possible, incompatible with the infraction that has just been punished. (If the child received a time out for hitting his sibling because he grabbed Thomas the Tank Engine, then the parent doing the time out should keep the siblings apart, especially if Thomas is still "in play.") During this redirect time, the adult should work to keep the child engaged. If the negative behavior recurs, there should naturally be a return to time-out. At the next time out, be sure the child really is finished with his bad behavior before beginning the redirection activity. The accompanied time-out is more labor-intensive, but is a viable way of increasing the effectiveness of the usually employed time-out procedures.

Physical Punishment. Is it OK to spank an autistic child? Is it OK to spank a typically developing child? Does it matter to the autistic child if you spank him? If it doesn't, what should you do? These are logical questions to which there are no absolutely right or wrong answers.

Teachers are simply not allowed to spank. That is a community value and in most places, law. Spanking at home, however, is a matter of a family's values. No child, however, including no child with autism, should be hit in anger, or hit without a clearly defined infraction having been committed. A spanking is designed as much to humiliate as to hurt enough to deter. For children with autism it sometimes only does one of these, and sometimes does neither. The humiliation of spanking for a typically developing child comes from the sense of failure the child has at having displeased adults whom he usually works to please. Spankings are typically accompanied with a litany of rules broken, feelings hurt, and disappointments created. Largely, this litany is not likely to have nearly as profound an effect on the child with autism as it would a typically developing child. Many parents would like to feel the child knows he's done wrong, knows he's been a disappointment, and feels remorseful, but given a child with autism who generally lacks empathetic or sympathetic responses to others, this likely is not happening.

If a spanking does not humiliate, does it hurt or startle the child enough to deter? Some children with autism, especially some of the youngest, some of the most hyperactive, and some of the most severely cognitively impaired have diminished pain reactions. For the typically developing child, the pain of the spanking adds injury to insult. If there is no apparent pain response, the overall deterrent value of the spanking is decreased, and if there is no humiliation and no pain reaction, then the spanking is basically useless, except for the deterrent value of restricting the child's physical freedom so the spanking can be administered. You'd be better off with a time-out.

Criteria for Spanking. My personal criteria for spankings are, first, that the spanking holds a deterrent value for the child, and, second, that it is reserved for those occasions when the child does something to endanger either himself or someone else. The issues of personal safety that I most often encounter involve darting away from a parent in a parking lot, darting away in the driveway while getting into the car, running out the front door of the house, and credibly threatening to injury a younger sibling, especially an infant. This should give a flavor of what I mean by "endangering," as there are many other situations in which the child's actions might make a sibling wake up or cry, or in which the child's behavior is incredibly annoying, like when he takes advantage of a parental lapse of vigilance to dart off to the cookie section of the market while Mom attends to a crying infant in a shopping cart.

STRATEGIES FOR HANDLING TRANSITIONS

A main area of adaptive dysfunction for many of those in the autistic spectrum is difficulty around transitions. This usually means that a child with autism shows marked behavioral resistance when a teacher or parent tries to move the child from one activity to another. Sometimes practitioners and parents talk about "problem with transitions" as if they are a neurologically based symptom of the disorder, like hand flapping. In fact, problems with transitions is what in chapter 2 was described as a tertiary symptom, a failure of the child with autism to be able to self-accommodate well to some aspect of his disability. In problems with transitions, the first problem is that the child prefers the current activity to the proposed new activity; second, the child does not fully understand what is expected of him or what will happen next; third, the child is unsure what's in it for him if he stops what he's doing. The child has failed to self-accommodate because he can't ask, "Where are we going? Why are we going there? What are we going to do there?" If he can't figure out what the transition is about from visual cues around him, the resistance is likely to be more marked. If resistance to unexplained changes and undesired transitions has been marked with protest, and the protest has resulted in parents or teachers desisting in making the transition, the child can be expected to quickly develop a rigid insistence on not making transitions. This is a purely behavioral response.

Many children with autistic spectrum disorders definitely tend to be on the rigid side, and many have irritable temperaments to boot. These factors, coupled with not understanding what transitions may be about or why they should be made is what makes for a problem with so many children with autism.

Lack of Desire to Please and to Model. Handling transitions requires an understanding of the child's autistic learning disabilities: First we need to help the child compensate for his lack of desire to please and get him to make a transition just because he was asked. Second, the child may lack a drive to imitate or model others, and so will not readily transition when other children do. To help the child compensate for these difficulties there should be some way to communicate to the child what is going to happen. For verbal children, simply telling them what they will need to do and then setting a time limit on the current activity can work. For other children, a written reminder is more powerful. For preverbal and non-verbal children who still think in pictures, not words, one way to show what will happen is with a picture schedule that can be used to show the child what he was doing just before his current activity, what he is doing now, and what he will do next. (Picture schedules were discussed in chapter 7.)

Keeping things routine helps a child understand predictability and realize that there are invariant aspects to his daily routine that his own efforts cannot change. Seat belts offer a good example of how well this can work. Many parents, knowing seat belts are the law and serve a valuable purpose, absolutely insist that the child keep his on. Children less often resist seatbelts than other routines.

Naturally, it is easier to established a high degree of day-to-day routine in a classroom than at home. Accordingly, some children have more problems with routines at home than at school. Parents who feel they must wait till the credits roll on "Teletubbies Take a Walk in the Meadow" (i.e., let the child's whims control the situation) will be less likely to stop the car and strap the child back in if he removes his seat belt. The parent who is afraid the child will injure himself or cause an accident if he is free to move around the car will insist on the seat belt and is more likely to persist until the appropriate behavior is demonstrated. It may take the other parent's sitting next to the child and holding the latch closed, but most parents are completely vigilant about safety.

Putting a child through any other transition is no more difficult (or easy). To accomplish a transition, whatever it is, the child just needs to be prompted and motored through the change of activities as much as needed. Along the way, he should be rewarded for baby steps if protest is high, or for simply completing the task if protest is only mild. Any resistance and tantrumming should be ignored. However, it will help significantly if the child knows what the transition is about—just like any child at the same level of development. Spoken or written words, as well as a series of pictures, should be used to alleviate anxiety.

Analyzing Transition Difficulties. Protest at transitions can be expected to be most severe, the greater the differential in reinforcement value between the activity being left and the activity being joined. Transitions can sometimes be eased by making the existing activity less rewarding. For example, a child meticulously hooking train tracks together might insist on finishing it by himself, not wanting to leave until each piece is perfectly aligned. If someone "helps" him finish, the added aggravation of a demand for social cooperation may make him much more willing to leave the activity. I have seen many children who will kick blocks, train tracks, or puzzles when "helped" along. (Of course, when this happens the child should always be asked, shown, or helped to clean up the mess he has made before starting the next activity—or before you know it, throwing the items will become the only way the activity can be terminated.)

Timers. Probably one of the most helpful ways to achieve any kind of undesired transition is to set a timer. It can be a kitchen timer, electronic sports timer, or an hourglass. The child is given his one-, three-, or five-minute warning—and when the time is up, it's time to stop. Getting the child to start the timer and turn off the ringer are ways of making sure he's aware of the limits and is as "bought in" as possible. A teacher or parent must be there when the timer goes off, however, so that an immediate transition can be clearly associated with the end of the allocated time for the activity. If the child doesn't like the timer and reasons that if he gets rid of it, he'll get rid of the time limits, put the timer where he can't get at it.

The key to success in teaching children with autism to deal with transitions is consistency and picking your battles: Although a child may have problems turning off the TV when the school bus arrives, it is likely easier to accomplish a transition in that situation because the need for the transition at that point is nonnegotiable. When it comes to turning off a video to start dinner, a transition may be harder to achieve because the limit is intrinsically more negotiable. While it is nice for a family to eat together, the battle to accomplish this may be disturbing enough to others to make it a less important "battle." Realistically, it is one thing to know how to accomplish a goal behaviorally, it's another to decide which goals are most important, and which can be deferred for at least a while.

Moving from Behavioral Methods to Behavioral Problems. So far in this chapter we have talked about modifications to behavioral techniques, like ignoring undesired behavior, restructuring time-outs so they are more undesirable, and understanding transition difficulties as the child's need to know and control what's going on. In the second half of this chapter, we will discuss specific areas where the child with ASD often needs application of behavior-management techniques. We'll give examples of how behavioral and communication methods can be used and combined in a framework of developmentally geared appropriate expectations for more desirable behavior.

DOMAINS OF ADAPTATION

It is widely recognized that many children with autistic spectrum disorders have peculiar eating habits, poor sleep, and no apparent sense of danger. These observations about children with autism are not diagnostic (as they are by no means unique to the autistic spectrum disorders), but the way concerns in these areas manifest themselves as problems in children with autism certainly does relate to the way autistic children perceive things and learn. In this section, we'll examine some specific adaptive difficulties that children with autism often have and relate them causally and in terms of treatment to their autistic learning disabilities. These areas of adaptation will be discussed in a roughly developmental sequence, starting with the ones mainly affecting the youngest children, and moving on to the ones mainly of concern to older children.

SAFETY OF SELF AND OTHERS

The number one issue for many parents and schools is the child's safety and the safety of others around the child with autism. As we discussed in earlier chapters, children with autism lack social referencing, they don't "check in" with caregivers while exploring potentially hazardous situations. Typically developing children can be counted upon to check back to see whether their behavior is acceptable or not—and then modify behavior accordingly. In addition, the majority of young children with autism are as well coordinated in motor skills as others their age, and so can run and climb as well as anyone their age. When a four-year-old child with autism also has moderate mental retardation, you are faced with a two-year-old's judgment in a four-year-old's body. A severely cognitively impaired three-year-old with autism is more like a twelve or eighteen-month-old in a three-year-old's body. Combine this problem with the child's having little or no receptive language, and it is clear why all sort of endangering behaviors occur.

The best response to children with a lack of social reference and a tendency to engage in endangering behaviors is simply to keep the child in situations that are not dangerous. This is especially important for the child who shows neither social reference nor instrumental reference. These are the children who do not look to parents either to show their activities off to them, or to determine whether they are about to get in trouble. (Instrumental reference can be understood as a more cause-and-effect behavior while social reference or joint attention grows from a desire to be noticed and gain approval.) Except through routines and limit setting, it is difficult to keep this group of children away from self-endangering activities. Essentially, they have little to no judgment, which is true for most children under a developmental age of three, *and* have no way of accessing the parental database on what is safe.

A somewhat different approach to deterring self-endangering behavior can be taken for the child who engages in more instrumental reference: Some children with autism who do not look to share attention for more purely social reasons will look toward parents to evaluate possible consequences of their actions to avoid undesired consequences. They are developed enough to understand which actions lead to which reactions, but substantially lack a desire to modify behavior just to please someone else. For these children some of the social "signal" about the prohibition—either the words, the facial expression, or tone of voice—is getting through. They may be getting mostly the negative content: the word "No!" a sharp tone of voice, or the gesture that precedes a spanking. If the child is aware of possible consequences, dangerous behavior should be easier to manage with clear consequences for specific violations if the child is one who can read cues that precede parental or teacher actions he wishes to avoid. Some of the best instrumental reference I see in little autistic children is in those with rather punitive, restrictive parents. These children have been particularly sensitized to the cause and effect of parental signals and undesired consequences.

EATING

Why Won't He Eat More? Many children with autism eat a narrow range of foods and refuse to try new foods. Parents often notice that the acceptable foods have something in common such as being crunchy, salty, or soft. If we think of the child with autism as someone who is not on the high end of exploratory, who prefers routines, and for whom certain sensory qualities may be preeminently desirable or undesirable, having narrow food choices is understandable, even expected.

In fact, many young children, autistic or not, are this way. With typically developing children, we have a strategy to overcome resistance to new foods that we don't have with children with autism—social pressure: "Popeye eats his spinach!," "Don't you want to get to be big like Daddy?" The child with autism will likely not care what Popeye—or even Buzz Light Year eats. The sense of strong identification with others is not in place—or there would be lots of spontaneous imitation of the mannerisms of others.

Behavioral methods are the most effective in changing diet. Before undertaking a diet-related behavior plan, there are several considerations: Is the child getting balanced nutrition through a vitamin supplement? If not, that may be the goal you wish to address. Is the child falling off his growth curve? If not, this problem may not be your worst one. Does the child selectively refuse vegetables and meats and eat just a few fruits and lots of carbohydrates? If so, this is not particularly atypical for children under five. Don't confuse a diagnosis of "autism" with a diagnosis of "childhood."

Diet and Behavior. Be aware that some practitioners have offered the idea that a child who eats a lot of one food is "craving" it for either some good or some bad reason. There is no evidence to support theories of these sorts. There is also no evidence to support the idea that children with autism have more food allergies or are more likely to react to foods with gluten (like wheat products) or casein (like dairy products). What "research" there is on these things is available only on the Internet and in books by parents who feel it "cured" their child or doctors who have "invented" a new diet. There are no reports in peer-reviewed scientific journals.

When a really well-controlled study of the effect of sugar on activity level was finally conducted, it turned out that sugar does not make children "hyper" (though exciting events like birthdays and Christmas parties at which kids eat unlimited amounts of sugary foods might logically be implicated). Children with autism naturally can have food allergies, but these would be manifested as they are in every other child—a rash, congestion, vomiting, or diarrhea after eating the food.

There are zealots promoting special diets, and there is real appeal for parents who want to do something that will make a difference. Clinically, my own experience with diets—the gluten-free, casein-free (GCF) diet, for example—stands as a strong example of a placebo effect: The first parent comes in and tells me the child's on "the diet" and is now hand-flapping less. A second set of parents is pleased with the GCF diet too; "the diet" has cleared up the child's diarrhea. The third set of parents has noted that since starting "the diet," there is more eye contact (although the child started speech therapy the same week as the diet and the parents wonder if that might have helped too). A fourth set of parents note language improvements. What drug in the whole field of medicine helps motor overflow, diarrhea, sociability, and language?

The "How could I not try this if it might help?" appeal is very strong and very understandable. If you try diets, try to keep someone like a teacher or grandparent blind to the start of the diet and, after a month, ask about any changes noted in the month prior to the diet and the month since the diet. Write down your own impressions of what may have improved before you ask the "blind" observer's opinion in order to collect an objective assessment.

Increasing Food Choices. Teachers and parents often note that children who will eat only a few foods at home will eat a wider array of what is offered at school. Why? Also, I see fewer eating problems in autistic children from larger families. Why? In school or in a larger family, children learn to eat what's put in front of them—or else the child next to them will eat it. The child who didn't eat it then won't have anything. This is a great way to teach the child to eat. Some parents defeat this natural tendency to eat when you perceive your food supply as threatened by sending snacks of the "only" food the child will eat with him to school and insisting that it be served as a special snack. My favorite example of this was Jagger, a four-year-old, 90-lb. boy with autism. Dad was a bouncer in a casino and it seemed that Jagger was marked to follow in his Dad's footsteps. His mother, a tall thin ballet teacher babied him, frequently picking him up and carrying him whenever he was a bit distressed. When it came to eating, he was her baby too. This pattern created tension between school and home until the teacher and the mother could agree on a feeding plan that worked.

Children will not starve themselves, though parents commonly believe the child has this degree of resolve. Using behavioral methods is a matter of taking advantage of the power of choice, in the same way as in the context of motivating communication or play. One way to do this is to offer the child a very small amount of a new food before offering the desired food, which should be clearly available. It can help if the new food is similar in texture, color, or taste to the familiar desirable food. Sometimes the child needs the new food put into his mouth. On a first try, extending a hand so the child can be allowed to spit it out is fine. Depending on the resistance, after a couple of tries, he should be expected to swallow the tiny bit of new food. As soon as the new food trial is over, the preferred old food should be noncontingently offered as the reward for trying. Over time, interspersing a few bites of the new food with the old food should be used before the old, preferred food is given noncontingently. When this goes OK, try a meal with the new food alone.

Sometimes, a non-preferred food may be offered when the preferred food is not available at all, such as when the child develops a preference for McDonald's french fries and won't eat the ones from Burger King. Parents worry that the child will give up fries altogether, and that he'll lose 90 percent of his daily caloric intake; don't worry. Offer other crunchy salty foods, and let the child learn that the world does not need to revolve around his food preferences.

What should be avoided though are protracted battles over food. Things can go wrong when there is an insistence that the child must finish a half-cup of milk or the rest of his rice before he gets dessert. In those situations, the child should simply have a choice: milk and dessert, or no milk and no dessert. Do not worry that everyone else is eating dessert and the child will be angry if he doesn't get his. While battles for widening food choice are going on, other foods should not be available for the child to take at liberty. If a child rejects the offered food, he should be given another chance a few minutes later to go through the choice process again. If the food is refused more than three times, the meal or snack should be over. By the next meal or snack time, the child will be hungrier, and this will change the balance of how horrible a teeny tiny bit of new food seems relative to again having no food at all.

Any plan to increase the child's range of foods should be done systematically, meaning one food at a time, adding foods that are close to acceptable foods, and making the presentation of a new food only a small event at each meal. The foods and the plan should be selected before the meal begins. The desired food should be ready to serve so the child clearly sees the relationship between his consuming of the new food and getting the old one.

While giving the child a sense of freedom by giving him choices is largely good, don't get carried away. If everyone is having hamburgers for dinner and this child eats hamburgers and hot dogs, don't give him a choice. Give him what everyone else is having. Children with autism give you enough extra work to do without adding short-order cook to your resume.

A related feeding problem is the child who won't feed himself and insists he be fed. This problem arises from mothers (and grandmothers) who are afraid the child will not eat enough if left on his own. (Cross-culturally, I see great similarities here between Chinese and Latino grandmas. Both groups of grandmas excel at the endurance event of chasing an autistic grandchild with a handful of rice.) While the dedication of such grandmothers is admirable, there is a point at which enough is enough Such children need to be started on a wide-scooping spoon—if they have no self-feeding experience at all—and helped, hand over hand, to feed themselves a few spoonfuls before being fed. It can be faster and neater to feed a child than to have him feed himself, but self-feeding is an unquestionably necessary life skill. For older children who are still fed but who have reasonably well-developed fine motor skills (for example, can trace letters and shapes), utensils should be required at all times. Usually the best way to get children who are accustomed to being fed to feed themselves is to first offer a spoon with desirable foods, like ice cream or yogurt.

SLEEPING

Many children with autism have sleep problems. One book with a chapter on sleep problems in autism notes that the problems experienced by children with autism are often among the most behaviorally intractable among all developmentally disabled children. There are probably two reasons for this. One is neurochemical. Serotonin, a powerful brain neurotransmitter, has often been reported as abnormal in autism, and some effective psychopharmacological agents include medications that affect the serotonin system. Serotonin also plays a role in sleep. It is not understood how serotonin regulation may affect sleep in some children with autism, but it is quite possible that it does.

In addition to biological causes for poor sleep, autistic children have significant behavioral causes for their poor sleep. This is the part we can do something about without resorting to sleep medicines. First, most typically developing young children don't like to be alone. When they wake up alone, they may call out, and if the parent makes a brief intervention, leaves promptly, and then responds less readily to subsequent night wakings, that pattern of response will promote better sleep. The typical child usually stays in his bed if he is confined to his room, because he may feel even lonelier if he gets out. If the child has a sibling in his room, he may climb into bed with the sibling and go back to sleep, or if he can, he may go to his parents' room and get in their bed.

It's different for children with autism: The child with autism usually does not hesitate to get out of bed. Loneliness and fear of the dark are usually not operative factors. Fear of the usual nighttime monsters that keep other children in bed are not a problem for the child with autism who lacks an imagination anyhow. The sleep patterns are most troublesome when the child regularly awakens others, wanders the house in search of preferred activities, or wanders randomly, getting into things like the knife drawer in the kitchen.

Getting to Sleep. Many children with autism have a hard time going to sleep. Bedtime should be at the same time each night and at a reasonable hour for the child's age. Parents should decide the bedtime, not the child. For a young child who does not want to sleep before ten, and who is still napping, it is time to cut out the nap. Doing this may require extra help in the house during the cranky period that unfailingly will replace the nap. Children who fall asleep on the way home from school should be awakened at that point, rather than being allowed to continue sleeping. The child may still need some quiet time, but cutting out the opportunity for deeper sleep should help achieve an earlier, quicker sleep onset at night, and possibly ensure longer bouts of sleeping once asleep.

All children need a high degree of routine for bedtime, and for children with autism this can be particularly important as the end of the routine signals the expectation that the child will remain alone in his room from this point forward. Parents who lay down with the child till he falls asleep should move this ritual from their own bed (if it is the parental bed) to the child's, and then gradually move away from being in bed with the child. One parent, for example, had the child's mattress on the floor, set up an air mattress for herself alongside, and gradually moved onto that so she could get up and leave without shaking the bed once her child was asleep. This is an excellent approach. Sleep research on typically developing children shows greater sleep problems in children who fall asleep next to someone else and wake up alone. The cues for onset of sleepiness include the closeness of that other person. As the child goes through the stages of sleep and rouses slightly (which is normal), he is much more likely to wake up fully if the "going to sleep" cues have changed. Sleeping on the floor or on another bed, patting the child, etc. would be better.

Some children with autism regularly sleep in their parents' bed. This is fine if all the children sleep with the parents or if the youngest child has always slept with the parent. If this is not part of a family's culture, then the child with autism should be helped to sleep alone too. If the child is a bed wetter or thrashes around at night, frequently waking parents, he should go back to his own bed. If one parent can no longer sleep with the other parent because of the child being in the bed, the child should go back in his own bed, even if at first it is in the parents' room.

Staying in Bed. The same rules for maintaining sleep should be used for autistic children as for typical children—short interventions that are not repeated, and a period in which the child "cries it out." Left to cry it out, typically developing children usually "get over it" in a few (miserable) days, but children with autism may take longer. Because children with autism are also more likely to wander around the house, and sometimes get into trouble, make sure that the house is childproof. It is also important that night waking is not rewarding (as, for example, when the child can go in the den and watch favorite videos). What probably works best is childproofing the child's room, putting away things that can be broken or pulled off the walls, taking out the TV, and confining the child to his room. One good way to confine a child without closing the door on him is to install two or three stacked baby gates and leave the door open. Some children with autism go to sleep (with or without a scene), only to wake up a few hours later and remain awake for an hour or more. The child with autism may not be able to sleep, but things should be set up to make being awake as uninteresting as possible. A few books and a few other nonexcitatory toys should be the only things accessible. This will help him return to sleep sooner rather than later.

Just like the battles about eating, there should be no "has to do it like this" standard for the child's sleeping habits. If one parent wants to sleep alone in the bedroom with the other parent, it can be done. The child's sleeping does not necessarily have to infringe on the rest of the family. It is a matter of training. Again, addressing sleep problems is another "battle" that parents must weigh along with the other things that need be addressed. This problem should be addressed before it becomes so severe that Dad is ready to sleep in the garage, or the child needs to nap through the first two hours of school each day because he's been up all night.

Medications. Medications are an important adjunct in treating sleep problems. A medicine that makes a child sleepy can promote sleep onset and leverage the effectiveness of any behavior plan. There are short-acting medicines with few side effects like, Trazadone (desyrel), common non-prescription pediatric medicines, like Benadryl for congestion, or health food store supplements like melatonin that may help promote sleepiness. (Generally, don't expect melatonin to be as effective as a prescribed medication, and also remember that "over-the-counter" doesn't mean that dosage and frequency of use don't matter.) Use of any medicine should be supervised by a pediatrician or child psychiatrist who is familiar with the sleep difficulties of children with autism so parents understand the effects of using these medicines, or the effects of any other homeopathic or prescribed medicines.

TOILET TRAINING

Many young children with autism are hard to toilet train. Here, as with eating, accomplishment of this milestone should be helped by an appeal to a sense of social conformity. For children with autism, such an appeal usually doesn't help. Usual parental ploys like "Don't you want to wear big boy underpants?" or "Pretty panties are only for good girls who don't make pee in them!" won't work. Instead, toilet training must rely on a series of tangible rewards and on the autistic love of routine.

When to Train? Some parents ignore toilet training for a long time because there seems to be so much other work to be done. The autonomy a child achieves when he can use the toilet himself is appealing to all kids, but it can be particularly appealing to a child with autism who has always shown the desire to do things for himself. Developmentally, toilet training for bladder can usually be achieved at 18 to 24 months, and for bowels, sometimes a little later. For children with autism, toilet training often occurs at only slightly later than expected ages for typically developing children if the parents use a toilet-training plan, and if the child appears to have basically normal non-language abilities. For more moderately to severely impaired children, a good rule of thumb is to wait until non-language mental age is in the 18- to 24-month age range. Once a child clutches at himself when he needs to urinate or has just urinated, or can indicate a desire to have diapers changed, it is time to toilet train.

Two-Tiered Toilet Training (the Four T's). One method for toilet training that can be thought of as the four T's involves a two-tiered reward system. This has been particularly effective for children who will happily sit on the potty, chomp down their M&Ms, watch a toileting video, or listen to the umpteenth reading of "Everyone Poops," and do nothing toileting-related. The first thing to do is to pick a period of a couple of days when you can be at home a great deal, and when the weather permits dressing the child in training pants or when he can run around with no bottoms. Make sure he has an idea of the toilet's function. Watching others of the same gender use the potty can help, though starting urination sitting down will work best with this method. If the child is terrified of the toilet, use a potty chair. If he insists on flushing, and not sitting, duct tape the flusher in place or unscrew it for a while. Pick a reward that is very, very high on the child's reinforcer hierarchy. Let's say it's Thomas the Tank Engine. Buy a new one. Take all the Thomas-related items in the house—Thomas books, Thomas trains, Thomas videos, Thomas bedspread, even the Thomas sippy cup—and put them away. The idea is to get the child Thomas "deprived." Put the new Thomas in a small clear plastic jar with a lid the child cannot open without assistance. Place the jar with Thomas in it out of sight in a childproof cabinet in the bathroom. When it seems a good time to use the toilet, take the child in, sit him down, praise the sitting, and immediately produce Thomas. If the child gets up, urge him to remain seated and to pee. If he gets up, immediately put Thomas out of sight. If he sits again, bring Thomas out. If the child tries to get Thomas, asks for the jar to "open," or angrily throws the jar because he can't have Thomas, respond by telling the child he will get Thomas for using the toilet. As soon as he does, praise him and remove Thomas from the jar immediately and let him have Thomas, no matter how little he has urinated. (If the child seems unsure how to urinate or what to do, try pouring a cup of body temperature water over the child's penis or vagina to simulate the sensation of urination and, at first, reward tolerance of that.) After five minutes in the bathroom with Thomas, put him back in the jar and say "Bye-bye Thomas, see you next time!" and return him to the inaccessible cabinet. If the child is taken on a schedule, and/or whenever he seems to indicate a need to urinate, he will get the idea of what he needs to do to get Thomas. Soon, the child may be requesting to go potty just to manipulate the parent into giving Thomas. If the child gets to the point where he produces one little squirt and then demands Thomas, the adult is not being manipulated, the adult has successfully taught bladder control! The critical part of this training procedure is that the child get a low-level reward (seeing Thomas but not having him) for the prerequisite act of approaching the toilet, but doesn't get the real reward until the potty has been successfully used.

This procedure is also useful for children who have been bladder-trained for a while, but still resist having bowel movements in the toilet. If the time of day or the child's behavior can serve as an antecedent to when to go to the potty, this can be a highly effective method. A food can be used as a reward, too, but if used, must be highly preferred and not available at other times during the initial intensive potty training period.

School versus Home Toileting. Teachers are often much more successful than parents at toileting programs because the routine of classroom life is well suited to going to the potty regularly. This first step of toilet training is called schedule training. The child is taken on a very frequent schedule, as often as twice an hour at first, to provide opportunities for the toilet to just happen to be the place for elimination. At school, where there are many activities that children do in unison, the presence of multiple toilets suggests the required performance. Even for children with neophyte imitation skills, the routine, repetition, and models are all helpful. Teachers, of course, can use the four T's method, too.

Parent-Teacher Collaboration on Toilet Training. Some teachers complain that the child is dry at school but wet at home. This is frustrating to the teacher who has worked hard to achieve continence. Parents then complain about the same thing: The child is dry at school but wet at home. This is frustrating for the parent who can't understand why the child would behave better for the teacher than for Mom. Understandably, it is much more difficult to preserve a routine at home that is as rigid as the ones that classrooms can use, but then, that's why we have timers. Collaboration between teachers and parents on other subtleties of the more successful toileting routine may help aspects of that routine be added to toileting procedures in the less successful location. Because children with autism tend to do just what they need to do to get by, many children can be completely toilet trained in one setting and not another if there is not a high degree of consistent expectations between the settings.

HYGIENE

Another area of adaptive difficulty for many individuals with autistic spectrum disorders is personal hygiene. We are generally motivated to bathe often, smell nice, and dress appropriately so that others will appraise us favorably. Not so the child with autism. Combined with sensory preoccupations with clothing labels, a claustrophobic feeling about wearing long sleeves, long pants, or turtlenecks— or the opposite—and you've got some potential for odd patterns of grooming. Children with autism often have no real drive to achieve independence in hygiene activities like dressing themselves, bathing, or brushing teeth.

Much of personal hygiene for individuals with autism is subject to the why-should-I-care conundrum. I was told a story by an amazing woman, Eustacia Cutler, who is Temple Grandin's mother, about how, as a teenager, Temple's clothes would smell so bad that they had to be washed separately from her siblings' clothes. When her mother told her this, Temple replied, "Well, just do my laundry separately!" This continued until Temple had a job at a meat plant that she really valued, and her boss told her to start wearing deodorant—or else. Finally, she had a reason to follow rules of hygiene, and she did.

Dressing. Typically developing children get interested in dressing themselves when they begin to care how they look in different clothes and how others respond to them because of it. Children with autistic spectrum disorders largely don't care, and so their parents pick their clothes. One way I can informally support a diagnosis of Asperger's syndrome is when a 16-year-old boy shows up at my clinic dressed like he just stepped out of a Nordstrom advertisement— wearing Dockers, a tucked-in Ralph Lauren Polo shirt, and loafers. No self-respecting 16-year-old would be caught dead looking like that—not even at his grandmother's Christmas party!

Clothing Sensitivities. When children with autism do care what they wear, it is usually because they are resistant to certain fabrics, to the feeling of zippers or buttons, or to things that are too tight or too loose. Within reason, accommo-dating these preferences is OK. When the insistences become rigid and maladap-tive, an intervention is needed. For example, Hadley insisted on wearing pajamas all the time and had been allowed (for years) to go to school with sweat clothes on top of them. By fifth grade, other children had noticed this and ostracized him further. It was then that this pattern was presented at the clinic as a complaint. There are other children who will only wear one shirt, and so it must be washed and dried while the child sleeps. Antonio insisted that each day's outfit include at least one Scoobie Doo or Mickey Mouse. Purchasing clothing similar to the preferred item and insisting that it be worn at least part of the day can be effective in dissolving the child's sense that things must be exactly as he demands.

Odd dressing rituals should be treated like narrow food choices already discussed. In both cases, the procedures involve a gradual desensitization to the thing that seems so all-important, until the importance loses its obsessive allure.

Bathing and Grooming. Typically, children begin to bathe themselves when they develop a sense of modesty and want to have some privacy in the bath or shower. Since a sense of privacy or modesty is based in a child's perceptions of how others appraise him, a sense of privacy or modesty is often missing in the child with autism. As such, having someone bathe you is a largely positive experience, irrespective of how old you are. To the extent that the person doing the bathing may insist on the use of soap, sponges, washcloths and the like, bathing may be less fun, however. This is the leverage needed to get the child with an ASD to bathe independently.

Bathing skills can usually be taught if the fun part of bathing is held out as a reinforcer for the "Why should I care?" parts of bathing. So, if a child loves to dump water on his head, he needs to be motored through shampooing before any object suitable for dumping water over the head is provided. Like everything else, independence in the tub can be introduced gradually, beginning with adults hand-over-hand showing all the cleaning procedures and backing off a little bit at a time.

Dental Hygiene. The same is true for brushing teeth. Many children with autism who resist brushing can have their interest in this activity renewed with the introduction of an electric toothbrush. Not only does the electric toothbrush do a better job with minimal effort, the sensory qualities of the toothbrush, not to mention the sensory qualities of the Water-Pik, can be quite appealing, especially if the child can begin by brushing his arm or Pik-king plastic Barney. Again, full-motor prompting with gradual prompt fading works to encourage independence, and a timer indicates the length of time needed to brush.

Some children with autism tolerate dental work when done by a gentle, patient pediatric dentist experienced with developmentally disabled patients. Some don't. For many, a short-acting sedative like chloral hydrate (the same thing that might be used to get an EEG or MRI) can make all the difference. No child with autism should be subjected to a dentist who has never really dealt with developmentally disabled children. No child with ASD should be subjected to an inexperienced dentist.

Hair. Hair care is another problem area, and there are many children with autistic spectrum disorders who only get their hair cut while they are asleep in their beds. One chain of kiddy barbers that is great for children with autism has a toy boat in the barbershop, and you have to put your seat belt on for the boat ride—and the haircut. (I'm sure a mock-up of Thomas the Tank Engine would work even better.)

Most parents come up with at least partly successful accommodations to dislike of the sensory experience of the barbershop. Buzz cuts solve the problem for at least a few months at a time. Then there's the "bowl" cut, which has a "Little Dutch Boy" appeal until about age five and then starts to look more socially stigmatizing. However, it's only when I see a long-haired, dreadlocked child with autism (whose parents don't look like that too) that hair is a red flag for the need to institute serious behavior-management skills training.

ADOLESCENT ISSUES IN ADAPTIVE BEHAVIORS
Sexual Interest

Most difficult for both teachers and parents is dealing with sexuality in children with autism. In the youngest children, masturbation in the form of sticking hands in diapers or underpants is common. Other children lay face down on the floor and rock back and forth on their genitals. It feels good, so why shouldn't they do it? Like other things, social disapproval doesn't quickly put the behavior in the closet and close the door.

Treating sexualized behavior in younger children is not as difficult as in older children and adolescents in whom the behavior has usually been going on longer and, in post-puberty, is more intensely gratifying. In younger children, it is usually enough to redirect the behavior by removing the hand and giving the child something else interesting to do with his or her hands instead. The whole idea of reward "valence" applies: This means that the replacement activity should be an equally desired activity if it is to be passed off on the child as a substitute. Other helpful ways to make masturbation difficult, and therefore less rewarding, is dressing the child in overalls, suspenders, or pants with belts.

Adolescents. Most adolescents with autistic spectrum disorders are quite autoerotic and will seldom try to touch another person sexually. However, adolescent boys with autism definitely will get aroused by scantily dressed females (including siblings), and this situation should simply be avoided. There seems to be much more uncontrolled sexual activity in boys with autistic spectrum disorders at the lower levels of functioning, possibly because masturbation is relatively higher on a fairly uncrowded reinforcement hierarchy. It can be very difficult to come up with a redirected activity that will be perceived to be as rewarding.

On the other hand, adolescent boys with Asperger's often seem almost asexual, with little enthusiasm for what turns on other equally intelligent boys of the same age. Some adolescent boys with higher-functioning autism can develop sexual fetishes. These can consist of touching the toes of women with open sandals, touching hair, or smelling for perfume. Usually the individual knows he is not supposed to do whatever it is he enjoys doing and may routinely recite "Don't touch hair!" just before or just after doing it. These kinds of acts range from socially stigmatizing to downright threatening if the woman approached is unfamiliar with autism or with the individual. Behavioral methods to redirect such behaviors can be used. Such fetishes, however, are often part of a larger picture of obsessive and repetitive behaviors that may interfere with other aspects of functioning. If this tendency becomes increasingly marked and behaviorally uncontrolled, it is another indication suggesting the child be assessed for a medication that specifically targets all obsessive, repetitive behaviors.

Parents and teachers need to realize that there is no real point in trying to end masturbation in an adolescent; one only needs to confine it to appropriate settings. When the adolescent is by himself, and others aren't around, he is, in any case, going to figure out that there is no one to redirect his masturbation.

For adolescents, identifying settings in which there is privacy, and masturbation is allowable can be helped by labeling the behavior with the query "Do you need private time?" and redirecting the adolescent to a private place like his bedroom or a bathroom.

THE NEED FOR INDEPENDENCE

In this relatively brief section, we will cover some of the issues facing older children, adolescents and the youngest adults as they approach the stage of life in which it is both normal and expected to gain increasing independence from parents. Adolescence is a hormonally driven stage —the same thing is happening to young people with autism as to their typically developing peers. There is a satisfaction in not being told what to do or how to do it, and in doing for oneself—when, where, and how one wants. Being thwarted results in amazing feelings of rage. Typical adolescents run out the door, slamming it, refusing to say where they are headed or when they will return. Adolescents with autism may do the same thing—only it's scarier knowing that neither they nor the others they encounter may know how to react when they face one another. (Sherman, a big 17-year-old with autism, got angry at his mother, ran away from his house, and ended up running along a freeway access road in his underwear. Fortunately, a car full of teenagers, mistaking him for a really drunk 17-year-old, stopped and pulled him into their car. After they realized they had quite a different situation on their hands, they took him to the local police station, which his frantic mother had already called.)

Giving older children and adolescents with autism the skills they need to do basic things for themselves, like prepare food and dress properly, can help reduce that infantile dependence that sometimes persists in the lives of people with disabilities, even when they possess the cognitive skills to take care of themselves. The difference is that since people with autistic spectrum disorders tend to be poor incidental learners, they don't learn to make Top Ramen, microwave popcorn, or hotdogs just by watching friends or siblings. The more time the adolescent can spend doing these little things for himself, the less time he spends being told when and how to do things.

Adolescents and young adults with ASDs lack motivation to do things just to be more like "cool" peers and so may not dress themselves well. While they may not pick up on the norms for dress by observing a group of kids their own age, a young person with autism may be more amenable to a sibling's going shopping with them (read: for them) than going shopping with Mom. As in the earlier example, young people with ASDs tend not to be very concerned about how others appraise them, so they don't care if their clothing stinks unless someone has explicitly taught them otherwise. Another adolescent might tuck his pant legs into his socks for biking, but not see the point in removing them between bike rides. These little things make an adolescent or young adult with autism appear unnecessarily peculiar. A peer life-skills coach such as a junior college-aged peer buddy can help with undoing these oddities.

SKILLS AT HOME

Life-Skills Curricula. We've just covered some issues about how to prepare the child with HFA or Asperger's for a fuller, adult life. What about the individual who has persistent cognitive limitations along with autism? When a life-skills curriculum is first offered, some parents express relief that their 15-year-old can stop being bored and frustrated by counting sets of objects he's been sorting for the last 12 years. Other parents express distress that the school is "giving up" on academics. Yes, that's true, if academics is narrowly defined as reading and writing and arithmetic. If school is defined as a place where children are prepared for life after they finish school, I'm much less sure.

When should we be teaching a primarily life-skills curriculum? To whom? A hundred years ago in this country it was not unusual for a particular child to be deemed not right for "book learning" and instead taught straightaway the many practical things that needed to be done at home. There were many more home chores to be done in a family, and someone had to do them. The reasoning was that it might as well be the one who it seemed would otherwise struggle to learn what the others were able to readily learn.

Home skills include cooking, housekeeping, and care taking outside the home. Not so long ago, every teenaged American girl took home economics; every teenaged boy took shop. Schools were responsible for teaching typically developing youth the skills they would need as adults in their communities. In those days, when pupils in special education were taught those things, it seemed acceptable because home skills were considered something everyone needed to know. It wasn't outside the mainstream, because all 16-year-old girls were learning to scramble eggs at school. With budget cuts in education over the last

30 years, these programs have all but disappeared. A small percentage of adolescents attend technical high schools. Now, instead, everyone is taught a core curriculum of math, science, and language arts.

What happened in special education? The same thing. Home skill and vocational programs disappeared; the core curriculum moved in. Most pupils with developmental disabilities are the least able person in their home and tend to get babied. They tend to be less expected to do chores than others their age or at their developmental level. Children with autism in particular tend to lack interest in developing home and self-care skills because of their lack of interest in the way others appraise them. So they don't have an opportunity to learn these skills either incidentally or at home.

When to Start? My predilection is for home skills to be taught at school for those pupils with autism who are moderately to severely impaired in overall communication skills and who are in the later elementary years and beyond. These are individuals who will not live independently, will engage in productive work on a limited basis, if at all, and really deserve the right to be as independent as possible, both in terms of self-care, and as a contributor to their immediate family group, whether it is a group home or their family home. The small space of a coherent family group provides many good opportunities for a person with autism to fit in but still have the routine and predictability that promote stable functioning.

Housekeeping. Some programs for teens work on skills related to washing dishes, doing laundry, making beds, and cleaning the floors. Depending on a young person's interests, there are usually one or more tasks with at least some intrinsic reinforcement value. A child with autism who really likes to watch running water can learn to do dishes well, as long as he's motored through the procedures first, and the water is turned off every time dishwashing ceases. For others, neatness is the thing, so making beds and smoothing the sheets, blankets, and bedspread one layer at a time may be very satisfying. Someone else might enjoy the sound of the vacuum cleaner: throwing white carpet freshening powder on the dark green carpet and vacuuming it till it's gone is a great way to learn to look for dust and lint. For sorters, there's the laundry—sorting by color to make loads, sorting by fabric to select temperature, sorting cleaned clothes by type of clothing, and matching socks. These can be done in a classroom. A classroom can be set up more as a studio apartment with places to cook, clean, serve food, do laundry, make beds, and have leisure time.

Leisure-Skills Development. Learning home skills means learning to carry out housekeeping tasks and become a fuller member of the family's culture. But all work and no play would make Jack or Jill dull. Life-skills curricula should include teaching adult play as well as adult work. This implies having things to do that are pleasurable to you and nondisruptive to the others. A life-skills classroom is a great place to develop and practice skills like listening to videos, CDs, and computers with headsets. Learning to take turns with equipment, use a sign-up list, or set a timer are all skills that can help a more severely impaired teen become a "good citizen" of an independent-living setting someday.

Insisting on Acting "Normal." The point of teaching adaptive behaviors to children with autistic spectrum disorders is twofold: First, the child becomes better adapted because he can dress more typically, eat more widely, and care for his own personal hygiene. Second, failure to gain adaptive behaviors, or development of maladaptive preferences in carrying out adaptive behaviors (such as failure to use needed deodorant, or dressing oddly), teaches the individual with an autistic spectrum disorder the wrong lesson: Allowing immature behaviors and peculiarities of appearance and routine to continue results in their self-reinforcement. The longer you are allowed to feel you can wear pajamas under your other clothes, the harder it will be to give up, because it felt so right and so good for so long. The more of the child's sense of reward that comes from maladaptive behaviors, the further he moves from being able to function in the mainstream. It is incumbent on teachers and parents therefore to teach adaptive patterns of behavior and to remediate and replace maladaptive patterns of behavior that are either outright dysfunctional or serve only to self-reinforce idiosyncratic behaviors that form a barrier to functioning in a range of otherwise accessible settings.

CHAPTER CONCLUSIONS

In the first part of this book, we defined autistic learning disabilities and autistic learning styles, explaining how it is that children with autistic disorders grow differently. In the second part of the book, we talked about specific areas of autistic learning disability, essentially how each symptom that defines the autistic syndrome carries with it connotation for how someone with the particular symptom may see and learn things differently. The profile of autistic spectrum symptoms that each individual has or doesn't have comes together to form characteristic patterns that influence the child's characteristic problems in communicating, playing, and socializing. In talking about each area of autistic learning disability, we have also discussed specific ways in which the existing strengths of a particular child can be used to compensate for a specific area of weakness, for example, using visual icons to supplement language, or using externally structured rewards of the child's choice to build motivation in place of an innate social desire to please and be like others.

In the third and final part of this book, we will look into different well-known methods for treating autism. In recent years, there has been great focus on name-brand treatments and heated debate about the fidelity of such programs. There is even more debate about which program is "best." There's a lot of debate about "how much" treatment is appropriate. In this book, rather than ask which method is better, we ask which aspects of each method address the various autistic learning disabilities we recognize. The idea is that since each child with an autistic spectrum disorder has different autistic learning disabilities, he needs treatments—or parts of treatments—that address his specific learning difficulties. The description of autism is not unitary, and it will be argued, neither should the selection of treatment method.

Methods of Teaching Children with Autism

How They Address Autistic Learning Disabilities and Autistic Learning Styles

Part III of the book deals with methods of teaching children with autism. Part III begins in chapter 10, in which we discuss the ways in which applied behavior analysis has come to be used as a treatment for autism. Chapter 11 describes the TEACCH curriculum and how it is used for children with autism. Chapter 12 deals with full inclusion as an educational approach to treating autism, including integrative education approaches. Chapter 13 brings together information on learning styles and treatment methods by describing different model programs and exemplary classes for children with autistic spectrum disorders. Chapter 14 further integrates all of the information presented by reemphasizing the need to put the "I" back in IEP by developing an individual child's treatment according to his specific autistic learning disabilities, and selecting features from treatment models that target those deficits.

PUTTING THE "I" BACK IN IEP

Most children with ASDs receive treatments informed by one or more approaches—whether or not the program is brand-named. In recent years, there has been a push to develop programs and classrooms with brand-named methods. While this impetus moves the discussion about how to educate children with autism forward a bit, no one "brand" is the be-all and end-all. A useful way to frame analysis of educational methods for autism is to think about how to put the "I" (for "Individualized") back into the concept of the IEP (Individualized Educational Plan). In searching for the Holy Grail of the one treatment that will "cure" autism, there has been a great deal of bloodshed on the road to Jerusalem. It has been difficult indeed to find effective autism treatments that serve individual children's needs. We are, however, no longer Crusaders of the Middle Ages, but scientists and clinicians with a bit more on which to base a rational understanding of the pros and cons of a treatment regime.

One fact that should be established first is that there are no data to support the contention that any one particular method of treating autism is more likely than the others to produce the optimal outcome. The data from comparative studies to answer such a question do not exist. It is not that there is *no* outcomes research, just that it is limited, much of it is single-case design, almost none uses random assignment to treatments, and none asks all the questions, controls for all the mitigating factors, and examines large enough groups of children to give us anything more than suggestions about what might be better than something else under specific circumstances. For every child who has made significant gains using one methodology in very pure form, there is another child who has made the same kinds of gains using a different methodology. Some methods may certainly be more powerful than others, especially at different points in development. At different points in development, the child's profile of strengths and weakness changes. A method that is good for one area of weakness may not be suitable for others. A newly diagnosed two-year-old with a minute attention span, no compliance, and questionable receptive language needs very different treatment than an eight-year-old who is verbal and performing within a year or two of grade level in most academic subjects, but has no friends and no interest in friends. Yet, very often, such children are offered very similar things. When he was two, the eight-year-old may have been the two-year-old just described. But what helped him at two is not necessarily going to help at eight.

EVIDENCED-BASED RESEARCH ON AUTISM TREATMENT

In the absence of all the data needed to assess the impact of different intervention methods accurately, the second strategy for systematic planning comes from relying on theory about how children with autism learn. By using the autism learning disabilities approach, it is possible to analyze learning strengths and weaknesses systematically. In Part III, we will survey model methods to see what kind of a job each model method can do to address a particular kind of autistic learning disability.

What Does the Research Really Tell Us? Treatment research on autism is not very advanced. A few reports of model programs, a few studies of groups receiving different methods of treatment, and some single case studies is all the evidence-based research we have. There is almost no longitudinal follow-up work. The research is fraught with enough methodological concerns and problems to make a whole book of its own. There are few randomized clinical trials—the gold standard of research designs, few studies done with untreated control groups (as that would largely be unethical), and little that has measured the fidelity of the supposed intervention. All this combines with the dearth of studies on responder characteristics: Is a particular method better for younger or older children? Does IQ predict response? Are there better outcomes for PDD, NOS than for autism? Does it work for children who start with some language, but not for those who are nonverbal? The evidence-based research done so far leaves us with much unanswered. That's why this book and so much developed curricula and treatment regimes for ASDs must depend on theory and clinical expertise.

Some reviews look at all of these studies and ask what commonalities there are among programs that get the best results. There are several agreed-upon principles.

Age of Initiation of Treatment. First, it seems that the best outcomes are associated with initiating treatment by two to four years of age with the most robust results on the younger side of this range. As we discussed in chapter 1, this relates partly to how malleable or "plastic" the brain is at younger ages. It probably also relates to what we talked about in chapter 2—that the younger the child is when intervention begins, the less he will have to unlearn (such as partly successful accommodations like screaming) and the more readily fully adaptive skills can be taught.

Intensity of Intervention. For interventions to be successful, they must have reasonable intensity. There is no agreement on exactly how intensity should be defined, but factors such as numbers of hours per week, hours per day, numbers of interactions, or child responses per hour, or the use of instructional methods across settings all seem to contribute to intensity. Intensity of initial interventions that include 25 or more hours per week for the first two years of intervention have repeatedly been supported by various studies, but the role of comparable intensity in older children is less well studied. As we review different teaching methodologies in Part III, we will see that different approaches emphasize different definitions of intensity.

Addressing a Full Scope of Deficits. Comprehensive curricula that address all the areas of deficit in a particular child have repeatedly been shown to be the most effective. The theme of this book is just this: All deficits and strengths must be inventoried, and curricula must be selected that address weaknesses and play to strengths to develop compensatory strategies.

Sensitivity to Developmental Sequence. Many successful programs are those geared to developmental teaching. This is the approach advocated and carefully explained in this book. Skills must be taught in the sequences in which they would typically arise for those skills to form the foundation upon which later-developing skills can rest.

Highly Supportive Teaching. Intensity is usually framed in terms of how much teaching is done. A closely related aspect is how supportive, contingent, developmentally geared, motivating, individually responsive, and mindful of opportunities to promote independent learning the teaching is. This is a hard-to-measure ingredient of excellent programs. Teacher excellence depends on excellent training, but also on excellent instincts and high motivation to get through to a child with autism. While these qualities can be hard to measure, most people recognize them when they see them.

Another aspect of superior autism treatment programs that relates to both curricula and teachers is the need for good systems of supervision of teaching and for good content. Teachers must be taught to teach. Teachers' aides must be overseen by a master teacher who is an expert in what the aide is trying to do. The content of what is being taught must be monitored to provide fidelity so that a program is not called one thing, but does another.

Parent Training and Involvement. Another critical feature of successful programs is training parents. Including parents in training workshops for home-based therapists and behavioral-skills training classes and using parents as co-therapists and treatment "reinforcers" during nontreatment hours have, as a group, been shown to amplify the successfulness of any treatment regime.

Reducing Behaviors Incompatible with Learning. A final agreed-upon principle of good quality programs is that it is necessary to have strategies for reducing behavior that interferes with learning. Broadly interpreted, this includes approaches for increasing attention and motivation and reducing mental downtime (evidenced by inattention and repetitive behaviors). Included here is the need for an instructional program to have methods for responding to outbursts and escapes during which, of course, instruction cannot be given.

FITTING AUTISTIC LEARNING DISABILITIES
TO METHODS OF TREATMENT

Finding the Answer. Treating autism is certainly more complex than deciding that a child needs to be plugged into Program A for "X" hours per week, and then—voila!—he will be much, much better in two years. The need to design sophisticated tailored treatments can be particularly overwhelming to a parent of a newly diagnosed child who just wants The Answer. There are people out there giving (usually selling) The Answer. Generally, they are trained and they are confident. They may only be trained to use the method that they claim is The Answer. This isn't a bad thing, but it means parents, as well as school administrators trying to decide who should train their teachers, must be wary.

Teaching children with autism is really hard work and requires energy and perseverance. Not everyone needs to understand multiple approaches to teaching children with autism to become the ones in the position of individualizing the child's treatment. A one-treatment specialist should be regarded as a technician. It is fine that such a person knows how to do one thing, and, one hopes, can do it well. But, in addition to the technicians, we need engineers to ensure that the parts are put together in a coherent, functioning whole.

I believe that the only ethical approach in treating ASDs, in the absence of definitive data validating one method as exclusively useful over another, is to consider the pros and cons of aspects of different methods. This includes acknowledging that there is no rationale for believing that there is only one way to educate a particular child with autism. This is not different from the assertion that if a typically developing child has the ability to learn to read, there are going to be multiple teachers and multiple curricula that can be used to teach him to read. Further, we know from studies of typical children that walking earlier does not mean you'll be an athlete, and reading earlier does not mean you'll be more intelligent. Earliness of intervention can have a powerful impact because of greater brain plasticity. The content, however, does not necessarily have to be geared to meeting academic objectives, but rather developing overall learning preparedness.

In chapters 1 and 2, we discussed all the reasons that early intervention is important. Early intervention is associated not only with learning skills that foster other skills, but also with preventing mental disengagement from learning experiences. There is still a lot we don't know about how much variance in outcome for children with autism is due to things like how early intervention begins, how severe and which initial symptoms of autism are present, how much mental retardation the child has, how much the home and family experiences informally support learning, and how much the type and amounts of selected treatment methods matters. There are data that suggest that all of these factors are pieces of the pie. Only some are ones that we can influence.

Is One Method the Best? To hear some people tell it, there is only one way to educate a child with an autistic spectrum disorder. Depending on with whom you speak, the one true way will be one or another of these ways. At this juncture, some readers are no doubt wondering which methods are considered "good" and which "bad." If that is the question you want answered, there is no need to read on, because the answer is this: Each of the methods that will be discussed and described are seen as being very good for some children some of the time. Each of these methods also has disadvantages for some children some of the time too. There are times when giving a child a treatment plan strictly implementing any particular curriculum may be absolutely suitable. Most often, however, there is no reason to believe that a particular child can't benefit from more than one kind of treatment plan. This certainly doesn't mean that it doesn't matter what you do. It doesn't mean that it doesn't matter how much (or little) you do. All it means is that both methods, as well as hybrids and combinations of methods, may be needed to serve a particular child fully.

Applied Behavior Analysis and Discrete Trial Training: Separating Methods from Curriculum

AN OVERVIEW OF HOW ABA/DTT WORKS

The purpose of this chapter is to provide a general overview of the methods of ABA/DTT, but is not meant to substitute for a manual or hands-on training on how to use ABA/DTT with children with autism. This chapter is also not to be taken as a recommendation that this is the appropriate method to use for any one particular child at any one particular point in development. There will be much discussion of when features of ABA/DTT may be particularly helpful and certainly appropriate as well as guidelines for ongoing reassessment of a child's progress using the method, to track whether it is accomplishing identified goals. This chapter is meant to be a way for parents who may be considering an ABA/DTT program to judge ways how it may be helpful to their child.

For classroom teachers, this chapter on ABA/DTT is meant to help IEP planning around when and how much ABA/DTT may benefit a particular child. In addition, the information here may be useful to alert teachers or home ABA/DTT therapists and tutors about potential pitfalls and some problem-solving strategies that may be worth considering. For school psychologists and parents, this section may be helpful in understanding when ABA/DTT is likely to be most helpful. It may assist in weighing considerations about how much ABA/DTT is likely to be helpful at a particular stage in development. We'll address likely cost benefits compared to alternatives. We'll also discuss how to balance issues of ABA/DTT as a home-based program that in some respects is "restrictive" against the mandate to deliver treatment in the "least restrictive environment."

Separating Methods from Curriculum. The title of this chapter is intended to direct the reader to keep in mind one key point about ABA/DTT as she or he reads. This is that applied behavior analysis is a science that studies how principles of behavioral conditioning can be applied to learning. Discrete trial training is a method of training that is consistent with principles of applied behavior analysis. Many aspects of good teaching rely on behavioral principles. Discrete trial training is just one way of using behavioral methods. What makes discrete trial training a special case of behavioral teaching procedures is that it has been shown to be an effective way to break down information so that children with autism can learn.

Neither the term ABA nor DTT implies *what* to teach. Over time, specific preschool-like content has become associated with applying principles of ABA/DTT to the teaching of young children with autism. This content has not always been sequenced developmentally, especially with respect to teaching language comprehension and expression. There is no reason why the curriculum content typically associated with early ABA/DTT programs must be used for the methods to be effective. What is provided here is a fresh look at ABA/DTT by considering various aspects of technique as well as ways in which more developmentally sequenced curriculua can be interjected. Given the research reviewed in the introduction to this part of this book, it seems incumbent on those designing programs for children with autism to ensure that concepts are taught in developmental sequence. Examples of revising ABA/DTT curriculum content developmentally will be given as we go along.

Making DTT Language Teaching Developmental. To some extent, such teaching was already introduced in chapter 5, when we talked about how children acquire semantic concepts through multiple examples of an object with the same label, not through learning one example of each of several object in a class. (This is to say, don't use five flashcards with a different barnyard animal on each card; use a bin that has five sections with three example of each animal in it.) Restructuring ABA/DTT content in ways that are as simple as introducing several different discriminative stimuli (SDs) for one semantic label simultaneously would be an example of more developmentally restructured curriculum. Similarly, using discrete trials to teach pre-linguistic and paralinguistic skills (as discussed in the VIA system in chapter 6) should precede discrete trials to elicit spoken words in a child who lacks both words and non-verbal facility.

Some History. The use of ABA/DTT methods to treat children with autism was pioneered in the late 1960s and 1970s by Dr. Ivar Lovaas at UCLA. Lovaas was well trained as a Skinnerian behavioral psychologist. At first he was interested in testing the power of applied behavior analysis methods in children with severe developmental and behavioral disorders, including severe self-injurious behaviors. Working with hospitalized children, he was able to stop self-injurious behaviors where others had failed. Encouraged by early results, Dr. Lovaas and his graduate students developed a curriculum based on the idea of clearly defined, repeated trials to teach a target skill. Each skill that was learned was seen as a small building block needed to move toward creating a normal, rather than atypical, repertoire of behaviors. This was the birth of the "discrete trial training" method. Behaviorists at the time saw all knowledge, including skills like language, as consisting of small components that could be learned piece by piece until a fluid whole was created. According to this theory, each specific skill needed to be explicitly taught.

In the late 1980s Lovaas published results on some children with autism whom he had treated during the 1970s and early 1980s. This study made a big splash because although fewer than 20 children were treated intensively (an average of 40 hours per week) with his discrete trial training methods, half appeared to achieve very normalized outcomes, something that was not true when the same method was used much less intensively (an average of ten hours per week). Nothing like this had ever been reported before in the treatment of autism, and the second California Gold Rush to find a Lovaas program was on.

Receiving less publicity than the Lovaas program were further careful experimental studies on teaching new behaviors to children with autism—many being carried out by behavioral psychologists who had been graduate students of Dr. Lovaas. The work of Dr. Laura Schriebman, Dr. Robert Koegel, Dr. Glen

Dunlap, and many others introduced new concepts in training children with autism, such as teaching pivotal behaviors (responses that potentiate other behaviors, like learning to ask questions), more natural and intrinsic methods of rewarding behavior (like using choice making), and incidental teaching (in which a child is exposed to natural models of behavior he may initially have learned in a more formal manner). These studies employed newer hypotheses and explanations about information processing in children with autism—like stimulus over-selectivity (which theorized that children with ASDs had difficulty calibrating the strength of basic incoming stimuli and therefore often over or under-responded to things around them). This work formed the basis for conceptualizations like the one in this book of "autistic learning disabilities" arising from innate problems in gating sensory and perceptual information.

Presently, a range of ABA programs for children with autism exists. Dr. Lovaas's programs are largely true to the method of treatment he reported in his landmark 1988 paper. Over the last several years, much of his research effort has focused on replicating the original findings—though no exact replication (or randomized clinical trial—which is the scientific "gold standard") has yet appeared in over a dozen years since the publication of the original study. One thing that has been learned as attempts have been made to replicate the original work is that fidelity to the qualities of the original therapy that was conducted at UCLA under Dr. Lovaas's supervision, and training of therapists was a key ingredient not easily copied. One study has shown that more severely involved children benefit relatively less.

There has been much debate about the reproducibility of Dr. Lovaas's original results, and to rehash the debate here might serve to dissipate the authoritative contributions that the work has made. Instead, it is more worthwhile to examine how Lovaas's original ABA/DTT methods plus the work of subsequent researchers can be regarded as a whole and best utilized as a vital, powerful tool in designing intervention for autism.

How Many Hours? One significant area of controversy that has emerged from Lovaas's own work is the issue of how many hours of ABA/DTT per week a child must receive in order to experience a successful outcome. Lovaas's number is 40. He compared it to 10. (What about 20? 30? What about children who have an ABA/DTT program 20 hours per week, and speech and language therapy, an integrated preschool experience with a one-to-one aide, and four other enriching activities each week?) Some work that has appeared since Lovaas's original study has looked at a number of treatment models and supports the idea that while intensity, such as a 40-hour-per-week program, is a key ingredient of a successful program, it is not necessarily true that all 40 hours must be ABA/DTT. A study that I completed suggested no differences in outcomes between children treated for 25 hours per week and those treated for 35 hours per week. It seems likely that parents with 25 hours a week of a home program have received just as much training and become just as aware of the need to structure their child's non-ABA/DTT hours meaningfully as parents with a 35-hour-per-week program. If that's true, it would be consistent with the larger reviews of numerous studies that suggest just that.

ABA/DTT and the Autistic Learning Disabilities Approach. Integrated into this description of the features of ABA/DTT methods will be discussion and analysis of how ideas raised in earlier chapters on individual autistic learning styles and autistic learning disabilities can be used along with a developmental framework to tailor intervention procedures that can primarily be identified as using the ABA/DTT model. This section is likely to be understood differently by a professional or parent already quite conversant with ABA/DTT methods compared to someone just becoming familiar with the range of options available for treating children with autism. For the reader interested in knowing more about more purely behavioral implementations of ABA/DTT methods, good resources are listed in the Further Readings section that corresponds to this chapter. The emphasis here however, will be to reexamine conventional ABA/DTT practices with the aim of reinvigorating them by drawing on ideas outside of behavioral psychology.

LEARNING TO LEARN

The single most influential aspect of the ABA/DTT approach to treating children with autism is what can potentially be accomplished in the first two to six months of an intensive focus on this type of treatment. The use of ABA/DTT can be regarded as an admirable learning-readiness program. Many of the earliest-targeted behavioral goals serve to establish competencies in fundamental skills such as cause-and-effect reasoning, paying attention, complying with instructions, and imitating. Each of these skills, in turn, is used in many ways to acquire other specific skills.

Development of Cause-and-Effect Understanding. In the very youngest children with autistic spectrum disorders, there is often a lack of clear cause-and-effect understanding. On its most basic level this means teaching the child that if he wants a food treat that you have, he first must do some small thing you ask of him. This is John Locke's "Social Contract" reduced to its essence, where evolutionary psychology starts in constructing an understanding of human society. It can't be reduced further than "Touch your nose, get an M&M." For some children, this is where treatment must start. Until the person teaching the autistic child has this power over him and this basic contract is established, the ability to teach is nonexistent. Most children with autism learn fairly quickly that you must do something to get something. It's easy to see how this is the most basic thing a child can be taught. It is also something that many children with autism do not clearly understand before they begin their first treatment.

Most initial diagnostic assessments include (often futile) attempts to get the child to point or touch pictures he is said to be able to identify, put together puzzles, nest cubes, or place pegs in a pegboard. Quite often, these materials are thrown at the examiner or swiped off the table. This may happen even if the child is offered a favorite food treat. The child may reach for the food treat with one hand while swiping puzzle pieces with another. This is a pretty good clue that the child has not yet developed cause-and-effect reasoning. (It also tells the examiner that she has not learned whether or not the child can do the puzzle, just that he doesn't want to—under these circumstances.)

For a child like the one just described, the first day of an ABA/DTT program can be a little like boot camp. There can be a bit of a rude awakening that he isn't going to get something for nothing anymore. Using discrete trials and full-motor prompting, the child is presented with a simple task (like "Touch nose"). One adult states what the child must do, while a second, (after a very brief opportunity for the child to touch his nose on his own), takes the child's hand and puts it on his nose. The child is then verbally praised in a lavish manner and the M&M (for example) is inserted into his mouth. Quite often, the child is made rather furious by all this intrusion, but another trial is quickly initiated. The adult again requests that the child touch his nose, and after the hand reaches the nose, the M&M is again administered. As the child gets the hang of this, with repeated "discrete trials," the child tends to protest less, developing an understanding that an M&M is not far in the offing. When this begins to happen, the adult who is moving the child's hand on his behalf gives the child a bit more opportunity to start or finish the act of touching hand to nose. (This is called "fading" the prompt.) "Touch nose," which is referred to as an "SD" or discriminative stimulus—that is, what the child must figure out, is then varied, and a related SD is also presented, for example, "Touch head." After a few days of this type of activity, the child has typically learned the rules of engagement—that he must do your "something" to get his "something." There only are a very few things that can get in the way of this procedure: Giving the child too much time to respond may make him feel that non-responding is a viable option. Or, the child may have difficulty if the adult fails to prompt enough or fades the prompt too fast. There can also be problems when using a food reward that is not all that desirable to the child, or that has reached satiation. With all these training factors taken into account, the more mental retardation the child has, the more slowly he will learn, but he will learn some things. The child who can interject alternative behaviors with a history of success in getting what he wants (like screaming and kicking) can be expected to be a bit slower to agree to this contract too.

Developing Attention and Compliance. The child does not know what he does not know. Through development of cause-and-effect understanding built through discrete trials, the child can now be engaged. This can be built upon quickly so that the child can be conditioned (through faded prompts) to look to the teacher for information and to learn as quickly as possible what it is he must do to obtain his positive reinforcer (be it an M&M, pretzel stick, or tummy tickle). When the child readily tries to figure out what he must do, he's paying attention. If the child consistently makes an attempt to produce the requested skill in response to the SD, he can be said to be compliant. (Compliance does not imply success, just an attempt to provide a correct response.) If the child is praised somewhat for attending and complying (as well as praised even more for succeeding), the child can be said to have the basics of cause-and-effect understanding, attention, and compliance—in other words, some important learning-readiness skills.

The child has gone from floating through a world in which nothing was particularly connected to anything else in a clearly discernible way to knowing at least a few things he can do to get predictable, desirable rewards. Done well, this pattern of learning disposes the child to learn more. Everybody likes more control over their world rather than less.

Instructional Control and Estimating a Child's Capacity. In an ideal world of autism treatment research, all children would be readministered any cognitive test that they had been given as part of an initial diagnostic procedure two to four weeks after starting this kind of training for cause and effect, attention, and compliance. Virtually all children would score higher at this point. Rather than swiping the blocks, pegs, and puzzle pieces, the child would eagerly look to see what type of food reinforcer was being offered. The child and examiner would now have a social "contract." If the child's IQ test score moved up from the moderately to the mildly mentally retarded range after a couple weeks of ABA/DTT, it is not likely because we have grown new neuronal connections in two weeks, but that rather we now have less error and more "true score" in our test results. The baseline of the child's abilities and disabilities obtained at this point should be considered a much better predictor of his capacities than the originally obtained data. At the very least, it is important to note whether initial testing of a child was marked by lack of cause-and-effect understanding, lack of attention, or lack of compliance, so that it will later be clear how much a new test score may be reflecting developmental change and how much may reflect acquisition of learning readiness skills. Both, of course are essential. Sometimes this second baseline testing reflects increased knowledge in a child who may previously have had untapped potential, blocked by his autistic defensiveness to new information introduced by others.

Development of a Concept of Imitation. Another major contribution to learning readiness that is a notable asset of the ABA/DTT method is development of the concept of imitation. Imitation, as discussed in chapter 4, is core to how young children learn. There are two major components to imitation—the mechanics of copying a model and the social drive to want to imitate something just because someone else is doing it. Early ABA/DTT programs are strong at teaching the first component of imitation. The second component is a harder nut to crack and requires additional techniques.

When a child learns how to copy a model, that child is learning that he can apply this copying "template" to anything interesting that is observed and try that action too. This process of making his own unique copy of the imitated action adds to the child's repertoire of "schema" or action plans. A schema can be modified or linked with other schema once it is assimilated (once the child knows it). The first type of imitation taught in ABA/DTT programs is typically imitation of actions (referred to as nonverbal imitations, or NVIs). Again, using the discrete trial format, the child can be fully motor-prompted to "Do this!" as an adult demonstrates an action like touching his nose. Gradually the prompts are faded until the child responds to the "Do this!" command by attending to the adult whenever cued (by having his name called, for example).

Generalizing the Imitation Schema. One of the factors to consider when teaching imitation is how mastery and retention of a new skill may be affected by being taught an activity that is intrinsically interesting versus an activity that, rather than being carried out for its own sake, is carried out because there will be an external reinforcer (food, tickle, verbal praise) when it's done. Which would be more reinforcing and memorable for a typically developing child? Would copying another child going down a slide head first belly down, or copying an adult who is repeatedly standing up and sitting down be more instrinsically interesting and therefore more reinforcing? The belly flop, most would agree. Much of what children are asked to learn in early ABA/DTT programs is more of the "stand up, sit down" nature. These "drills" are manualized in curriculum materials for ABA/DTT programs. They are absolutely fine for initially establishing a concept of imitation, but for the child to get the idea that imitation is a schema he can generalize, he's going to have to be taught something more fun, that is, something with intrinsic or direct reinforcement.

This takes just a little imagination: Standing up and sitting down on a beach ball would be more fun (and therefore more intrinsically rewarding) than standing and sitting on a chair. Using a chair initially, changing to a ball, moving to a foam block, pretending to sit on a dollhouse chair, or sitting on Elmo keeps things lively. Furthermore, it builds in what in behavioral terms is often referred to as "generalization." Nowhere is it written that a child will not be able to learn to imitate a second action if he doesn't master the first one with 90 percent accuracy over four trials a day for three consecutive days. (Actually, it *is* written into many IEPs, but it's silly!) Children can be taught this way, but it does not parallel how concepts like "sit down" or "stand up" are acquired in typical development. By teaching using only one SD, a new problem may be created. Narrow, rigid patterns of behavior are definitely appealing to many children with autism—and so introducing them and encouraging them may indeed speed (narrow, rigid) mastery of an action like standing up and sitting down in a particular chair. However, the action is a meaningless skill unless the child realizes that the skill is actually a schema he can generalize (in this case, that he can "sit down" on many different kinds of things).

Administering Discrete Trials and Collecting Data. This kind of thinking turns some of the ABA/DTT system for doing things topsy-turvy. It might make it very difficult, for example, to keep a running tally of "mastered" and "failed" trials of an SD if the tutor runs around the room sitting down and standing up on anything the child seems interested in. We don't keep this type of data in the course of teaching new things to more typically developing children, and it is not clear why every single trial needs to be monitored for children with autism. We certainly don't want to sacrifice meaningful (spontaneous, contextually relevant) teaching of skills to data collection. There are in fact, a few studies now that support more periodic, rather than continuous, data collection procedures anyway.

It is important to have periodic criterion testing of how readily a child is acquiring a concept like "stand up, sit down." Whether we learn more from collecting such data every time a child is asked to do something, or whether we might learn just as much by collecting criterion data once every two days, or even once a week is a research question that needs to be studied. It doesn't happen to be one that has already been answered as is sometimes implied by the standard design of ABA/DTT programs that are structured to include data collection on all trials.

Making ABA/DTT Language Teaching Developmental. Another thing that is seen in the initial stages of a good ABA/DTT program is whether a particular child with autism is one with a good rote memory. Rote memory, memorizing whole chunks of information, is how some autistic children first get a grip on conversational language (through echolalia). Good rote memory is often in evidence in early ABA/DTT programs as an effect of over-drilling. Over-drilling is when the child has had the same material taught together as a set so consistently that concepts of the set have not been generalized or assimilated individually, but rather chunked together. This is why some children working on early receptive commands like "Touch nose," will first touch their ears, then their eyes, and finally their nose, when asked to touch their nose. The child has acquired a schema, but it is a rather imprecise schema that tells him that touching any body part is somehow part of the same "something" that will eventually get him his desired reinforcer.

In chapter 5 it was described how a typically developing child acquires the idea of touching his nose by touching your nose, his nose, and other noses, then coming to the realization that other body parts have names too. This allows for specific concept (of a nose) formation, rather than rote memorization. Rote memorization may serve the child with autism well as a compensatory device in the future, but in the youngest children, encouraging the child to learn in a manner that more closely simulates typical language may build a more solid language foundation. To avoid label acquisition that is a reflection of rote memorization rather than comprehension of a concept, multiple SDs must be taught simultaneously. A horizontal foundation for language (many examples of one thing) more nearly reflects typically emerging language than a rotely memorized "vertical" vocabulary list of one example of each object in a category like body parts, animals, vehicles, or colors.

This doesn't mean that early language concepts shouldn't be introduced with discrete trial training; they certainly can be. They should be subject to repeated practice (repeated trials) too. Acquisition and mastery should be externally reinforced if a context for direct and intrinsic reinforcement is not obvious. The method is certainly valid, but the organization of the teaching content can be structured more to simulate the foundation of imitation and receptive language that develops in typical children.

Home-Based ABA/DTT as Parent Training. One of the tremendously advantageous and not well-studied aspects of ABA/DTT programs is that they are often conducted in the homes of the youngest children. This means that the parents most often receive formal training in the use of ABA/DTT methods themselves through initial and follow-up workshops designed to train all staff working with the child. For a parent who, just prior to the child's diagnosis, may have been really struggling to have any sense of control over the child and communication with the child, this can be a welcome relief. Basically, the parents are taught applied behavior analysis's ABCs of childcare. Parents learn to systematically analyze what may trigger an undesirable behavior and to provide consequence to reduce it. Parents are also gratified to learn how to teach the child, and may, for the first time, experience real efficacy in parenting the child. In addition to directly teaching parents through in-home workshops, there is often help implementing behavioral plans. This assistance comes in the form of senior therapists, case managers, and program managers visiting the home to monitor program fidelity.

Social Support from a Home-Based Program. Folks who choose to be ABA/DTT trainers are generally a young, friendly bunch, and many parents describe the wonderful respite they get from tutors who drop off and pick up siblings from school on the way in or out of the home, give them time to nurse the newborn in peace, or always start a pot of coffee. Some research on parenting stress found there was less stress in parents with home ABA/DTT programs compared to parents who had children attending a school-based program. For parents who can make use of this type of support in their homes, it is wonderful when home-based services are available in their child's early stages of treatment.

School-Based ABA/DTT Programs. Some families, however, prefer their privacy and may not be comfortable having a group of friendly young therapists frequently present. Some families have infants, twins, or other children with special needs that conflict with the demands of a home program. (The father of one family that lived in a rather rough neighborhood stated that they couldn't deal with a home program because of "business associates" visiting at odd hours.) Often, both parents must, or prefer to, work outside the home and prefer not to have to worry about the remote management of the arrivals and departures of tutors when they are away. For such families, school-based ABA/DTT programs may be a better fit. (This said, it is still important for parents to remain informed about the child's program so that they can provide needed natural practice of emerging skills during non-treatment hours.)

Increasingly, early-intervention programs for children under three, as well as preschool special day class programs may include an ABA/DTT component, or provide ABA/DTT exclusively. Some agencies or schools have a mix of at-home and at-school teaching. If the very young child gets the one-on-one teaching that is needed to establish learning readiness skills, there is no reason to believe that the ABA/DTT services must be delivered at home. There are different models for doing this.

Mixed Home and Center-Based Treatment. There is a strong case to be made for a combined service-delivery model. A part-time home program can provide valuable parent training as well as ensure that all adults in the home understand the methods of teaching new things to the child with autism. Center-based hours can be used for supervisory check-ups, periodic criterion data taking, planning of revised drills, and specialized related services like speech and language therapy and occupational therapy if those are needed. A school-based component can also allow some opportunities for peer contact on a one-on-one facilitated basis, through peer tutoring, or through free play.

ABA/DTT Classrooms. Some schools (usually preschools) that run ABA/DTT classes have four, five, or six separate carrels, each designated for one child and one adult. The child can have a carrel that is his alone (so records of his work can stay in a fixed location), or children can shift carrels as they work on a variety of activities requiring different materials. There are advantages to this group setting in that teachers and aides can see and hear what is going on with other children and have frequent contact with one another. Teacher and aides can keep abreast of who's having a good day and who's having a bad one. Children can have the experience of shifting among staff the way they would experience the shift among tutors at home. Another possible benefit of school-based ABA/DTT is that a credentialed special-education teacher probably has a more broadly developed base of teaching skills and strategies than a senior therapist or case manager who oversees a home-based ABA/DTT program. Aides in such a specialized ABA/DTT class have typically been through the ABA/DTT workshop training and have had the additional (though admittedly often minimal) training required to become a teacher's aide. Often the teachers for such classes are former ABA/DTT case managers who have returned to school for a broader early-childhood special-education certification.

Giving Parents Behavioral Expertise and Specific Strategies. Some classroom-based models for ABA/DTT have been able to build in other program design features that are more difficult to achieve in home-based teaching. Features can include bringing the parent into the classroom one day a week to work as a classroom assistant. This can be an invaluable experience: It is interesting how many parents want to learn more about young children by signing their typically developing preschooler up for a parent coop program, but how little of that there is in special education. However, parents can learn by trying out skills with another child under a teacher's supervision—just as they would do in any parent coop preschool. The parent has a chance to understand methods she has been taught with a little more objectivity than she might be able to apply to her own child. Since every parent will want her child to receive good-quality intervention when he is worked with by another parent assistant, parents are likely to be as well trained and at least as motivated as many instructional aides.

Some programs introduce parents to their in-class parent training model by having a professional and a parent watch the classroom together through a one-way mirror before beginning direct classroom work so that the parent understands what's happening and why. This way parents can learn what to do, but also develop an appreciation for why a teacher does things the way she does.

Concept of Learning in a Natural Environment. One thing that is clear from the research is that children learn through a variety of experiences and in a variety of settings. A child can have a full-time ABA/DTT program at home, but if parents who have little or nothing to do with the program come home at the end of the day, and the day's "work" for the child is not carried over into what he must do to communicate and to show his newly emerging understanding to those in his home environment, much of the significance of the day's treatment will be lost. This means that even when parents may not have the time to participate as tutors in their child's home-based ABA/DTT program "officially," they have to have enough ongoing contact with those providing the program to know what the child is learning, what needs practice, and what is now sufficiently well learned that the child can be expected to evidence the new skill on a regular basis.

Educational law sets up a bit of a contradiction for providing programs for the youngest children (those under three years old). On the one hand, there is a mandate to teach the child in natural environments. Some might interpret this to mean that the child must receive services in the home. (We know, however, that a significant proportion of children under three spend large portions of their day in day care, so group-based settings can be a natural environment too.) Educational law for children over three says the child should be educated in the least restrictive environment. This is widely interpreted to be a classroom-based service rather than a home-bound service and, if appropriate, inclusive placements should be preferred over special-education placements. What this boils down to is that, in our culture today, there is no one right or wrong place for a very young child. If the child can benefit from inclusion with other children (using criteria such as those that will be discussed in chapter 12), then he should be included. If the child needs intensive and one-to-one or one-to-two special education, then he needs to be with staff who can provide that. If the parent feels that out-of-home educational placement is not what she wants for her toddler because she would prefer to be a stay-at-home mom, or because she prefers a home-schooling approach, then a home-based ABA/DTT program may be the best fit.

CONSIDERATIONS IN SETTING UP AN ABA/DTT PROGRAM

Whether you are a parent or a school administrator, there are many things to consider in setting up a successful ABA/DTT program. Here we will review considerations to ensure the success of a program whether it is school-based and designed to serve a number of children, or home-based and designed for just one child. Not all ABA/DTT programs are equal. Because ABA/DTT programs are a much newer innovation in the special education of children with autism than special education itself, the programs, where they exist at all, are usually mainly or exclusively self-monitored for fidelity. There are people offering ABA/DTT programs who learned their methods directly from Dr. Lovaas as one of his graduate students, and there are people hanging out a shingle as a "behavior skills trainer," "behavioral tutor," "autism trainer," or "behavior management specialist in autism" who may never have completed any coursework on typical or atypical child development, but once worked for six months under the supervision of a woman who the previous summer did a workshop with a graduate student from Dr. Lovaas's research group. The former sounds better than the latter, but there are past doctoral students of Dr. Lovaas running very lucrative businesses who really haven't incorporated new ideas into their work in ten years. They don't have to—the demand for their services is that high, even if their product is not very good. There are also local speech and language therapists, teachers, resource specialists, and parents who have read widely, gone through many kinds of training, kept their minds open, and are bright enough and intuitive enough to work incredibly well with children with autism. There are similarly educated parents who began by building a program for their own child and go on to offer programs for other people's children, who may or may not have similar learning needs. Because there are formally and informally trained treatment providers who range from excellent to ridiculously bad it is not an easy job to the gauge quality of ABA/DTT providers. Even an ABA credential does not mean everything, but it doesn't mean nothing either. In shopping for ABA/DTT programs, caveat emptor definitely applies.

The best way to research the qualifications of a potential therapist or teacher is to watch that person in action. Bring along a more knowledgeable, experienced friend or therapist currently working with the child, or ask for a videotape of a sample session with a child who is like the child you intend for your program to serve. Try to have a choice to make. Many parents, in particular, who are desperate to start "the earlier the better," and "before the window of opportunity starts to close" can be very vulnerable. Bad programs are not better than no program at all. A child who is turned off to learning by an overly strict, punitive, or rigid therapist who consistently misses communicative signals initiated by the child and only knows to go "by the book" (treatment manual) may be well worth passing by. You as a consumer of this teacher's, tutor's, or therapist's services should feel that this person likes children. We don't want to leave the dalmations to the whims of Cruella de Ville. The only way to know if someone really likes kids is to watch them interact with kids. Even a new young tutor who has never been to a training workshop should be able to do *something* with even the most self-isolating autistic child that looks like a moment of connection when they first meet.

Tutor-Technician Training. A number of nonpublic agencies offering ABA/DTT services maintain a core of case managers and senior therapists, but are less able to attract and retain a core of one-to-one tutors needed for a home-based ABA/DTT program. Parents may be advised to find their own one-to-one tutors, and when three or four are identified, the agency provides a two- or three-day training workshop in the home, plus supervision by a senior therapist and case manager. Amounts of training, quality of training, follow-ups to training, and ongoing supervision can all have an enormous impact on quality control in the program. (This is precisely why Lovaas is taking so long to replicate his findings of 15 to 20 years ago.)

The one-to-one tutors who are identified are often young women who are either recent college graduates or community college students. Most families are able to find tutors who have either completed some coursework in child development or education or who have had practical experience working with children in a daycare, camp, or preschool setting. This can work out fine, but it is important to consider the limitations of this job pool. First, most such tutors are not yet parents themselves and often have a limited point of reference as to what is age-appropriate behavior and what is autism. It is important to know the difference between a cranky two-year-old who needs a nap and a noncompliant two-year-old. Specific example: I recently read an assessment declaring that a particular child met the criteria for autism, citing routines and rituals like needing an adult to lie down with him to fall asleep and needing to have his four favorite stuffed animals with him for this! Not particularly odd to anyone who's parented a two-year-old. Not surprisingly, the evaluator was not a parent.)

Some families initially recruit helpful relatives and neighbors willing to contribute hours. Most of the individuals in this pool (including the parents being trained) may know more about typical development, but likely know no other children with autism. This means that training needs to include something about what autism is.

Manualized instruction such as is used by many nonpublic ABA/DTT agencies needs to be tailored to the specific learning strengths and weaknesses, as well as interests of each child. This can be difficult if there isn't at least one supervisory person who has close ongoing involvement and experience with many different children with autism as well as treatment besides ABA/DTT.

Senior Therapist and Case Manager System. An admirable asset of most nonpublic agencies offering ABA/DTT services is that they have adopted the quality-control model initiated by Dr. Lovaas in his original work, in which each program has a senior therapist who is on site on a regular basis each week and who is overseen by a more experienced case manager who can be a liaison between the family, tutors, senior therapist, and the agency providing service. Weekly team meetings that, ideally, involve all of these staff as well as the parents are designed to monitor the learning of new skills, potential emergence of maladaptive learning, and opportunities to revise and add to drills, introduce and individualize teaching materials, share insights, and develop consistency among all staff. They also provide needed social support for individual staff members who often work alone one-to-one with a child in his home and benefit from ongoing contact with their colleagues. Without team meetings, programs can grow stale and the child may be exposed to too much unvarying demand that can promote a growing disengagement from the program over time. Team meetings also serve as in-service training for the more junior staff so that they can become active problem solvers themselves. It's an apprenticeship system.

What the training most often lacks is opportunities for the tutors to read about autism, behavioral analysis, or development. These would all have to be free-time activities, which, unlike a teacher-training situation, would result in neither course nor internship credits. As a result, most one-to-one tutors in ABA/DTT programs are more like technicians than teachers in certain respects—knowing what to do, but not always knowing why an activity is done in a particular manner. This lack of the larger picture should not be a major problem in a good quality program with substantial supervision. In cases in which families are considered "satellite" families who receive very episodic contact with case managers or the supervisory agency, however, it can result in unintentionally poor quality programs because of "drift."

Setting Up an ABA/DTT Program through a School. In many parts of the United States, more schools are starting special day class programs with significant or exclusively ABA/DTT curricula. There is no reason that an ABA/DTT program must be conducted exclusively in a child's home. There are great classroom-based ABA/DTT programs in rural areas and poor areas, as well as in urban areas and academic centers around the United States. In more rural areas, it may be more feasible to focus treatment resources in one center that service providers can get to and bring children to that site. Having senior therapists and case managers spend 20 hours per week in cars, shuttling between sites does not result in as much quality programming as having eight or nine children treated at one site at which the case manager or program manager is located. Similarly, I have seen children not be able to access early ABA/DTT programs because they live in neighborhoods in which it is simply not safe for 23-year-old tutors who do not know the neighborhood to walk from place to place alone.

There are a few special considerations in setting up an ABA/DTT program through a school. Sometimes teachers selected to organize such programs have been senior therapists or case managers with a nonpublic ABA agency for a while, but may have fewer years in the field of education than most credentialed special-education teachers. There are wonderful possibilities for collaborations between such new ABA/DTT trained teacher and a more experienced teacher, plus school-based speech therapists, school psychologists, or resource specialists. One brings behavioral expertise and an understanding of one-to-one instruction; the other can adapt the curriculum content to some group-based activities and/or to the multiple-child setting of a classroom, even if all work is one-to-one. The only necessary ingredient is a willingness on the part of the collaborating parties to learn to speak one another's languages.

Collaborations do not always get off to a smooth start. Some schools with ABA/DTT classes initially formed these programs under duress to stem the flow of dollars to expensive home-based ABA/DTT programs that are often given carte blanche after acrimonious administrative court hearings. Court-ordered collaborations often turn out like bad arranged marriages. It is imperative for professionals who find themselves in new and unexpected collaborations to just focus on the common goal of helping children learn and try to put aside what was said during the court procedures.

ABA/DTT Tutors as Classroom Aides. It can be particularly difficult when home-based ABA/DTT therapists come into special day classes as a one-to-one aide for the child with autism. The one-to-one aide is virtually never as trained in special education as is the classroom teacher, but may be very well trained to use ABA/DTT methods, which essentially encompasses one-to-one work. A classroom, by definition, offers the child with autism an opportunity to develop group-based learning skills. The one-to-one aide can serve an important function in helping the child transition into becoming a group member, but the group, the aide must remember, is the teacher's group. The ABA/DTT aide needs to show respect for the new "culture" she is joining. The teacher will very likely not use the same SDs that the aide has been taught to use. That's fine. The teacher should have an understanding of how the child has been taught up to this point and know his existing response repertoire but should really be there to provide an opportunity for the child to begin to learn in a less restrictive, more incidental, more generalizable manner. (If he is not yet ready to take instruction from anyone other than a one-to-one aide, he's not ready to be meaningfully included in a classroom.) Some of the class time might be spent in one-to-one DTTs with the one-to-one aide, but if the child is in the class (special day class or inclusion class) for no other reason than to have a change of scenery for the DTTs, the educational value of such programming must be questioned.

FEATURES OF THE ABA/DTT MODEL

Use of Motor Prompting. A major feature of learning via DTT, initially, is motor prompting, or physically moving the child through all or part of a requested response. There are both advantages and disadvantages to be considered in using motor prompting as a teaching technique: When a new kind of performance is requested of a child who may have neither the receptive language nor the motivation to carry out the performance simply to gain adult approval or attention, motor prompting may be a beneficial strategy. In these two respects, the use of motor prompting can be seen as a very tailored accommodation to two key learning deficits often present in young children with autism. Motor prompting in the context of DTT is often also used to produce "error-free learning," the idea that the child can always succeed if given enough help. The art of using this technique is in giving enough help to ensure success, but not so much help as to inhibit the self-guided part of the learning. Another interesting benefit of motor prompting is that it gives the child the opportunity to associate the person prompting him with his achievement of the targeted goal—and his subsequent experience of a reinforcer. This can help the child become less resistant to situations in which teaching adults want to do things with or for him in order to teach him. For example, many parents of young children with autism note that their child likes books—but only to look at on his own; will not accept having a book read to him. As a child is desensitized to adult participation in a goal-directed activity, it usually becomes easier for the child to tolerate, and even enjoy, such joint learning activity during non-treatment hours.

Prompt-Dependence. Disadvantages of motor prompting can include the passivity that is part and parcel of someone else's showing you what to do rather than more spontaneous and independent problem solving. In cases in which the child, left to his own devices, would not likely initiate goal-directed problem solving (might instead spin puzzle pieces and not place them in the puzzle), motor prompting can refocus behavior and make it more functional. On the other hand, children can also learn to remained disengaged, waiting for the motor prompt, with the understanding that getting an adult to take them part way to a task's completion is likely to be quicker and more accurate, and require less mental effort—all contingencies working toward reinforcing passivity. Sometimes, this pattern of behavior is referred to as "prompt-dependence," a condition in which a behavior is not spontaneously initiated because the child has become overly accustomed to getting help to achieve his success.

This pattern of prompt-dependence can be particularly notable in higher-functioning children with autism who rather readily figure out the prompting "game." Once in a group-based instructional setting, such a child may hold back from starting a task until he has a "personal invitation." This can maintain the child's expectation of having a one-to-one aide present long after her help is needed for the child to comprehend and complete activities. Conscientious efforts to fade prompting as quickly as possible can be very effective in stemming development of this pattern.

Methods and Schedules of Reinforcement. Understanding schedules of rein-forcement is integral to making any ABA/DTT program (or any behaviorally based program) work well. Reinforcement schedules were discussed at length in chapter 4 as part of understanding motivation in children with ASDs. They will be recapped here as they apply to different stages of ABA/DTT programs. Using reinforcement schedules well involves understanding the relative power of different intervals of reinforcement counterbalanced by a sense of how much effort a child has expended to reach an immediate goal. Gauging this second factor is a skill that comes with experience. (For example, if a child writes the first three letters of his name readily, but dallies on the fourth, it can make sense to administer a reinforcer after the fourth is completed to get the action back on track, rather than waiting until the whole name is complete.)

Fixed reinforcement schedules are the most basic way of administering a reinforcer. This means that the child gets a reward at a regular interval, like getting one M&M for each puzzle piece correctly placed. One-to-one reinforce-ment schedules are often used in the early stages of training compliance and attention. As soon as the child develops some mastery of the requested tasks, however, the level of reinforcement can usually be successfully pulled back—

maybe with an M&M after every second puzzle piece. It is easy to teach a new tutor to follow such a plan.

More powerful, however, are intermittent reinforcement schedules. An intermittent reinforcement schedule is like the example given above wherein the child is never sure when the next reinforcer will come. The theory is that the child will work harder to hurry to the time when the next reinforcer will be administered. If the administration of the intermittent reinforcer is tied to getting oneself back on task after a lapse, the child should learn that it can be particularly rewarding to refocus.

For children who are more adept or older, reinforcement strategies can usually include use of a "token economy." A token economy is like a child's version of a paycheck. After a period of time, he is paid—in a token (it could even be a penny). After accumulating some number of tokens, the child can trade the tokens for what he wishes to "buy"—like his own bowl of popcorn at snack time. In introductory token economies, the actual reinforcer, like a piece of popcorn, can be dropped into a clear closed jar each time the child "earns" a piece. At the completion of the task: snack time!   In more advanced token economies, the child can save tokens all day or all week. Coordination of the token economy across home and school is always a good idea. Letting the child post his own rewards as he earns them is a good idea, like having pennies with Velcro backs that the child can be given to place on a token board. (Active sensory motor involvement in the reward increases its sense of immediacy and value.) Letting the child choose in advance what he plans to "purchase" so he can be reminded of his goal and can gauge his progress as he moves toward it enhances the value of the system to the child too.

Advantages of High Levels of Reinforcement Used in ABA/DTT. ABA/DTT programs are often noted for their high levels of reinforcement. With younger children and children with more severe impairments, there tends to be more reliance on favorite foods as reinforcers. These are usually paired with verbal praise and physical praise (hugs, tickles) so those experiences become desirable by association, if they aren't already. In using these procedures, the child learns to respond to a wider range of reinforcers, including reinforcers that are more typical for any child of the same age. Once a child responds to social praise, he's a step closer to benefiting from instruction in a setting like a classroom, in which social praise (and not M&Ms) is the coin of the realm. The use of high levels of reinforcement and constantly getting rewards tends to make the child more amenable to learning experiences. (You can see this as either learning to love to learn, learning to love high levels of reinforcement, or both.)

Drawbacks of High Levels of Reinforcement. There are also potential drawbacks to administering high levels of reinforcement. The most important of these is that receiving a high level of food, sensory, or even social reward may detract from the experiences that reinforce typical children in many of their learning experiences: work for its own sake. When a child builds with blocks, arranges a dollhouse, or sets out a meal of pretend food, the typical child may look for praise when he's done, but will likely do it even if no adult is in the immediate vicinity.

Children with autism will do the same thing. Often the play they find most intrinsically rewarding is repetitive (and so is labeled self-stimulatory). By this definition, even the typical child who is laying out a play meal when no one is there to watch is engaging in self-stimulatory activity. But we recognize the self-directed, creative aspect of the meal play as appropriate and desirable in a way that the repetitive play of a child with autism usually is not. What it does mean is that the child with autism does have a concept of selecting and carrying out an activity for its own sake. It needs to be built upon. It's up to us to help that child gain self-reinforcement from his more appropriate activities (like completing a puzzle) by giving only a mild external reinforcer when it's done, so most of the reinforcement is his self-satisfaction, not our external stimulation.

Sometimes, ABA/DTT programs, in an attempt to make the work really fun for the child, instead end up over-stimulating the child. Here's what could be called the "UCLA-basketball-overtime-winning-point-reinforcer": The child, after much effort, completes a five-piece form board. He's told, "Yeah! Good doing puzzle! All Right! High Five! Low Five!" followed by a tummy tickle and a head squeeze. (Goodness! It's just a five-piece puzzle!) Watching the child, it may be possible first to see a brightening at completing the puzzle, followed by a slightly anxious or avoidant or overwhelmed look. Reinforcers can be too much of a good thing at once. It the child becomes over-aroused, it will be more difficult to segue to the next task. Also, when excessive levels of reinforcement become the norm, the child can feel unsatisfied by milder levels of reinforcement for later tasks.

Sometimes there is an overreliance on tangible food rewards. While the child may desire a particular food reward highly and never seem to become satiated, it is important to keep in mind that administering reinforcers is intended to organize a motivational system. Over time, the goal is for the child to be able to function in a teaching environment that is less restrictive than the one in which the teacher must wear her apron with the pretzel-sticks pocket.

Exposure to Short (Discrete) Trials. Discrete trials may be particularly beneficial for young children with short, underdeveloped attention spans. It allows tasks that are presented to be kept simple and for success to be easily within reach. As has been discussed, this format can make a crucial contribution to developing attention, compliance, and cause-and-effect reasoning. Trials can be kept varied and short to increase attending.

Discrete trials should really be thought of as a technique that is relevant as long as a child has a short attention span and needs many practices to learn to perform a skill independently. Most children who benefit from DTT may, after six months or a year, be able to learn without successive trials of the same task and without the repetition of serial trials of closely related activities (like receptively identifying all body parts, all farm animals, etc.)

Moving beyond Discrete Trials to Deliver Intensity: Additional Techniques. Discrete trials are not the only way to deliver one-to-one instructional intensity. Over time, the role of the adult as successive initiator of all teaching should naturally give way to the adult's being able to follow the apparent interests and queries of the child. This can include addition of explicit features of the pivotal response training (PRT) model in which the child learns to asks questions or needs to provide an answer before the next interesting thing can happen. This may include having the child choose among drills that allow for more self-initiation of program activities. Constructive visual schedules of drills serve the same purpose.

Naturalistic Models for Preserving Intensity and Increasing Initiative. We hope and expect for the content of curriculum to move closer to the form in which teaching is carried out with other children at the same developmental level. However, many children may still be receiving instruction in a one-to-one format, still be receiving (much more limited) motor prompting, and still be receiving external reinforcers for task completion, even after other aspects of the initial methods are no longer needed. Are such teaching sessions discrete trials? Not any more. It's great when a child has made progress beyond the point of needing such highly specified teaching.

In the course of discrete trial teaching, the tutor or instructor must be very alert to any sign of the child's showing initiative. If the child lingers on a puzzle piece's shape, repeating "circle," have that child quickly draw a circle or discriminate a circle from a square that you draw. If a child identifies a bear on a flashcard as "Pooh," ask him to name Pooh's friends. Typical children learn through joint attention, which is essentially showing adults what they are interested in at the moment. If we want to make DTT teaching more developmental, it is important to look for such opportunities in the child receiving discrete trials in order to afford him those same opportunities for child-directed learning that a typically developing child has.

It's always interesting to me that many parents will still describe any one-to-one teaching as discrete trials, something that initially may sound inappropriate for a child who is now known to speak in sentences, make choices, and complete multistep assignments with only a little assistance. I'm not sure if parents think I won't think the teaching is important if it isn't called discrete trials or what. Typically I will say that I can't recommend discrete trial teaching for this child any longer because he needs more naturalistic teaching. It is only then that I learn what is really going on. It's sad to think that parents of autistic children can come to believe that their children will only be able to learn though contrived means like DTT and fail to notice the child's becoming more of a typical learner. I find it thrilling to see incidental learning emerge.

The point is that it is important to know whether a child really is receiving DTT and if he has developed a capacity to move away from it in order to consider how to add one-to-two (one adult-to-two children) instruction, small group instruction, a focus on more direct (non-external) reinforcers, and other systematic steps to further ready the child for entry into a more mainstream setting.

The *Sesame Street* Syndrome. When a timely transition from pure DTT to more child-initiated learning is not capitalized upon, some disadvantages of the DTT method may become evident. The first of these might be called the seventies' *Sesame Street* Syndrome. In the early years of *Sesame Street,* segments would be developed from a matrix of curriculum goals and methods of instruction.

Segments would be then be "test-marketed" by watching the eye fixations of a selected preschool-aged audience. Segments for which children did not show sustained interest were not aired. This methodology came under criticism when the first *Sesame Street* generation went to kindergarten and it was found that the teacher was not as interesting as a mop-topped insect singing "Letter B." There was concern that these children had become overly passive learners, waiting to be entertained more each day. Similarly, children receiving prolonged DTT learn to act passively ("sit good," "look at me") and think that then some fairly new fun activity will likely materialize within arm's reach. This is very different from more enriching learning experiences in which a child selects (or is guided to select) a preferred activity. If a child with autism begins to show spontaneous and additional interests in his instructional materials, and the interests are ignored and not incorporated into teaching, that tendency for self-initiated learning can be extinguished. This is the place where discrete trial teaching begins to require much more of a natural sense of teaching and less technical skill. The tutor eager to do "good" by getting all the drills done twice will likely be missing out on spontaneous teaching opportunities.

Consequencing Attempts versus Successes. A related problem occurs when the child becomes increasingly lethargic about discrete trials and often seems to be responding almost randomly, even with "mastered" material on "maintenance." In an admirable effort to keep instruction upbeat, incorrect and correct trials may (unintentionally) not be consequenced very differently with "Good try" and "Good touching alligator!" both said in a positive tone of voice. Especially if the child has limited receptive language and mainly comprehends the "good" or the tone of voice, he may respond as if on an intermittent reinforcement schedule— for making any responses since eventually some will be correct. In the bad old days, Dr. Lovaas recommended that a higher vocal contrast be drawn: a sharp, loud "No!" for a wrong response and a more buoyant voice for a correct one. For some children with whom this indiscriminant responding presents a difficulty, a sharper contrast still may be a helpful approach, especially in early stages of mastery.

ABA/DTT Burnout. A potential problem with an ABA/DTT program is the child's starting to burn out. Sometimes, parents have an intuitive feeling about this. A teacher may feel that DTT is a bad fit for this child. Taking some estimate of the child's likely degree of mental retardation into account when analyzing any increase in negative behaviors in the context of an ABA/DTT program is crucial to avoid over-drilling. The more mental retardation that is present, the more slowly the child will learn. A child pushed beyond capacity may suffer symptoms of burnout, developing aggressive and other resistant symptoms that emerge when instruction begins or when tasks grow more difficult. Treated simply as noncompliance, the symptoms will persist and the child's sense of helplessness at not being able to stop the task demands can generalize into defiant, resistant behavior across other settings. We all have things we can't learn. Some of us will never navigate with a map, play piano, or competently complete a tax return. Some children with autism will never learn colors or to talk. Persistently teaching piano to someone with no interest whatsoever in it is like continuing to use discrete trials to teach a concept beyond a child's developmental capacities. It is simply not true that anyone can learn anything if it is taught correctly. All of us, including children with autism, have our limitations.

Sometimes parents, at the suggestion of therapists or teachers, present the burned-out child for a medication evaluation to address the agitated behavior. (This is what, in chapter 2, was referred to as a "tertiary symptom"—and one that can best be addressed by changing aspects of the teaching that originally brought on the behaviors. Pulling back on the instructional content and intensity associated with the appearance of the undesired behaviors is likely the answer if the undesired behaviors abate when the program is slowed. Bad behaviors may have been the child's only way of letting us know he had reached his limits. Pushing beyond this point can create intractable behavior problems.

ABA and Problems "Operationalizing" the Concept of Mental Retardation. The "mental retardation" part of autism is often the hardest part of the diagnosis for parents to handle. This is made especially more difficult because of problems in measuring the exact extent of mental retardation. Mental retardation is not a fixed trait like a mitral-valve prolapse, but is a clinical state that can be ameliorated with treatment. It does not mean that the child can't learn. It does not mean that as soon as the child can demonstrate that he has learned something that a diagnosis of (some degree of) mental retardation is wrong. Behaviorally oriented psychologists do not always acknowledge mental retardation as a viable concept, since it is not a discrete behavior, but rather a collection of behaviors that, as a whole, constitute a qualitative state, the way a collection of behaviors make "toddlerhood" a qualitative state. Some parents are told by behavioralists that the decision to use an ABA/DTT approach doesn't hinge on whether or not the child with autism also has mental retardation. This is correct in the sense that the same behavioral analysis principles apply irrespective of the presence or absence of mental retardation. However, the rate at which new skills can be expected to be acquired and spontaneously used in functional contexts (the rate of development) will vary according to how much mental retardation is present. This is important to know because parents will often visit a couple of ABA/DTT programs before deciding to opt for one, or will go to a lecture at which videos of DTT are shown and assume that their child will acquire skills in the same manner as other children they may have seen. In reality, all children grow at different rates, and it can be very helpful to have a realistic idea of the growth that can be expected for a specific child for whom a program is being designed. The idea is not to discourage the parent of the more moderately or severely mentally retarded child with the limits imposed by the degree of disability, but rather to set up a calibration for progress so that there is a way to know whether a given program has been effective or continues to be effective. Without an expected developmental trajectory, any progress at all can be taken as a sign that a program is successful. All children will continue to progress, to some extent, due to developmental change alone.

Use of Task Analysis. A key feature of ABA/DTT methodology is the use of task analysis to examine and revise treatment procedures continually. Sometimes task analysis is referred to as "doing the ABCs" (antecedents, behaviors, consequences). Every response can be said to have an antecedent. The antecedent is what the child was asked to do to produce a response or behavior. Every behavior has a consequence in addition to having an antecedent. If the child produces the wrong response, the antecedent should be altered. The antecedent could be the level of prompting, but it often includes an analysis of the response made in error. Did the child respond because the object he was asked for was on his right, and he always responds with a choice of the object on his right because he reaches with his right hand? If so, a task analysis would suggest moving the object to the left 50 percent of the time, or holding the child's right hand so he must respond with his left. As tutors work one-to-one with children in ABA/DTT, they are trained to note errors so these can be discussed at weekly team meetings for task analysis. This is a very systematic and helpful approach to revising instruction.

Taking Data. One of the by-products of task analysis is the taking of continuous data during all discrete trials. Dr. Lovaas initiated this procedure with experimental subjects as he developed principles for teaching and revising his curriculum. One tutor worked directly with the child, while a second recorded results. In that context, his procedures were experimentally rigorous.

It is less clear, however, whether all tutors forever after need to take data on all trials of all tasks they teach. In chapter 6 we discussed how taking data during DTT or during any one-to-one teaching may disrupt the development of language pragmatics. Earlier in this chapter, we talked about newer studies that support more episodic data collection. If a child's response rate to a given receptive language drill is 50, 55, and 52 percent across three administrations in a day, taking data once a day may be all that's needed to indicate that further work on that particular drill should continue. If a child builds a block design with 12 blocks and gets 11 right the first day, 10 on the third, and 11 again on the fifth, taking data once in that week might have told us that the child is almost, but not quite, there. Narrative notes from a single weekly criterion test might be as useful for revising instruction as daily data sheets. Some information would certainly be lost, but would loss of that information have a momentous impact on the continuation and revision of ensuing instruction? When resources for developing a program are limited reduction of data taking may be a viable way to conserve resources. When a child learns slowly, the "shape" of his data will change slowly too, and collection of data can likely be reduced with minimal loss of fidelity. So there really are two concerns about continuous data collection in ABA/DTT programs: First, data collection can interfere with a natural interaction between child and adult; and second, absent a single case study, much data may be excessive.

ABA/DTT FOR TEACHING SPECIFIC SKILLS

Discussion to this point has focused on the use of ABA/DTT to develop methods of instruction for children with ASDs. It is clear that ABA/DTT techniques are very useful, can be very powerful, and if done well can move children from an initially very disorganized, learning resistant state into much more malleable, teachable little creatures. We did discuss several ways in which use of this powerful set of methods can go awry. Like a powerful medicine, it should be in the hands of professionals who understand teaching, child development, autism, and mental retardation—people who can diagnose problems that may occur in the administration of the treatment.

The reliance of ABA/DTT programs on lower-level tutors who usually have gaps in their knowledge of one or more of the above-mentioned areas is the real potential weakness in the model as it is most often implemented. On the other hand, many tutors are well trained and well supervised. Many, if not most, are better qualified than many classroom special-education aides who are also spending substantial amounts of one-to-one instruction time with children. (But, there are many classroom aides with broader bases of experience than many, if not most, DTT tutors.) The point is that the training and experience of those that have the most direct contact with the children will be a key determinant of a program's effectiveness.

ABA/DTT can be examined not just in terms of methodology, but also in terms of how well specific educational objectives are addressed by this model. Several of these objectives have already been mentioned, but we will now briefly focus on each to identify ABA/DTT's strengths in addressing specific autistic learning disabilities.

Advantages in Teaching Imitation. As part of initially developing compliance and attention, the child with autism is taught to attend to and copy the actions of another. This was discussed in terms of developing a template or action-schema that the child is subsequently able to generalize to other imitations. Certainly the first imitative act is hardest to teach, and each subsequent one is assimilated by the child more readily. Moving from imitation that occurs under instructional control (when requested) to imitation that occurs when the child sees something new and interesting is a second, and at least as big, a step. Getting a child to draw some new shape with a crayon, roll a different truck, or slide down a slide the way someone else did requires the use of stimuli that are very interesting, and a situation in which copying the other action is the main interesting thing to do.

These situations are much more difficult to contrive than a nonverbal imitation drill. However, for many children, the teaching of the first step (like nonverbal imitation) primes the second step (like object imitation), and the second step in imitation arises more spontaneously. Motor imitation is virtually always easier to teach first in a preverbal child. Once the concept of imitation is in place with actions, it is a smaller step to develop verbal imitation. However, many preverbal children with autism don't seem to understand that they control their sound production, which may be intermittent and arise at unpredictable times, as described in chapter 5.

ABA/DTT, however, can still be an effective method for bringing vocalization under instructional control in the preverbal child if the teacher or tutor is prepared to drop everything and run to a mirror with the child as soon as he vocalizes, reinforcing each repetition right away with a high-value reward, repeating the child's vocalization, and showing him that she wants him to "Do this!" (as she imitates the mouth movement she just saw in the mirror). A full-motor prompt in this case might involve shaping the child's lips for the sound and then reinforcing any attempt on the child's part to respond by moving his lips upon request. While vocal imitation isn't speech and certainly isn't language, it opens the door for teaching both. Once spontaneously vocalized sounds are under instructional control, a lexicon of sounds, and then expressive words, can be developed.

Developing a Template for Receptive Understanding. The next objective addressed by ABA/DTT is often development of receptive understanding. For many children with autism, it is a big breakthrough when they realize that each and every object has a label. ABA/DTT methods are strong on using visual prompts for these identifications, a method that is very compatible with the most typical learning style of a child with an ASD, which is to compensate by attending more strongly to concomitant visual stimuli rather than auditory stimuli. A picture is produced, and the child is asked to "Touch bird"—at first with a picture of a bird, and then with pictures of a bird and of a dog to choose between. The subsequent step, which can be more difficult to teach, is helping the child understand that all actions (not just objects) have labels too. By demonstrating actions, ABA/DTT teaching can make these visual as well.

Disadvantages in Teaching Verbal Skills. One of the chief educational controversies surrounding the use of ABA/DTT to teach verbal skills focuses on how much the child is learning *speech* and how much he is learning *language*. Language learning occurs when a child has a general and abstract idea of a word meaning, a template that can be fitted against new possible examples and then judged to meet criteria for being an example of that thing. Speech occurs when a child utters a word that is associated with a specific example of a thing, but not when other versions of the same thing are presented. Obviously, we want children to learn language rather than speech. Speech and language therapists make this distinction, with the "speech" part of the work focused on articulation, clarity, and volume, and the "language" focused on semantics (words), pragmatics (communicative use), and grammar (sentence structure).

Behaviorists, on the other hand, often refer to "nonverbal behavior" or "verbal behavior." As was said earlier, such terminology originates in the theory that language is no different from any other complex amalgam of behaviors—like driving a car, which it would be argued, can be broken down into steps and taught, one component at a time. However, most experimental scientists now agree that language is qualitatively different from a behavior and underpins the ability to think in a uniquely human way. Language consists of an infinite number of combinations of words, all of which obviously cannot be taught. So what can children learn from behavioral approaches to teaching nonverbal and verbal behavior?

ABA/DTT teaches a lexicon, a dictionary that is being given to the child through specific examples rather than through general concepts. Just as is the case with developing spontaneous imitation of others, some children with autism are able to use the skills taught through ABA/DTT as a taking-off point for more spontaneous language use. If you were helped to memorize enough vocabulary words in a new language, your ability to "listen" in that language would improve and so then would your ability to speak that language. For some children with autism, the behavioral teaching of lexicon is just what they need to get started—and all that they need. For others, verbal expression becomes stuck at the point at which the child is described as needing to "generalize" his language, that is, to understand many examples of the word and when it can be used. Strategies for addressing this difficulty will be discussed in the section that follows this one as part of an examination of how developmental theories of language might be used to recast behavioral ones.

Language Pragmatics and Discrete Trials. In addition to knowing words, language consists of knowing how to use them: when it is your turn, what the topic is, what is considered a related comment, whether you need to clarify, and whether the individuals in conversation with one another are understanding each other. These conversational competencies are often referred to as "language pragmatics," and even in the highest-functioning individuals with autism or Asperger's syndrome, language pragmatics is the hardest part of language to handle because it is the most social part of language. There are curricula for teaching language pragmatics to an individual or to a group, and curriculum for "conversational drills" (an oxymoron). Indeed, once a conversation has been scripted, much of language pragmatics has been lost. However, for some higher-functioning individuals with very good rote memories, this kind of work may provide tools to improve social appropriateness of language in a limited way.

Advantages of Teaching Play. ABA/DTT is also used to teach children how to play appropriately with toys. Again, in some respects, "teaching play" is an oxymoron. Nevertheless, it is important for the development of representation, language, and socialization that children engage in play. (This was discussed in much greater detail in chapter 8.) By teaching specific play schema through nonverbal (and verbal) DTT imitation drills, the adult can introduce the child to new actions, ideas, words, and whole activities. This has the potential to broaden the child's repertoire of interests by introducing things the child might earlier have ignored or actively avoided. As the child learns functional and appropriate ways to use different toys, he is also becoming a more interesting and inviting playmate for other children—who may imitate or join him—even if he does not yet have the skills to spontaneously imitate or join in with others.

It is much harder to teach true imaginative play than to teach more concrete play (typical of children under three years old and in the sensory-motor stage). As is the case with other skills, ABA/DTT lays a foundation that enables some children to further develop. One of the reasons that more spontaneous play is hard to embed in any kind of a DTT format is that, by definition, it is something that comes from the child's self and is innovated as the play proceeds. Scripted play in the form of board games is certainly amenable to teaching in a DTT format, but more open-ended narrative play is less DTT-compatible. Once the adult takes the role of structuring and directing the play, it is no longer based on the child's imagination. (Some good examples of moving from DTT-taught toy use to scripted play were, however, illustrated in chapter 8.) Some of the best ways to move toward innovative spontaneous play involve teaching a script that is revised a bit each time it is played—a bit like improvisational theater. When children play, and especially when they play together using language as a guide, they often do completely silly illogical things like having the mommy make spaghetti for lunch, and then having the boy eat his lunch and then ride his spaghetti to the ocean to kill bad dinosaurs. Most adults don't play like this, and adult-scripted play tends to be tamer, especially in a DTT format, in which there's a script to follow. In the case of teaching play, imagination is where the utility of DTT ends and the need for peer teaching models kicks in.

ABA/DTT as a Springboard. It is clear that there are many uses for the ABA/DTT teaching model beyond developing attention and compliance. Basic aspects of imitation, verbalization, and play can be introduced to help the child develop a toolbox of words, activities, and actions. Some children with autism take these fundamentals and go on to "generalize" them, but development of the capacity to do this is only partly under the therapist's or teacher's control. Equally operative are the capacities of the child. For some children, the stopping point is the point at which ABA/DTT methods give way to more incidental learning. For other, lower-functioning children, the stopping point is the point at which the learning-to-learn skills of compliance, attention, and imitation have been established, a basic receptive and expressive (verbal or nonverbal) vocabulary has been established, and functional play has been taught. Rather than transitioning to learning from more typical and incidental models, these children are ready to use those skills in less restrictive environments and to achieve more independence through their ability to learn through task-analyzed teaching.

ABA/DTT and Inclusive Education. Most often, ABA/DTT agencies recommend placing the child with an ASD in a preschool with age mates. The idea is that exposure to age-appropriate models provides the opportunity to engage in the same behaviors spontaneously. A one-to-one aide who is an ABA/DTT tutor typically accompanies the child to serve as a shadow, an individual who can prompt the child to apply the specific behaviors he has learned through DTT.

Providing this opportunity to learn spontaneously as well as to use existing capacities to function more independently and in a less restrictive environment is definitely the way to go. Selecting the exact environment in which to provide these opportunities is a more complex matter than just selecting a preschool with peers of the same chronological age. In chapter 12, we'll talk more about inclusive-education models and considerations. For now, suffice it to say that the guiding principles for success in such inclusive experiences absolutely need to incorporate a couple of things: First, "priming"—using DTT to initially pre-teach things the child will see and do in the inclusive setting—-is needed. Second, you must select a setting in which one-to-one peer training and integration with a classmate can be achieved prior to school entry. Third, the child with autism needs to be included with developmentally comparable peers, especially language-comparable peers, in order to comprehend and benefit from the school milieu.

INTEGRATING A DEVELOPMENTAL PERSPECTIVE
WITH THE ABA/DTT MODEL

Developmental School Placement. A good place to start talking about how a developmental perspective can be used to inform the ABA/DTT model is to start where we just left off—integrating the child into a setting with peers. A capacity to imitate others is probably the most critical skill acquired in an ABA/DTT program that is a prerequisite for any successful group-based educational placement. After development of some imitation capacity, a shadow-aide can support the child in imitating others instead of just imitating the tutor in the ABA/DTT program. (In chapters 4 and 8, which concerned development of play and social skills, there were more ideas on how to do this.) For the purposes of the present discussion, suffice it to say that one should consider what kinds of imitative models will be present when a program is selected as an opportunity for a child with autism to start to learn imitatively from others.

The smallest incremental step that we can arrange for a child with autism with respect to learning imitatively from peers is placing the child with peers who engage in play like the child's own. Most children with autism who have developed some early play skills are not yet playing with toys the same way as others their age, but usually more like a somewhat younger child. It can make sense, therefore, to provide an opportunity for the child to be placed with others at their *developmental* age rather than their chronological age, at least to begin. This will allow the child to focus on imitating peers instead of an adult, and imitating without a discrete trial prompt. In terms of intrinsic reinforcement, imitating familiar and preferred play should be more self-sustaining than imitating unfamiliar and developmentally more advanced forms of play.

Developmental Language Teaching. A major remaining challenge for those using ABA/DTT to teach children with autism, and especially to teach them functional language use, is what is often referred to as "generalization difficulties." This means that the child has mastered an SD and sometimes even multiple SDs for a particular object, but still doesn't seem to have a "general" idea of what constitutes that object, so when a new example arises, the child has difficulty identifying the object.

This generalization problem manifests itself in either receptive or expressive word use. In this case, the child has problems moving beyond scripted sentence use, such as "I want ___, please, mom" or " A ___is an animal." These types of sentences may have been taught with 20 fill-ins (SDs) each. So, the child may know that "a (pear/hamburger/cheese/orange juice) is a food," but not be able to say, "Mom, I want food," or "Mom, I want something to eat," which would be a novel combination of specifically taught elements.

One way to promote generalization would be to reorganize how ABA/DTT receptive and expressive language drills are constructed so that the teaching of vocabulary more closely resembles how a lexicon is established in a typically developing child. A typically developing child can be characterized as developing a lexicon "horizontally"—learning many different examples of a concept in close temporal proximity. A child in an ABA/DTT program acquires vocabulary more "vertically," learning many examples of a classification via one kind of stimulus at a time (like flash cards of parts of the face, or a box of rubber farmyard animals, or a kit of life-sized plastic fruit). An example of "horizontal" language acquisition that builds in 'generalization': A typically developing 11-month-old Sarah is in the bathtub. Sarah gets soap up her nose in the course of having her hair washed and looks like she's going to cry. Her mother distracts her by wiping the soap bubbles off her nose with a washcloth and makes it into a game, saying, "I've got your nose!" The ploy works and Sarah giggles, so her mother reaches into the tub, puts bubbles on her own nose and then wipes them off, saying, "I've got Mommy's nose!" Since Sarah has watched with interest and, after a delay, smiled at this sight, her mother takes the washcloth and wipes Sarah's nose again, this time exclaiming, "I've got Sarah's nose!" This goes on for another five turns, and Mom is getting a little bored, though Sarah is still into it. So, Sarah's mom grabs Bathtub Barney, dramatically piles soap on his nose, and then wipes it off saying, "I've got Barney's nose!" After the bath, Sarah is having a story read to her before bed, and in the story sees a reindeer with a big red nose. She spontaneously points to it, looks at her mom, and says, "Nuh-nuh." Her mom says, "That's right! The reindeer's nose! A big red nose!"

In this example, nose was learned from a live three-dimensional example involving the self (Sarah), another (the mother), a three-dimensional object (Barney), and a two-dimensional object with yet another identity and a different-looking kind of nose (the reindeer). The initial mastery of the concept was begun with four different SDs (thinking of it in ABA/DTT terms), and the concept to be taught proceeded from an interest demonstrated by the child, not from a list of receptive vocabulary to introduce. Assuredly, the mother did not finish putting Sarah to bed, and run and tell Dad that Sarah had mastered "nose," and then said, "What body part do you think we should do next?" Yet mastering one or two words at time with just one SD is, essentially, how vocabulary is taught to children in ABA/DTT programs.

It is possible to use the DTT format to maintain the intensity of the teaching and the shaping of the responses when doing receptive and expressive vocabulary drills, but change the structure of the content. Multiple objects could be presented, and the one that seemed to receive the most attention ("What do you want?") could then become the subject of a drill. If the child chose a small rubber Barney from a bin of figurines, the drill might be to find Barney's nose for several trials. Then a bin of face puzzle pieces might come out and the "nose" discriminated from a choice of two—or even presented by itself. Next, a picture book (in which someone is bound to have a nose) could be used to find some noses there. Generalization could be tested by reversing the process: After introducing and practicing the names for numerous body parts, new two-dimensional and three-dimensional examples of each body part could be used to test whether the child had indeed formed a concept of each body part.

ABA/DTT as Method but with Developmentally Based Teaching. The common theme of the two foregoing discussions of "developmental" school placement and "developmental" language teaching is the ways in which central elements of the ABA/DTT model might be informed by what is known about how typically developing children develop skills. The hypothesis being advanced is that if we can start children with autism learning the same content as typical children (though the methods used, the DTT needs to be there to compensate for learning style differences), we may be able to create the momentum needed for subsequent learning to be self-generative, taking advantage of some of the same internal motivators that organize typically developing children at the same states of development as they start to see "general" patterns.

WHAT'S APPROPRIATE FOR THE YOUNGEST CHILDREN?

Another developmentally oriented question about ABA/DTT is how intervention can be made meaningful for the youngest children. As awareness of early signs of autism grows, and awareness of autism increases, children are being identified earlier. In one study going on in my research group, we serendipitously ended up with seven children each of whom was the second autistic child born to their parents. Needless to say, these babies had been watched with eagle eyes from day one, and some these children showed enough specific signs of autism to be diagnosed in the first half of the second year. A couple of these kids had older siblings (three- or four-year-olds) in ABA/DTT programs. In one case, the parents' first response to the diagnosis was to put the newly diagnosed 13-month-old, Jack, into an ABA/DTT program right away. Is this what should be recommended? If it were recommended, how would you do it? How much?

Jack's diagnosis was based on lack of eye contact, lack of social reference, lack of reunion comfort after separation distress, lack of pointing, and narrow, repetitive play activity. Jack also had very limited receptive language and very limited vocalizing, but that could be a language disorder as seen in up to 25 percent of siblings. He had a history of poor attention span—even for a 13-month-old—but that could be infancy. Jack still took two solid naps each day.

I was not comfortable with an ABA/DTT program because Jack was not a preschooler; he was really still just a baby. No one should expect a typical 13-month-old to sit in a preschool chair pushed up to a matching table, so why would that be appropriate for a child of the same age with autism who has even less understanding of what "work" and a table and chair are supposed to mean?

Gearing Way Down Developmentally. What do kids do before they sit in chairs? Young toddlers are supposed to explore on their own in a fairly undirected manner. That's a starting point for modifying an intervention plan. Ideas for very early intervention can be drawn from a number of methodologies, and those will be discussed as we discuss each of those methods. As far as using discrete trials, the demand for attention and compliance really should be indexed to the child's developmental level. Developmental level will be hard to estimate in a young autistic toddler, but likely it will be less than chronological age. If we now think of a 13-month-old with autism as an eight-, nine-, or ten-month old, what are likely to be meaningfully understandable activities changes even further. In the second half of the first year of life, developmentally, the child is just getting started with sensory-motor experiments, just starting to learn cause and effect (think busy boxes and pushing a button or turning a dial to see Elmo pop up). Appropriate intervention should consist of these same kinds of early causality toys, but perhaps with massed trials that ensure that the child has a more intensive learning experience than he might have from his own undirected play.

There is no point in having the toddler "Stand up!" to teach compliance, because most babies at the eight- to ten-month developmental level can barely, if at all, understand such requests. Teaching receptive vocabulary to babies can hardly be considered remedial either. At this age, babies and toddlers are engaged with the primary inputs coming from their senses, things that can be used to make sounds, things that produce different textural experiences, things that move. Using a discrete trial format to teach the child to choose and control stimuli of these sorts, without allowing for the formation of perseverative patterns, may help entrain exploration and decrease the self-reinforcing tendency for perseveration found in autism.

Sensory-Motor Learning: Choice, Motivation, and Self-Initiative. At the beginning of this chapter, there was discussion of how many (though not all) ABA/DTT programs can trace a direct lineage to Dr. Lovaas. Here in California, most DTT tutors and virtually every senior therapist or case manager in an ABA/DTT program is connected to Dr. Lovaas's academic "family tree"—though some removed by several generations. A lot of tradition in practice has been handed down. The majority of non-public agencies providing ABA/DTT services are much more influenced by this apprenticeship tradition in learning to do DTT than by fresh interpretations of the literature or by ongoing research. Nevertheless, key behavioral research centers produce ongoing work that has changed the treatment practices of a growing number of providers. As educators adopt ABA/DTT practices, they have been particularly willing to implement new ABA research ideas along with longer-practiced ABA/DTT methods.

Pivotal Response Training. One major contribution has been work on pivotal response training (PRT). Many of the methods are the same with massed trials, shaping, and task analysis. The content, however, is organized a bit differently. The guiding principle is to teach things that will help the child learn other things.

For example, heuristics. If a child, through DTT, can be taught to ask "What is it?" (and when he's told can repeat the object's name and then play with it), he will likely ask for it by name again later because asking for it by name is associated with the object's desirable use. Francis, age four, sees his tutor is holding an interesting new helicopter that launches its top propeller when you pull a rubber band. He watches; she plays with it. She prompts him to say, "What is it?" She replies, "It's a helicopter!" She says, "Francis, what is it?" He replies, "It's a helicopter!" His tutor gives him the helicopter for a moment. In a related activity, the tutor might wait until Francis tries but fails to use the rubber band to launch the propeller. The tutor says, "Francis, do you need help?" Francis has been previously trained to say "Help, please" when he cannot complete an activity, so he says "Help, please"; the teacher helps him pull the rubber band and launch the propeller.

Another example, a teacher has a pillowcase full of stuffed animals that feel very different—a snake, a giraffe, a porcupine, etc. First, the teacher reaches into the pillowcase and retrieves an animal, asking, "What is it?" and responding with the label of each animal as she removes it. Then, she hides one animal in the pillowcase and has a child stick his hand in the pillowcase; when he grabs an animal, she asks, "What is it?" and prompts an answer. Later, the activity is reversed, with the child putting an animal in the pillowcase and asking another pupil, "What is it?" The second pupil, with the teacher's help, is prompted to respond. This type of teaching preserves the repetition of the massed discrete trials but teaches the child a *heuristic*—a way to ask a question to continue an interaction, a useful skill that from the beginning has general applications.

CHAPTER CONCLUSIONS

The ABA/DTT approach presents several advantages for children with autistic spectrum disorders. It uses clear behavioral principles to establish a learning "contract" that for many parents of children with autistic spectrum disorders provides them with their first opportunity to teach their child directly and effectively. ABA/DTT addresses imitation deficit, and takes advantage of good visual spatial and visual motor skills, as well as good memory. For some children, this really gets the ball rolling. For others it develops initial learning-readiness skills that allow the child to benefit from exposure to education in other less restrictive educational settings.

In the next chapter, we will examine one of the widespread classroom-based methods for educating children with autism, the TEACCH approach. Like ABA/DTT, it is build around core autistic learning disabilities, but addresses them in different ways that may be viewed as a stand-alone method of intervention for some children, as a developmental progression beyond ABA/DTT for others, or as part of a combined approach that draws on various methods as needed.

CHAPTER ELEVEN

The TEACCH Curriculum

TEACCH AND AUTISTIC LEARNING DISABILITIES

A major organizing force in the development of classroom-based curricula for children with autism has come from the work at Project TEACCH at the University of North Carolina in Chapel Hill. Spear-headed by Dr. Eric Schopler, who founded and for many years edited the *Journal of Autism and Developmental Disorders,* this approach to teaching children with autism was the first to utilize what, in the terms used in this book, are autism learning disability-specific methods. TEACCH is an acronym for *T*reatment and *E*ducation of *A*utistic and Related *C*ommunication-Handicapped *Ch*ildren.

TEAACH is built on exploiting the relative strengths and preferences of individuals with autism by creating learning, working, and living environments that might be called "autism-friendly." The guiding philosophy of TEACCH is to create learning and living environments that, as much as possible, are in synch with who children and adults with autism are. Many features of TEACCH take advantage of what children with autism do best—like organizing their worlds visually. Other features of TEACCH take potential limitations of the child with autism and turn them into strengths—like creating a very routine-based school day that appeals to children who prefer rigid, predictable routines.

STRUCTURED TEACHING

TEACCH, like the ABA/DTT methods that have already been discussed at length, are based on the use of principles of applied behavior analysis. Rather than a more purely Skinnerian application of ABA (like DTT), TEACCH emphasizes the use of known rules and predictable consequences when the rules are followed. In the case of the TEACCH program, the rules can pertain to learning adaptive behavior—like where to put your coat and lunch box when you come in a classroom. Rules can also pertain to how classroom work is completed—like where you look for a new assignment, and where you put finished work. It is always possible for the child to have some visible structure to which to refer, so that he understands what he should be doing at a given moment. The visible structure may take the form of picture-based schedules, placement of curriculum materials in particular locations in the classroom, or work assignments with the same structure (like a basket with a file folder of pictures to organize in some way) but varying content day-to-day.

COMPARING TEACCH AND ABA/DTT MODELS

Structured Teaching versus Discrete Trials. The term "structured teaching" is often associated with TEACCH classrooms. Structured teaching refers to procedures that make instruction systematic and predictable in organizational or temporal structure. Unlike the concept of "discrete trial training," there usually is not as much micro-management in "structured teaching." Discrete trials are structured virtually second-to-second, with frequent prompts to keep the child actively engaged with the materials. By contrast, the child in the TEACCH model is also continually under instructional control, but in the sense that there is always a task he should be doing or a place for him to be. Structure may be provided by adults, materials, physical organization of the environment, or routine. In the TEACCH model, there generally is more leeway for the child to self-initiate action with teaching materials. The child is always given an opportunity to figure out what he should be doing or how he should be doing it, and, if at all possible, the chance to get going under his own steam. This contrasts with DTT, in which, after a fixed (and brief) interval, prompts at predetermined levels are administered. If the child derails or falters in the middle of a task, a TEACCH-trained teacher is more likely to give the child longer to repair his own off-task behavior and refocus himself. Acquiring the ability to self-direct and to revise a problem-solving strategy is rightfully seen as a critical part of the learning process. An ability to engage in and monitor one's own self-direction is seen as key to independent learning, and increased independence is seen as an overarching goal. This type of approach can be contrasted to ABA/DTT, in which the child is more "scaffolded" by a higher level of prompting and redirection. ABA/DTT likely leads to a higher rate of tasks being fully completed with accuracy, but with more prompts and therefore less independence and self-reflection in reaching a solution. In TEACCH, there is more room for independent problem solving in assimilating an understanding of a new idea or problem.

Self-Initiative versus Compliance: Which Takes You Further? Another way to characterize differences in the internal thinking processes that accompany TEACCH versus ABA is to say that TEACCH is a way of solving problems from the "inside out" rather than in discrete trials, which is more of an "outside-in" process. Solving from the "inside out" means the child's actions are guided by his internally motivated actions as he attempts solutions to a problem. Solving from the "outside in" means using the shaping procedures of ABA (like motor-prompting) to move through a problem, gradually fading "outside" help until the task is independently mastered. In many ways, the processes set in motion by the TEACCH procedures more closely resemble how a typically developing child solves a problem on his own—in fits and starts, with increasing accuracy and perseverance as the task becomes familiar and is fully mastered. Imagine the parent of a five-year-old who is good at puzzles presenting the five-year-old with a 50-piece map of the United States and letting him work it out, while the parent stands by to answer any questions the child has or to respond to any comments the child makes. In an ABA/DTT model, the child is first given the puzzle one piece at a time, perhaps north to south, east to west, with the parent providing verbal instructions like "New Jersey goes under New York." Let's assume that both children develop the ability to independently complete the puzzle accurately within a week of receiving it. If I had to guess, I would guess that the first child, who mastered the puzzle on his own, had more fun, and the child, mastering the puzzle with lots of parental guidance, learned to do the entire puzzle without help more quickly.

One of the greatest challenges of teaching children with autism is their lack of motivation to do all the things that other people do just because other people do them. The first parent in the above example allows the child more self-initiative, and the eventual reward of completing the puzzle serves as a positive reinforcer to that child for that initiative. The second parent has allowed fewer opportunities for self-initiative and more opportunities for successfully following directions. The child's eventual success in that case serves to shape a learner who follows directions and is compliant, but may not be as able to operate successfully when the situation demands independent problem solving.

The foregoing example was of two typically developing children. Here's an example of how a task might be taught to a child with autism using TEACCH versus DTT. If Bernard, age three was completing a new form board in a TEACCH setting, he might reach for a form board, which would have been placed in a specific location he had come to know as the place to look for his first task of the morning. This would be the first of his three work baskets. He would put the puzzle on the table in front of himself independently, and decide independently which piece to place first. He might solve by trial and error, sliding the piece (say, a trapezoid) around until it fell in the correct cutout, or he might look at the trapezoid first, orient it, and decide on the correct cutout and place it directly. He would likely not be verbally prompted during this process as long as he appeared to be actively problem solving. If Bernard were being given the same form board as part of a DTT task for the first time, his tutor would place the puzzle in front of him and likely choose the trapezoid for him. If Bernard did pick up the trapezoid piece within, say, five to ten seconds of being told "Put it in!" he would likely be motor (and verbally) prompted to "Put it in," his hand guided through the first successful placement, after which he would be verbally praised. He might even be praised with a food reward. The timing of initiation of an attempt to place the trapezoid would be up to the tutor, not Bernard. The tutor would likely keep the pace of instruction brisk and engaging. Let's say that placing the trapezoid was a relatively difficult task for Bernard. When he did the puzzle using the TEACCH method, it might have taken him three or four times as long to place the piece the first time. On the surface, it might seem that there was less learning with the TEACCH model because it took longer for the child to place just one piece. The instruction might be judged to be less "intense." Working with a one-to-one tutor using the DTT method, Bernard might have gotten all three pieces of the form board completed in the time he would have taken to complete just one piece on his own. However, with TEACCH, several key things happen differently, just like in the example of the typical five-year-olds doing the maps of the United States. There is more opportunity for child self-initiative with the TEACCH method. The task doesn't start until the child does something. (Had he not started independently, or seemed confused about what to do next, his TEACCH instructor could have cued him by pointing to his first assignment containing the form board or helping him place it on the table in front of him, and then stepping back as soon as it seemed that he could take over. Self-directed behavior is further reinforced in the TEACCH method when the child finishes the form board: He puts the puzzle back in its basket, places the basket in the place for finished work, and takes up the next basket of work. In the DTT model, by contrast, the successful child tends to do the things he has been most reinforced to do: He sits passively when the task is completed, waits for praise and other reinforcers that might be used, and then waits some more as the tutor clears the puzzle from the table, and sometimes waits while the tutor takes data, before she introduces the next task.

Often, observers seeing a TEACCH task like the one just described for the first time, see it as a less intensive intervention than an ABA/DTT administration of the same tasks. While it's true that the teacher is usually more active with the child in the ABA/DTT model, the child is having the experience of being more independent in the TEACCH model. Since one TEACCH task can follow another with no pause for changes of material or data taking, the actual time the child spends using each approach is likely comparable. Some of the child's time in the TEACCH model, however, is spent organizing—getting out his task and putting it away. This part of the activities, in a strict sense, is "extracurricular," but it is, arguably, a functional, adaptive part of learning to learn.

ASPECTS OF THE TEACCH CURRICULUM

In the TEACCH model, interactions between teacher and child resemble those in a classroom for typical children at the same developmental level, with the teacher stepping in when the child seems to get stuck. The intensity of the learning experience comes from the inclusion of tasks specifically tailored for the child, the breadth of tasks that over time increases duration of independent work periods, and the specificity of each task, structured in a way that makes clear when the task is finished.

Visual Schedules. One of the key aspects of the TEACCH method that is particularly advantageous for children with autism, particularly for the preverbal or nonverbal child with autism, is the use of visual schedules. Visual schedules very much reflect the inner mental organization of the child with autism who can "think in pictures." Each picture can and should serve as a "freeze-frame" of the child's internal video that guides goal-directed behavior. The prototypic visual schedule is a long, vertical strip of Velcro mounted on a piece of poster board, topped with the child's photo with his name written on it. The most informative work schedules have each child's Velcro strip mounted on its own color poster board to provide an additional cue to help a young child, or a child very new to TEACCH, find his personal schedule accurately. Pictures of major daily activities are itemized using a series of pictures that attach to the Velcro in the order in which the events will occur.

In a TEACCH class, the pictures could be photographs, Mayer-Johnson icons (graphics), or written words. Each of these kinds of icons represents increasingly symbolic and visual ways to represent an object or action. It is important that the kind of icon used with each child corresponds to how symbolic his thinking is. Icons that are much more symbolic than how the child thinks don't represent exactly what a child has "in mind." The match of the right kind of icon is important for "talking in pictures" in a way the child will readily understand. If icons are too abstract, it can be confusing, and therefore less motivating, to children with more marked communication difficulties. My predilection is to err on the side of being too concrete rather than too symbolic in the selection of icons, so as to make being successful with the picture schedule as easy for the child as possible.)

Some TEACCH programs have all pupils' daily work schedules in one location in the classroom. In other classes they are spread out, such as at each child's workstation. Each child comes to know the location of his work schedule. A daily work schedule for a kindergartener might show his cubby with his backpack and jacket in it, the reading center (where he can go after arrival and before circle time), his chair with his name on it for circle time, a small group work table for a group task that will follow that day's circle, his workstation, the snack table with snacks laid out, the bathroom, the playground with a picture of a preferred playground toy, another workstation picture, a picture of his speech and language therapist to indicate when he'll go to speech therapy, and a picture of a special closing circle activity (like the cassette tape player to indicate music). These pictures would represent activities of 15 to 20 minutes' duration each and cover the morning's activities. The schedule could be individualized by day (for example, there would be a picture of inside recess on a rainy day), by pull-out services to be received (a picture of the occupational therapist rather than the speech and language pathologist), or by goals on that child's IEP (perhaps a couple extra bathroom breaks if this was a period for focused potty training).

The teacher in a TEACCH classroom like the one just described periodically announces transition times with a bell or clean-up song indicating that it's time to start cleaning up, and another bell a few minutes later when it is time to "Check your schedule!" for the next activity. Children take their icons from their work schedules and carry them to the pictured location as a way of remembering what they are in the midst of doing.

Visual Schedules and Types of Icons. Initially, most children need schedules with photographs (or even three-dimensional objects) to know what to do and where to go. In the early days of using this a system, children may need full motor prompting to move from one activity to another. They learn the system of taking their photo (icon) from their personal activity schedule to the location at which the activity will occur. The icon, like the activity schedule and the schedule board at the location of the activity will also have bits of Velcro attached to it so that the child can remove his icon from the schedule to its new location. The teacher later collects the icons that the children have placed at the activity location. At circle, there might be a board that says "We came to Circle today . . ." with a Velcro strip for all of the children to place their personal icons that show each child sitting at a chair or mat. Alternatively, for those children who are still very isolative and unaware of routine beyond their own immediate world, a place to attach the "circle time" icon to the chair or mat they use for circle time might make a clearer connection between the activity and the icon representing it. Within a class, different children, according to their abilities, might use different kinds of icons. In one class I visited, some children had photo icons with words, some had color or line drawing icons with words, and some had cards with written words only. By the time he reaches the "just words" stage, the child is basically just working off of a "To Do" list, like any organized person. The idea of picture schedules is to lend as much structure as necessary, but not more than is needed.

Visual icons can be used in different ways to promote independence and to move children toward preparedness to enter the organization of a typical early elementary class. For example, one TEACCH class of 12 children was divided into three groups, the "Blues," the "Greens," and the "Yellows." The teachers had prepared a board for each group of four children, with a picture of one child in each quadrant. Below their picture, she had placed an icon depicting their next assignment. At the conclusion of snack, she first asked all the "Blues" to raise their hands. (They had been given blue squares.) The Blues were dismissed first, and went to their "Blue" poster to get their respective assignments. While the dust was clearing from that transition, the teacher handed the "Greens" their green triangles. The Greens were asked to raised their hands and were then dismissed to their "Green" poster to check for their next individual assignments. The process more closely resembled the end of snack and the beginning of reading groups or some similarly tracked activity in a regular second-grade class than a "Check your schedules!" call in a TEACCH class. (This class contained a substantial number of children who were already partly mainstreamed, including some who were slated for a transition to full inclusion for the following school year.)

TEACCH and PECS. As we discussed in chapter 6, the PECS (Picture Exchange Communication System) model is a curriculum designed to teach preverbal communication skills to children with autism. Basically, PECS, or adaptations of PECS like VIA (Visual Interaction Augmentation—described in chapter 6), are ways to use visual icons to augment receptive or expressive meaning of spoken words in children with receptive and/or expressive language difficulties. A TEACCH class is a very compatible setting for a PECS or VIA program. PECS or VIA involve specific strategies like giving an icon to receive the corresponding object or activity. This fits closely with the TEACCH picture-schedule strategy of using icons to indicate activities that are about to be undertaken, are now finished, or may be planned. For a preverbal child, using both together makes a great deal of sense, and icons that sometimes might be placed on a picture schedule could be used interchangeably as PECS or VIA icons at different times, just like words are used in different situations. As long as adult-child contact around the icon also involves the adult's using the icon as a prop for verbalizing a word or phrase depicted by the icon, both methodologies can serve to increase receptive language and prime initial verbal approximations. As was pointed out earlier, in using either a TEACCH picture schedule or another visual icon for communication augmentation, it is always essential to support oral and paralinguistic communication simultaneously so that "augmentation" does not become "substitution."

Workstations. A central feature of TEACCH programs is the use of workstations. A workstation is a small, somewhat confined area within the classroom in which the child has access to a set of assignments (usually three at a time). The workstation has a place to sit, a place for the work to be spread out, a place at which assignments waiting to be completed are kept, and a "finished" basket in which completed assignments are placed. The idea of using three tasks to comprise a single workstation assignment is that this configuration constitutes a "beginning," "middle," and "end" to an assignment, allowing the pupil to comprehend in a straightforward way when he is "getting started," "in the middle," and "almost finished." Children (Western children, anyway) learn to use workstations from left to right to prepare them for the concept of reading.

Each of the three baskets of work is coded with a picture card such as a blue square, a red circle, or a green rectangle. When the assignment in the "blue square" basket is complete, the child puts the blue square card on a "Finished" card attached to his workstation, and places the completed work in a finished basket. In this manner, the child can represent to himself, as well as to a supervising teacher, where he is in the completion of his assignments. In some classes, the icons used on each work basket are ones that are particularly interesting or motivating to the child, such as Winnie the Pooh characters, dinosaurs, or race cars. This way, the child has a chance to interact a bit with a favorite object as he does his work. The icons on each work basket might also foreshadow the content of the work, with Winnie the Pooh indicating a page from a Winnie the Pooh math worksheet or a picture of Piglet indicating a Piglet-decorated reading assignment on which lines are to be drawn between a dinosaur name and a picture of that species of dinosaur (something more interesting to many children with autism than a simpler assignment on which lines are drawn between the name of a color and a patch of that color).

Physically, workstations consist of a small self-contained work cubicle with the pupil facing a blank (non-distracting wall); there is a small shelf directly above, or to one side of, the pupil. The work space often resembles a child-sized library carrel. (Many of them *are* library carrels, as elementary school libraries have largely replaced their carrels with computer workstations.) Typically, the carrels are placed at 90-degree angles from one another so no one is constantly within the personal space of anyone else. A classroom might have an eight-foot square area walled off by a couple of those partitions now so popular in the world of adult work cubicles, with one carrel placed on each of the three solid sides of the cubicle. The idea is for children to learn to work independently without becoming distracted by nearby activity. As each of the three tasks are completed, finished work is placed in a "finished" bin (often a plastic laundry basket) for the teacher to check for accuracy later, if need be. Often, and especially with the youngest pupils, the work is monitored on an ongoing basis so there is no need for checking later. On the other hand, older pupils who may be completing a language comprehension or math worksheet may have to wait, (just like they would in a typical elementary class), to have their work checked before being dismissed for a break. Skills like raising your hand to let the teacher know you are finished help prepare a child for rules they may encounter in an inclusive educational setting.

When children are working at workstations, the level of supervision and prompting needed is likely to vary enormously as a function of how familiar the child is with working at a workstation, how developmentally advanced he is, and how difficult or new his work is. All those factors being equal, most classrooms will need one supervising adult for every two (or perhaps three, more advanced) pupils at workstations. Initially, some children will need one-to-one supervision to learn to self-monitor at a workstation. This may be especially the case for children coming from programs with substantial periods of one-to-one teaching. Such children may have developed a degree of prompt-dependence with a teaching adult and need gradually fading assistance to become more independent learners.

The adult supervising a student at a workstation is there to teach: redirect, prompt, correct, and praise success. Teaching intensity should be high enough to keep the child engaged with the teaching materials, but not so high as to "motor" him through his task. This use of highly structured teaching results fairly naturally from how a class's workstation area is set up. (However, I have visited classes with poor implementations of TEACCH. In one, a child at a workstation stared quietly into space, not looking at work materials for more than five minutes while a rather sedentary aide sat directly behind him, also staring into space. Finally I asked the aide when she might engage this pupil, and she replied, "He's doing TEACCH—you're not supposed to help: It's an independent work time." How this woman thought this child was supposed to learn, I don't know.) Teachers (and aides) need to teach, meaning, among other things, that the teacher needs to intervene when pupils really get stuck. TEACCH offers a structure for promoting and organizing that learning in which there is opportunity for both independent learning as well as guided learning.

Gradations of Structure in a TEACCH Class. After the child working in a carrel has learned to complete three assigned tasks in a row with little difficulty in staying on task, he can be moved on to a less restrictive and more social workstation arrangement. In one classroom, pupils who had "graduated" from carrels were moved to cooperative work tables, the type usually used in elementary classrooms for four to six pupils at a time. At the first table, the pupils still had workstations in the form of corrugated cardboard boxes in which three sides out of six remained; these sides, each two-and-a-half-feet high, were attached to the table with duct tape, creating four distinct workstations at which pupils sat close to one another, but could not see one another's work or see one another working as they leaned into their assignments. At a second table, the same arrangement was in place, but the teacher had cut the three-sided boxes from to a height of about six inches—just enough to keep each child's workstation separate from the next child's. At a third table, separate "workstations" were indicated only by the presence of masking tape dividing the table into quadrants. As the routine of the workstation became ingrained, the pupils gained skills in self-directed, sustained independent classroom work. This system allowed pupils to move into increasingly less restrictive learning situations for individual seat work.

TEACCH and Individualization of Instructional Content. A core advantage in a TEACCH classroom is that individual baskets of work at workstations allow classroom staff to individualize curriculum content to that student's pace and interests. In a special day class, children are typically at different ability levels in different areas of learning. One student may sight-read, while another may read phonically. One student may have emerging one-to-one correspondence (learning that the number "2" corresponds to two objects, not three), and another student may be working on three-place subtraction with borrowing. Pupils with autism can have dissimilar degrees of disability in certain areas but may all have only single word or phrase expressive language—so there are some activities they can work on as a group. In areas in which an individual pupil has special challenges, the pupil will need a more intensive focus, and this can be accomplished at his workstation. In areas in which a pupil has special talents, these can be addressed with opportunities to move ahead in that area while completing tasks at his workstation. Using the workstation system, tasks can readily be individualized in a way that addresses weaknesses as well as strengths.

Addressing Motivational Issues. Individualizing instruction by individualizing curriculum content is just one way to think about "individualizing" and educational planning. TEACCH does a very good job of this in the context of a special day class in which the biggest concern of parents is often that the overall level of teaching is going to be "too low" (or "too high") for their child. The time spent in workstations solves the problem by devising individualized tasks—just as can be done in an ABA/DTT program.

Content is one major aspect of "individualizing." Another is individualizing the motivational system that propels the child through the instruction. The TEACCH workstation approach addresses this motivational concern to some extent through allowing the child to choose which of his three work baskets he will complete next. Some children may spy a preferred puzzle and do it first; some may see a dislikable handwriting task and do it last. The idea is that having the ability to choose is what motivates the child.

Another approach, which will be discussed in more detail when we review model programs, is the "activity schedule" approach developed at PCDI—the Princeton Child Development Institute. Briefly, the child uses a loose-leaf notebook with poster board pages to select and order icons from a shelf lined with work baskets and then completes the work in the selected order. Unlike TEACCH, the "activity schedules" concept does not work in groups of three, nor does it necessarily involve work at individual workstations.

TEACCH AT HOME

More Formal TEAACH Programs at Home. In the 1970s when TEACCH was first developed, a prominent innovation was its inclusion of parents as co-therapists. At the time, this was a big breakthrough. Treatment for autism was just emerging from the "bad old days" when parent psychotherapy to "defrost" so-called refrigerator parents was essentially the only route for involving Mom and Dad. When psychoanalytic theories of the origins of autism hit the trash bin, TEACCH was the first to define a positive role for parents. Over the years, however, while TEACCH continues to emphasize collaboration with parents as integral, surprisingly few see or use TEACCH as a home-based teaching program. There is no reason that implementation of features of TEACCH should be restricted to classroom use. There are a variety of circumstances in which it might be very helpful to use TEACCH methods at home, whether or not the child is placed in a TEACCH program at school.

TEACCH can work at home at least as well as a home-based ABA/DTT program. Having shelves of work baskets at home that can be selected for workstation tasks, as well as using picture schedules for daily home activities (like dinner then homework) can help the child consolidate the requirement for being responsible for himself both at school and at home.

Where Access to Special Education is Limited. For families far from any reasonably well-designed special-education services, home TEACCH programs can be particularly advantageous. Moms I've worked with—some from countries that have yet to implement the concept of special-education programs—have been able to teach their children at home using these methods.

A home-based TEACCH program can be set up just as it is in a classroom, with a small area of the home set aside for structured teaching. Parents of some children, especially those who live in areas in which there are limited special-education services specifically for pupils with autism, may find home workstations a particularly relevant approach for the child who has outgrown ABA/DTT and needs more opportunity to become less prompt-dependent and more self-initiating with his learning.

Project TEACCH at the University of North Carolina in Chapel Hill runs brief summer institutes to train teachers from overseas, giving them firsthand opportunities to see TEACCH classes in action and to get experience using TEACCH under supervision. These programs are often invaluable to families with little other access to special-education training.

Less Formal TEAACH Programs at Home. The most natural transition to implementing TEACCH methods in the home probably occurs when the child has become familiar with them at school. A home workstation can add time to the child's instructional hours and it can make the child more comfortable following more structured rules of behavior at home.

Home workstations are also a great answer to the "How do I keep him engaged and still make dinner?" question. Many parents who spend after-school hours in direct teaching tasks with their child feel overloaded or guilty when pulled away to make dinner or attend to other tasks, like helping siblings with *their* homework. It is, let's face it, not realistic to administer discrete trials while cooking dinner—even if you're the Microwave Queen. On the other hand, a workstation in the kitchen, where the child can work on a structured series of familiar tasks or do homework, can be a much better fit for a family's schedule at that time of day. Occasional supervision and assistance on workstation tasks can realistically be given if the child is engaged in tasks he knows and usually prefers. This doesn't have to be a formal arrangement, just a way of monitoring the child so he doesn't slip into mental-downtime activities. A dinner-time kitchen workstation may be a particularly nice counterpoint for a child who has had more structured DTT teaching in school or at home during the day and needs an opportunity for more self-directed activity.

Workstations can work well if they are an activity that can be carried out near siblings who are working on their school assignments in a quiet, calm atmosphere (meaning no TV, computer games, pop music, or other distractions). The advisability and practicality of using workstations in this manner will, of course, vary with the child and the family. For many families, it makes much more sense to use dinner preparation time or sibling homework time to allow the child with autism a video choice for a half hour or an hour to increase the likelihood that the other family activity is uninterrupted.

PICTURE SCHEDULES AT HOME

Picture Schedules for the Extracurricular Hours. A child who has a picture schedule at school can readily understand and use a home picture schedule that might show his after-school schedule as snack, computer time, outside play, a homework session, video, dinner, bath, and bedtime. Parents can put the schedule in a central place like the kitchen, and use small Velcros in each room in which the child would take the appropriate icon after "checking his schedule." This can help keep a child organized in several respects: It can show him what to expect, can help him listen for key words about an activity as it is about to begin, and can help build flexibility in dealing with small daily changes like no outside play because it is raining.

Picture Schedules to Design Routines and Assign Responsibilities. For those autistic children who are quite anxious about changes in routine, children who are not verbal, or children who frequently test limits and attempt to do prohibited activities (like turning on the TV at dinner time), this is a way of introducing and enforcing the idea that households need to have rules and that children need to follow them. It is really easy for parents of a child with a disability to feel sorry for the child and express it by not expecting at least as much from that child as from siblings at the same developmental level. This is no favor to the child or siblings. Picture schedules at home can also be used for siblings who may find it fun, especially preschool-aged siblings. A picture schedule that helps siblings negotiate difficult issues like planning a choice of videos: whose turn it is to choose, how many can be watched, and in what order to view the videos can be visually scheduled.

Picture schedules at home are a good way of using the power of choice making to develop a child's feeling of having some control over his life. This is especially important for the child who receives numerous and intensive interventions that fill many hours. For example, if the child comes home from school, like the child in the example above, and snack, computer time, outside play, a homework session, video, dinner, bath and bedtime are things that will happen during the rest of the day, the child might be given a choice about placement of all but his work session, (assuming a tutor arrives at a given time) and bedtime. If possible, letting the child choose whether he wants computer time before his snack, or wants to go outside after a video rather than before, allows him to take an active part of the process, not just be a passive recipient. As the child becomes aware of, and interested in, making these choices, the child simultaneously becomes more engaged in what is happening around him—because he has a role in it.

Involving the child in choosing the order of activities should not only make him more aware of what will be happening, but can be expected to drive the desire to communicate about these activities in broader ways. This means that even a child who can talk may benefit from a picture schedule at home because it gives him a (physical) framework for conversation about something he considers important, namely, what he has chosen to do.

Picture Schedules and the Routine-Bound Child. Picture schedules can be used to smooth other frequently occurring rough spots at home: A common one is going out in the car. The child may have a distinct preference about where he wants parents to go and may become upset when a change in route suggests that the destination is not what he has in mind. Placing a long strip of Velcro across the back of the car seat that the child sees from his own seat, and showing the order of stops to be made on a particular expedition from home, provides a way for the child to know what will be happening and to better listen to any discussion of the destination. This can be especially helpful if a route is changed. The child can "see" what is happening by referring to the picture schedule, and it can be used ahead of time to prepare the child for any change. Changes in routine depicted on a car picture schedule can be used to make the needed changes more inevitable. On other occasions, by giving the child some choices in organizing it, like on a Saturday, when he could choose whether to go to the park after MacDonald's or after the grocery store, can make using the schedule more acceptable. If there are siblings, letting each child make a choice is a nice way of teaching all children that they have an equal vote. Once a child makes a choice in the order of activities, he has made a sort of commitment to doing those things, and at least you know that he has a basis for anticipating them; this can only make compliance a bit easier and the likelihood of extended protest a bit less likely.

Picture Calendars. Sometimes, adapted picture schedules can be used at home to show main activities day by day for a week at a time: Some children, for example, have a hard time on Saturday because they get into the routine of going to school and seem to think that if they just find their backpack and lunch box and put it by the door that the school bus will come. A calendar by the door that shows the whole week and shows a school bus on the days that the child goes to school and some key activity on the days he doesn't can help resolve this sort of misunderstanding. When the child gets home from school each day, the picture of the bus (or school, or teacher) can be put away for that day. When there are no more buses left on the calendar, then there's no more school. This sort of system is also helpful in developing a concept of days, weeks, and months, which otherwise remain quite abstract for some children.

TEACCH AND INCLUSIVE EDUCATION

TEACCH for Integrated Preschools. To the best of my knowledge, the TEACCH model has not yet been implemented in typical preschools. It should be. Typical preschoolers love routine. They love being in control. They love knowing what's coming next. They love little baskets of things. These aspects of the TEACCH model have essentially already been popularized by Montessori schools. Montessori does not use picture schedules but many preschoolers would love these too. They would love all the Velcro.

Three- and four-year-olds are industrious and enjoy doing simple things that adults will see as successful and praise them for. While the Montessori curriculum is associated with specific materials designed to stimulate the development of specific kinds of mathematical and lexical understanding, there is no reason that the same or very similar materials could not be used as content for workstations in addition to common preschool-age TEACCH curriculum materials.

TEACCH and the Integration of the Child with High-Functioning Autism. Many higher-functioning children with autism do not really need a special day class because they are far enough along in age-appropriate academics, but are not yet ready to truly integrate into a group-oriented preschool. Preschools are very social places, and that's what the child with autism or PDD has the most difficulty. In a preschool class that interspersed workstations with free play, or workstations with cooperative activities (perhaps using workstations to "pre-teach" the cooperative activity task for the child with autism), the child with PDD or autism would have a better chance of participating more independently in the program. Picture schedules and routines would ease adjustment into a setting in which language is the coin of the realm.

Especially if some of the adaptations to the TEACCH model described earlier, like reducing the size of workstations gradually, are used, a child with autism could be systematically prepared for full inclusion in his preschool rather than just plopped into it with his shadow aide (or personal handmaiden) who may or may not really appreciate the challenges of integration. (We will talk more about this in the section of this chapter dealing with inclusive education.)

TEACCH AND THE ADULT YEARS

One strength of TEACCH is what the developers of TEACCH themselves sometimes refer to as a "cradle to grave" service delivery system. TEACCH methods can be adapted in content and procedure to be developmentally suitable for children at an early age and can continue to be adapted to provide structure for adults in a work setting, or those challenged by daily living. Parents of the youngest children, of course, are not likely to be as interested in this formulation as are parents of teenagers or adults, who have arrived at a stage of understanding what their child's full capacities will be and are thinking ahead to supporting the happiest, most independent lifestyle possible for their child as he moves into his adult years.

TEACCH for adults is often associated with supported employment for moderately disabled adults and with teaching daily living routines for more severely disabled adults. Adults with ASDs as well as adults with other developmental disabilities can benefit from methods that have been developed by TEACCH.

TEACCH and Adult Social Life. The TEACCH model has also been used quite successfully as a job-coaching model for cognitively unimpaired adults with high-functioning autism or Asperger's syndrome who have difficulties understanding and adapting to explicit and implicit rules at work or in higher education.

In North Carolina, where TEACCH is based, there is an extended community of adults with high-functioning autism or Asperger's syndrome who form a social nexus for one another, supported by key personnel from TEACCH. Like a community for seniors, the adults with HFA or AS come together for regular meals, recreational activities, or other social activities. Most have come to a point in life at which they recognize that they are most comfortable being around others with concerns similar to their own. Members of this group are at peace with their choice of primary reference group—just like seniors living in an assisted-care community. These individuals with HFA and AS may do many things independently, like drive or work in the community, but they have as their foundation, their community's professional staff to oversee and anticipate problems that might occur in the general (non-autistic) community in which they interact with non-ASD individuals who are not therapeutically trained to deal with them.

Job Coaching. TEACCH has a well-developed set of procedures for ongoing social contact with the TEACCH professional staff who make regular job-site visits to monitor how things are going and modify work schedules to help work go smoothly. A TEACCH job coach might explain autism to a job supervisor, negotiate adaptations in the workplace, and see that the adaptations benefit rather than inconvenience an employer. The TEACCH job coach might remain on site, full time for a day or two, or a week or two, depending on the job. All individuals being coached get at least weekly visits from their job coach—unlike some programs that provide higher levels of initial coaching and then pull back until a problem arises. Some sites employing multiple TEACCH clients have a full-time job coach on site. The TEACCH job coaching/supported employment model is more proactive and more social than anything else I've seen done with autistic adults who are most often clustered with other developmentally disabled individuals at home and work. The interactions between the job coach and the person being supervised function more like an employee-work supervisor relationship that a pupil-teacher relationship—more consultative than didactic.

Adaptations for ASD in the workplace include avoiding placing ASD workers in jobs in which there are hard-to-"read" social cues like being a food-server and having to realize when a customer might need something. However, work in a cafeteria line in which you ask a customer to choose a vegetable and then respond would likely come off much better. Quiet workplaces, like an office in which there is filing to be done, or in a store in which the worker might move stock would be preferable to a workplace where others might play a radio or chat about sports scores as they work. Jobs with strong routines, like starting each day by pouring soup into steam trays, then washing all the soup pots, and finally, washing all the steam trays are preferable to those which require that the person wash different kinds of items each day.

An individual who does filing, for example, might arrange to come to work very early and leave early to avoid times when many others are milling about. Another individual might work fewer hours, or take a shorter brief lunch to avoid socializing. The job coach might arrange for the work cubicle to be at the end of a row so that extraneous noise is minimized, and there's not a lot of traffic. TEACCH work schedules in the form of detailed daily "To Do" lists that might be put together jointly by the job coach and the employer. Employees are placed in jobs in which they can perform productive labor, not just do busy work. Doing a good job on a task selected to complement an individual's interests is seen as a major part of the reward. TEACCH job coaching is carefully fit to the individual so that on-site, one-to-one participation by the job coach is minimized. If the task must be taught hand-over-hand, it is not a good "TEACCH" fit, just like full motor prompting is discouraged for an elementary pupil learning to learn at a workstation.

Support for the More Challenged Adult. More challenged workers need more support. This might include working in a setting in which contact with others is minimized. For example, one TEACCH work site is in a high-technology park cafeteria. Most TEACCH-coached workers (and a few graduates) worked in the part of the kitchen in which they loaded, washed, or unloaded dishes, silverware, and glasses. A couple cleaned the enormous pieces of cookware used to prepare the food. One man had started out in the TEACCH-supported employment program, but for a number of years had washed as many pots as well and as quickly as other workers and was unionized, and being given a regular salary with benefits. After talking to him, it became clear that he was certainly autistic and that his language skill was likely around the five-year level. What was wonderful was the pride he obviously took in the cleanliness of his pots, the condition of his work room, and the performance of his job. Newer employees in the dishwashing room had picture schedules posted to show them that forks had to be loaded into the silverware basket first, then spray washed, and then loaded into the dryer. Another icon showed plate scraping and plate loading.

An icon showed where in the sequence of work tasks the lunch break would come. During lunch, the TEACCH cafeteria workers gathered at one table to eat and hang out with their on-site job supervisors who brought along each worker's pre-selected lunch leisure activities like a Game Boy or a coloring book. The idea that any of these individuals would be better served by taking a lunch break at a table with others not from their work program is anathema to the TEACCH philosophy. Everyone clearly was comfortable eating lunch together and being left to do their own thing. Occasionally, a job coach would point out the upcoming end of someone's lunch hour or the need to bus a tray, but virtually all of this happened independently.

What was most impressive about the TEACCH adult work program was that these adults were simply living their lives. There was no push to make something of themselves that they were not and demonstrated no interest in being. Most were adults in their twenties and thirties, probably in the mild range of mental retardation and also autistic. There was no press to structure a conversation among them, to make them sit at tables with non-handicapped fellow cafeteria workers, or to select "age-appropriate" leisure activities. They were accepted for who they were by their job coaches, and they accepted themselves.

A CRITIQUE OF TEACCH

Up to this point, the general principles of how a TEACCH curriculum functions have been described. But what are some possible concerns about TEACCH, as a treatment approach for autism?

The "Culture" of Autism. TEACCH comes from a philosophical perspective on autism that says, "This child sees the world differently. It is up to us to understand those differences and teach this child with an understanding of who he is, helping him emphasize his strengths and compensate for his weaknesses." The TEACCH philosophy is aimed at helping each individual fulfill his potential by learning to do things he can do well and that can provide self-satisfaction. By contrast, we could say that the "philosophy" of ABA/DTT is to normalize the child, to make him understand and value the same things as the rest of us, because we assume this will be his best shot at happiness. Proponents of TEACCH talk about the "culture" of autism. The "culture" of autism is a different world, in which it is OK for social interactions to be rather instrumental and kind of one-sided, in which there is no chitchat, and in which something is not likely to be fun just because you've never done it before.

This view of a culture of autism can be compared to work on the culture of deafness wherein some deaf individuals prefer the company of other deaf people, as exemplified by those at Galludet University in Washington D.C., the only deaf university in the United States. Many deaf individuals, some of whom have grown up in hearing homes (and felt "outside" of a subtle verbal joke, a parenthetical comment, or a comment modified by tone of voice) and some who are from families with two deaf parents, consciously choose to go to a deaf university in which interactions with friends, as well as instruction, is in a language they fully understand. These individuals do not see deafness so much as a handicap as a difference. If TEACCH is the center of an "autistic culture," is that good or bad? For individuals who want a choice (or families who want to offer a choice to their adult children), TEACCH is a valuable and unique resource. Others see it as segregationist and think it bypasses the presumed advantages of inclusion and integration. It is both, and clearly for some adults it is the right choice, and for others it is not—but it's hard to view having a potentially advantageous choice as an unqualified bad thing.

TEACCH and the Promotion of Verbal Communication. For younger children who receive TEACCH curricula in the preschool and elementary years, there are elements of a "culture of autism" too. One criticism that is leveled at some TEACCH programs is that the visual augmentation available through picture schedules is so advantageous for children with autism that it lowers the verbal "press"—the need to understand a word to know what to do, or to use a spoken word to express communicative intent. Just as there are better and worse ABA/DTT programs, there are better and worse TEACCH classes. In a good implementation of the TEACCH methodology, there is no less emphasis on language than in any other class for children with the same language develop-ment difficulties. The visual augmentation is a means the child can use to better understand what is going on, but it is intended as a bridge to supporting improved receptive and expressive skills. An inadequate implementation of a TEACCH curriculum on the other hand might allow a child to function without needing to listen to words or trying to express himself verbally even as the capacity to do so emerges.

Since TEACCH is not as "oral" an instructional milieu as other classes designed for children with autism, TEACCH programs are able to serve the most severely affected children with ASDs—those with functioning in the lower end of the moderate to severely mentally retarded range and with receptive language levels around or below the one-year level. For these children, especially ones in the older elementary years and above, the world of spoken words is beyond their grasp. For these children a more "silent" TEACCH class is not disadvantageous, as it might be for a younger child, with higher potential for spoken language development.

TEACCH and Opportunities for Imitative Learning. TEACCH worksta-tions are sometimes criticized as isolating, keeping the child from imitative models. If the child has not yet developed spontaneous imitation skills, this is not a real concern. If the TEACCH class has, and all do have, activities in addition to workstations, there will be plenty of opportunity for group participation with an adult (or peer model), such as singing and dancing at circle time. It is at these times that the relative isolation of one-to-one work is counterbalanced with ample opportunities to acquire imitation skills. In contrast, children in home-based ABA/DTT programs have no opportunity during instructional time to imitate peers (although they may imitate adults), and when placed in a typical preschool with chronological age mates, they often are deprived of this further by being presented with imitative models that are too sophisticated for them.

Many children with autism need the visual and sensory focus that the isolation of the workstation provides. Compared to an ABA/DTT program in which there are no opportunities in the program for modeling of peers, the TEACCH model can be seen as a step toward including peers as a learning model by interspersing individual with group work times.

TEACCH and "Intensity" of Instruction. A final criticism is that there is not as much one-to-one interaction in a TEACCH program as there is, for example, in an ABA/DTT program. This may be true. However, TEACCH classes undoubtedly have more intensive teaching ratios than non-special day classes, and often have more intensive teaching ratios than other classes serving children with autism. So, such an appraisal is relative.

In classrooms for typically developing children, a major challenge is learning the ways in which the teacher is different from your mommy. The classroom teacher is not there to anticipate what you will ask, know what you mean by what you say, or even understand your solipsistic way of relating your experiences. Part of the challenge for typical children in learning to be part of a class is to figure out how to wipe their noses—before others make fun. Having Mommy rush up with a tissue may have seemed so much simpler and more efficient. Similarly in a TEACCH class, the loss of constant one-to-one contact can be seen either as a loss of Mommy (who can make your every effort into success), or a baby step into meeting the challenges that arise when you need something and it looks like the best answer might be to try to help yourself. Children with autism are usually quite resourceful when it comes to helping themselves get something they want. TEACCH gives the child some opportunity to do this. Natural reinforcers are the breaks the child receives after the task is done.

Summing Up TEACCH. At this point in your reading, if you sit back and compare what has been said about TEACCH and what has been said about ABA/DTT, at least one theme will emerge: One is not always "better" than the other. There are times when one may be more appropriate than another. TEACCH may be appropriate as a step for a higher-functioning child with an ASD when he leaves an ABA/DTT program and is preparing to function independently in a mainstreamed class. This type of TEACCH class might use picture schedules and workstations, but also emphasize learning to work independently, follow directions, and participate in small-group learning. Another kind of TEACCH class may be appropriate for the child who has developed the basic skills of learning readiness from an ABA/DTT program, but has not been able (or ready) to develop oral communication and can benefit from a more visually organized teaching regime that takes a next step in learning by promoting the use of visual supports to move the child into a more independent, less prompt-dependent learning style. TEACCH can continue to be a relevant educational model for the nonverbal child with an ASD throughout the school years because of visual supports and routines—compensatory strategies naturally employed by nonverbal children. TEACCH can also be adapted to support employment and job-coaching strategies for adults, providing support through continued use of picture schedules for more verbally challenged individuals and through a wraparound "culture" of autism for higher-functioning adults with ASDs.

CHAPTER CONCLUSIONS

TEAACH, like ABA/DTT, is a method based on principles of behavior learning theory. In both methods well-defined contingencies and a high degree of fairly invariant structure are used to direct the child's learning. Both models are special-educational methods particularly tailored to some autism-specific learning difficulties. However, not all special-education services are delivered in the context of home- or school-based special-education programs. Sometimes specialized instruction is embedded in educational settings attended by typical peers. When a child with autism is put in the mainstream and given necessary accommodations so he can benefit from an inclusive educational placement, typically developing peers are seen as part of the treatment milieu. This third approach to educating children with autism will be discussed in the next chapter.

CHAPTER TWELVE

Mainstreaming That Works: Too Accommodating, or Really Including?

WHERE DOES INCLUSION FIT IN TREATING AUTISM?

Two main approaches for teaching children with autism have been described so far. Both the ABA/DTT approach innovated by Lovaas and the TEACCH approach innovated by Schopler are in widespread use in therapy and education programs seeking primarily to address the specific learning needs of children with autism. Not all children with autism, however, are in autism-specific programs. Not all children with autism are treated with just one modality. Not all children with autism are in special education.

In chapter 14 there will be discussion of curricula and treatment programs that involve combining different methods, such as classes that contain both DTT and TEACCH instruction units, or children home-based programs that are combined with special education. Other children are in general special-education classes with a variety of resource and therapy services.

Definitions. Increasingly, more eclectic programs draw on multiple approaches to teach children with autism by using a component of inclusive education. Inclusive education means that the child is educated alongside peers who are without developmental disabilities. Inclusive placements may be part-time or full-time. One type of inclusive placement, usually referred to as an "integrated" placement, includes a balanced mix of children with special needs and typical children. By contrast, the term "inclusion" is more often used when there are not more than one or two special-needs children in a classroom for typically developing children. There are schools that "include" children with autism just for non-academic activities like recess, physical education, assembly, music, or art. There are also schools that only "include" children with autism for academic subjects. This partial, selective inclusion is what, in the past, was more commonly referred to as mainstreaming. In this chapter the terms "mainstreaming" and "partial inclusion" will be used to refer to situations in which a child with autism is not fully included. The term "full inclusion" means just that—a child who spends all his time in general education, and none in a special-education class.

There is no single way to bring inclusion into the special education of a child with autism. In this chapter, we will consider how inclusive placements can work, when they may be the best choice and, if used, when and how they are likely to contribute to a child with autism's learning. Unlike ABA/DTT or TEACCH, the idea of inclusion has not been specifically devised to meet the treatment needs of children with autism. It is a tool for the special educator that is used under various conditions to serve children with the full range of educational, emotional, and physical disabilities. The fundamental principles of inclusion were not worked out with the needs of children with ASDs in particular in mind, as was the case with ABA/DTT and TEACCH, but have largely accumulated through practice, model programs, and theory that indicates ways to develop effective programs.

UNDERLYING LEARNING PRINCIPLES

Just as TEACCH has an underlying philosophy that involves accommodating the individual with autism's natural style of learning, and ABA/DTT is based on principles of applied behavior analysis with a focus on principles of gradual, error-free learning and strong reinforcement paradigms, inclusive education can also be described in terms of basic underlying principles.

Imitation. A key element to inclusive education is that placing a child with a disability alongside typically developing children will provide an opportunity for the child with the disability to model or imitate the more appropriate, more adaptive behavior of typical peers. This is a particularly interesting and central assumption to evaluate with respect to the learning difficulties most often associated with children with autism. A specific area of autistic learning disability for many children with ASDs is in the area of imitation. Difficulties in spontaneous imitation of social behaviors are universal across the autistic spectrum. Early failures in social behavior, as in an infant who does not play peek-a-boo or a preschooler who does not copy the way Mommy walks in shoes with heels can be construed as failures due to lack of imitation. From the beginning, the child with autism is one who learns things differently because of imitation difficulties. ABA/DTT programs start out with the teaching of more formal (non-social) imitation skills in the form of nonverbal imitation ("Do this!") drills. Presumably, the child with autism who doesn't imitate would imitate if he could, or would imitate if he found what others were doing to be something interesting that he wanted to do himself. It certainly makes sense to teach imitation skills to a child who doesn't imitate, as it is definitely a central modality for learning in the toddler and preschool years.

Arguably, an intervention method based on imitative learning is not as likely to be effective in a pre-imitative child, any more than group instruction is likely to be effective in a child who doesn't yet even attend during one-to-one instruction. Imitation tends to be specifically impaired in autism—meaning that the developmental level of imitation skills is often lower than the developmental level of other non-verbal skills. For children with learning difficulties outside of the ASDs, this is less often true, and so inclusion may well be more appropriate for such children if they are provided with imitative models at their developmental levels. When we look at how learning is supposed to work for a particular child with autism who is being placed in an inclusive setting, we need to take a good look at whether this child has developed imitation skills, what kinds of imitation skills they are, and, developmentally, to what kinds of imitative models he will be exposed in an inclusive setting.

Imitative Learning versus Cause-and-Effect Learning. The flip side to assuming that an autistic child will learn to imitate good things in an inclusive placement setting is the assumption that the child will learn to imitate bad things in a special day class placement in which other pupils may exhibit signs of autism that are not currently present in the child for whom a placement is being sought. Since one component of what underlies the lack of imitation in children with autism is a lack of desire to do or be like others, the child with autism is not likely to imitate something bad just because others are doing it. A child with autism who does not, for example, flap his hands when overexcited isn't going to see another child with autism flap his hands and say to himself, "Hmmm, that looks fun. I'll try it too and maybe the other guy will notice and want to come over here and we can flap together!" Sensory symptoms such as hand flapping, toe walking, and spinning objects are not something that children with autism have learned from one another. These are "hard-wired" problems (as described in chapter 1). All over the world, children with autism who have never met one another, and who have never seen another child with autism, flap the same way—just the way typical babies all start off with "high water mark" walking the same way.

One possible exception to the "doesn't-imitate-others" rule is when a child with autism experiences the bad behavior of another child to be very instrumental and useful to that child's getting his way. The child with autism may learn that bad behavior, not so much through imitation as through simple cause and effect. So, putting a seven-year-old boy with autism in a class with another student who regularly dumps his desk and is removed from the room may result in the seven-year-old boy with autism's learning that dumping your desk is an effective way to get out of class. This will be especially true if leaving the class means sitting in isolation outside the room on a chair, avoiding an assignment, and getting away with running down the hall to play in the water fountain as soon as the teacher goes back inside.

Putting a child with autism with other children who are autistic is not going to teach him to be autistic, just as simply putting the same child with typical children is not going to teach him to be more typical, especially if he lacks imitation skills. There are ways to foster imitation both in and out of inclusive placements, and this is an important topic that was discussed at length in chapter 4. However, the point here is that presence or substantial absence of imitation skills is an important factor in considering the developmental appropriateness of inclusion in a typical educational setting.

Developmental versus Chronological Inclusion. Sometimes people assume that a child that is developmentally delayed should be placed with chronological age mates so he can learn to act his age. On some level, this might make sense: If you are going to learn something you don't now know how to do, you might as well learn to do it the way you are expected to be able to do it. This reasoning is based on a very behavioral model: Any new skill (like acting like a six-year-old if you're six) can be learned if it is broken down into parts. The problem is that if you are six and autistic, you may play with Buzz LightYear like a three-year-old, flying him around making noises. That's fine, but a six-year-old who's flying his Buzz is likely chanting "To Infinity and Beyond!" jumping off things alongside Buzz, and scripting the play, saying things like "Come on Potato Head—let's rescue our pal Woody!" This is going to be over the head of the six-year-old with autism. If you are playing like a three-year-old, you must first go through the stages of playing like a four- and five-year-old before the things the other six-year-olds are doing catch your eye.

Play Integration with Chronological Age Mates. There are effective ways of getting the autistic six-year-old and typical six-year-old to play together. However, this won't happen simply by placing the children together. A typical six-year-old is relatively unlikely to choose to play with a typical three-year-old on a playground without some outside encouragement, reinforcement, or ideas about how to get the three-year-old to play along in a way that will be fun for both of them. If there are children his own age and gender around, he'll likely find them to be more attractive playmates. There are ways that adults encourage six- and three-year-olds to play together—like when a six-year-old cousin is stuck with his three-year-old cousin for the afternoon with no other options. The strategies an adult might use in that sort of situation is closer to what can constitute meaningful implementations of inclusive-education strategies when developmentally different children are brought together.

UNDERLYING SOCIAL POLICY PRINCIPLES

Where did inclusive education get started? What are its uses? How does one decide when an inclusive versus a special day class placement is the "appropriate" placement? What are the laws and precedents that support its implementation as an educational approach for children with ASDs?

Historical Background. Only a little more than 25 years ago, there was no mandate for special education in the United States. In 1975, PL (Public Law) 94-142 was passed by Congress and became know as "IDEA" (the Individuals with Disabilities Education Act). For the first time, a law guaranteed children with special educational needs three basic rights: a free and appropriate public education (sometimes now referred to as "FAPE"), an individualized educational plan ("IEP"), and education in the least restrictive environment ("LRE"). This was a tremendous breakthrough for families of children with special educational needs because, up to this time, a school district could simply say they had no program to serve a child they deemed particularly difficult or exceptional to educate. Such a child might receive minimally supported home schooling or nothing at all if the child was seen as profoundly impaired. Up until the promulgation of PL 94-142, there were special-education programs, but they were not universally available. There were private special-education services, but no way for a family to have such services paid by a public agency, even if there were no public services whatsoever.

Where did the push for IDEA come from? The special-education rights movement descends pretty directly from the civil rights movement. The tenets of IDEA were readily accepted by most Americans opposing segregation and unequal treatment based on race. As laws and court decisions began to bolster full racial equality, advocates for the physically and mentally disabled demanded equal treatment for them as well. It is likely that these movements trailed behind the civil rights movement because the disabled are less often able to speak on their own behalf—and vote. The physically disabled (who undoubtedly vote in greater numbers than the developmentally disabled) began to push for equal treatment in the form of public access and job accommodations for the handicapped. In the 1980s, handicapped restrooms and ramps, and wider doorways came to be expected. Closely following these developments were increased efforts to provide accommodations allowing the developmentally disabled the same inclusion in mainstream society that the physically handicapped now were experiencing. Through the late 1970s and 1980s, special education itself had grown with more and more programs to serve the increasing numbers of children being identified as having developmental problems. Any neurobiological condition deemed to have deleterious effects on educational outcomes must be accommodated. In many states (such as California), there is separate, related legislation that specifies that children with mental health needs are entitled to school-based services to address those needs if the condition may limit the chance to make educational progress. However, in the early 1990s, the special-education movement and those seeking rights for the physically disabled joined forces with more promotion of individuals with educational disabilities into the educational mainstream. It was considered not enough to provide "separate but equal" access to education, but access to education alongside those not needing special accommodations. Over the last ten years or so, law has codified these rights.

It is essential to note that the legal right that grants access to mainstream education to any child whose parent chooses it comes from a law primarily driven by policy rather than educational or developmental research. There is little disagreement that the moral standard underpinning inclusion law requires provision of all necessary supports to "make inclusion work." However, if inclusion is not appropriate because of the developmental differences between a child and his age mates or near age mates, many feel that all the supports in the world cannot make inclusion work. It is one thing to accommodate a mildly mentally retarded autistic six-year-old in a kindergarten class; it is another to try to include a severely retarded ten-year-old in a fifth-grade class meaningfully.

From a developmental perspective, it makes the most sense to start with identifying accommodations the child needs to best fulfill his potential. If one of the things that could benefit the child is inclusion, great, do it. Figure out what supports are needed to do it right. Maybe the child needs support imitating peers. Maybe the child needs to have peers trained to initiate social contact with him. Maybe the child needs inclusion because he is academically at or above grade level in a particular area. Inclusion should be a *means* for developing skills. Inclusion is a method. Inclusion should not be regarded as an *end*. A child should not be in an inclusive placement simply because it is his "right." If the child can be benefited by a mainstreamed placement because it will provide stimulation he can use, then it's great that the law is there to support access to such service. Things get mucked up however when the child is included just because the parent wants inclusion or hopes inclusion will somehow help, or the school feels it is the politically correct thing to offer. In such cases, the down side is that the included child is essentially being deprived of the special education he needs because of time spent in a general education setting. We wouldn't put a five-year-old math genius in high school calculus because he has a right to learn calculus. Instead, we would acknowledge that he needs to learn other math skills first, and then take calculus. The situation for some children with big gaps between their functioning and that of classmates may not be much different from putting a bright five-year-old in calculus. If the bright five-year-old hasn't been taught to multiply fractions yet, he's not going to magically assimilate calculus.

The current educational standard allowing parent-choice inclusion has essentially become a civil rights standard. But "equal access" in civil rights terms cannot be superimposed on special education without the possibility of depriving some developmentally disabled children of the right to an appropriate education. I argue (and others may disagree): The child's right to an appropriate education should take precedence over the parents' right to select inclusion if experts deem that appropriate education is impossible or very unlikely in the inclusive setting.

The Medical Standard: "Do No Harm." In medicine, the Hippocratic oath is to "Do no harm" to the patient. This means that even when the doctor may not know how to cure a patient, he or she is not free to experiment on that patient in a manner that may be detrimental. Special education, too, is bound to "do no harm," and in most cases will also fail mostly unrealistic expectations to "cure" the child. But in many cases special education will provide some degree of remediation. For some, remediation that is not a "cure" is seen as a failure, black and white. If parents enter the world of special education aware that "cures" are unlikely, they are better prepared to accurately weigh progress (and appreciate shades of gray).

Delivery of Special Education in the Inclusive Classroom. The reality of inclusion is that needed special services are usually provided in a classroom of typical peers, primarily by paraprofessional aides. These individuals, while virtually always well meaning, are, by definition, not as well trained as a special-education teacher. The further the included special-education student is from his typical classmates developmentally, the more time he is likely to spend under direct instructional control of his aide. In this situation, the child who needs the most special education, may get the least. This shortcoming can be viewed as particularly egregious when the child might otherwise benefit from features of a special day class that cannot be duplicated in a mainstreamed setting, like small group size, physically isolated work areas, and imitative models at his developmental level.

The Psychological Standard: "In the Best Interest of the Child." In the field of children's rights law pertaining to noneducational aspects of child welfare, such as mental health and family disposition, a widely adopted standard is making a decision "in the best interest of the child." Articulation of this standard is not consistently used, however, when selection of an inclusive educational placement is at issue. If we assume that "best interests," in the case of a child with an ASD, is access to services that are understood to directly remediate or help him compensate for his difficulties, this could sometimes favor selection of a special education class rather than inclusion. For a particular child this might be the case if inclusion did not seem developmentally and educationally to meet criteria for "FAPE" and "LRE."

The IDEA Standard: "Free and Appropriate Public Education." Most interesting is that the choice of inclusion can at times contradict what otherwise might be considered an appropriate educational method. The confusion here stems from the fact that some regard inclusion as a method, while others regard it as a setting wherein a variety of methods, including any method used in a special day class, is possible. If inclusion is regarded as a setting and not a method, then it must be argued that some methods are more readily, fully, naturally used in a special day class than in a mainstreamed class.

In educational planning, there is a case to be made for putting the child's needs first, the methods to address those needs second, and the appropriate placement in which to execute the methods third. In this way, assessment of the child comes first, development of a treatment plan comes next, and strategies to accomplish the treatment follow. Strategies for accomplishing the treatment need to include consideration of who will treat and where treatment will be carried out. The reason for this taxonomy will be given in the next section, which describes particularly contentious educational litigation.

The Civil Rights Standard: "Necessary Accommodations to Be in the Mainstream." Louis was an eight-year-old boy with autism and moderate mental retardation. At eight, he was noted to have severe dysarthria (almost unintelligible speech), very limited receptive language, and single-word language he mainly used when presented with a visual icon of something he wanted. After a couple of years of modest progress in a special day class with similarly disabled peers—in which his limited, but functional language first started, he'd learned to use icons, developed one-to-one correspondence for small quantities, and been potty-trained; his family opted for mainstreaming in second grade. The family had great admiration for the second-grade teacher, as she had taught Louis's older sister and really made an impact. Louis had a full-time, one-to-one aide in second grade, as well as access to a resource room and its' teacher with whom he met for one-to-one instruction for about 30 percent of the instructional class day. Many IEPs had been held to adapt the curriculum for Louis, but there were increasing behavior problems. During penmanship, as other children practiced capital and lower-case m's on individual chalkboards, Louis received hand-over-hand guidance to copy a simple shape onto a white board with a marker. Many other adaptations of this task more closely resembling what the other second graders were doing had been tried but, in fact, Louis did not yet appear to have fixed handedness, let alone an appropriate grasp on a writing instrument. He did not even look at the board as his hand was helped to write on it, despite verbal and physical redirects of his gaze. Teaching episodes like this were accompanied by Louis's loud vocalizations, disruptive to other pupils. A prissy girl whined, "Teacher, can you ask Louis to be quiet?" At other times, when instruction held little functional value for Louis, he would run to the bookcases and excitedly dump books from the shelves or push over a chair or desk. Only when he saw his resource teacher did he verbalize any words or complete any requested task. The contention was that Louis had an inadequate behavior plan in his second-grade class, but that inclusion was the right place for him, if only someone competent enough could be found to do it effectively.

From my perspective, Louis was being deprived of access to developmentally appropriate education during his time in the second-grade classroom. With his resource teacher who structured language tasks at the 18-month receptive-language level (at which he had consistently tested), he showed no behavioral difficulties. In fact, there were no behavioral difficulties reported in the resource room in which he received one-to-one teaching with appropriate materials. In the resource room, Louis would either be alone with the resource teacher, or there would be one or two other children, at some distance, working independently on something else.

There were so many things this little boy needed—to develop more vocabulary, to improve articulation, to develop handedness so that he could use a spoon and fork well on his own—but these were not part of the second-grade curriculum or any adaptation of it. Should the resource teacher simply have provided all her services within the second-grade class rather than the resource room? Is a classroom within a classroom really inclusion? What are its benefits? Louis never watched or participated in the activities of his second-grade classmates unless motored through the activity. This little boy deserved a peer group, but one at his developmental level, engaged in activities he could recognize and have the potential to join.

In a case like this, the inclusion itself can be seen as the antecedent to Louis's negative behaviors. No amount of accommodation or task analysis of learning style or teaching methods would change this.

After a contentious hearing, it was indeed found that Louis's inclusion was essentially an abrogation of access to needed special-education services. This resulted in a finding that a developmentally appropriate special day class would be the least restrictive environment for Louis's access to a free and appropriate public education. It had been shown that "necessary accommodations" could not be made in the second grade class. Attempts to make them had resulted in disruption of the learning for the typical second graders. This decision was appealed, and an automatic "stay put" order allowed Louis's family to keep him in the second grade for another year. I saw him again at the end of that year. Aggression to teachers and peers had increased, and Louis had twice been suspended for unprovoked attacks resulting in injury to classmates. I saw Louis approach a classmate a head taller than he: He first hugged her then, more roughly, "chinned" her sternum. The girl looked fearfully to Louis's aide who immediately redirected him not to touch and to move away. It has now been agreed that next year he will enter a special day class. The second-grade teacher required to take Louis for an additional year is moving on to higher-grade elementary teaching. A federal appeals court decision that could reverse the lower court and return Louis to inclusion if his parents choose, is still pending.

Inclusion Can Work. It's cases like these that can give inclusion a bad name with some educators. The bottom line here is that inclusion can work, but it's not for every child, even if the law says it can be. In the sections on inclusion that follow, we'll thread our way through some of the issues to consider in deciding whether inclusion may be a useful educational method for a particular child, and if so, what accommodation is needed to make the placement as beneficial as possible.

INSTRUCTIONAL SUPPORTS

In the practice of inclusive education, a major determinant of success is support given the child. All kinds of supports are needed to modify the general education setting so that it can offer the advantages of the special-education setting while not cutting the child off from the unique compensatory advantages of experiences gained only in the mainstream. Key among these supports are staff—teachers, aides, speech therapists, occupational therapists, resource teachers and inclusion specialists—to provide the special adaptations needed by a child with autism.

Teacher Training. Many regular-education teachers, especially kindergarten and early elementary teachers, are enthusiastic about trying inclusion and generally have a positive attitude about acquiring new skills to serve a special-needs child in their class. However, what many parents don't realize is that it is not uncommon to find that a regular-education teacher has not taken even one special-education course in her training. She may never have been exposed to a child with autism before. Usually she will start out by doing the things she knows and will quickly identify what she needs to learn.

It can be difficult for a general-education teacher to figure out how she is supposed to relate to the one-to-one aide who initially often accompanies an inclusively placed child with autism. Regular-education teachers in the early grades usually have some experience deploying parent classroom volunteers, a general classroom aide who is there to help all pupils, or a teaching intern. Often, though, the aide comes with her own agenda, especially if she has been trained by a nonpublic agency, like an ABA/DTT program. On one level, this is a relief for the teacher who has 16 to 31 other pupils to instruct. On another level, the teacher may be left feeling she's not doing her job, or questioning why the child is in her class if the aide seems to be running her own little program for the child.

While a teacher may have difficulty with an aide who has her own agenda, parents may have difficulty with the aide who has no agenda (that is, no training or experience with autism). There are some ways to accomplish a productive middle ground when putting a special education aide in a general education class.

Home to School Transitions with a One-to-One Aide. In the best cases, the teacher and the aide will learn how to work with the child with autism by meeting him before he comes to class. One good method is for the teacher and aide to visit a home program or class and see the child in action. Later, the teacher can meet with the classroom staff or attend a program team meeting to get a clear idea of what the child can and cannot do and what it might take to get him to do it. When there is a home program, an aide should spend time watching the program and be given supervised opportunities to work with the child in the home program so she can learn as much as possible from the tutors. In some cases it may also be helpful for a senior therapist or case manager to come to school to watch the aide and give suggestions for a transitional period.

Making inclusion work under these conditions requires that the aide and any teachers, tutors, or therapists previously experienced with the child respect the fact that the classroom is the teacher's turf. Suggestions about where Carson's desk might go, where Carson could be taken for a time-out if needed, or stating that Analisa would be the best peer buddy to take Carson to the playground should remain just that—suggestions.

Once outside care providers start to lobby for their curriculum adaptations by suggesting to the parent that the teacher is wrong because she doesn't want to do things the way the home-based teachers suggest, the teacher-parent relationship can easily be undermined. From then on, the teacher is always in the position of having to prove herself to the parent because someone the parent has trusted (the home-based teacher) has told her that the teacher lacks needed expertise. Creating such rifts is not likely to be in the best interest of the child. Instead, a group meeting after school (in the classroom, if this is about what goes on in class) is less confrontational and acknowledges the teacher's central role. Often, home-based providers come from a behavioral perspective while teachers come from a developmental-educational perspective. The involved parties need to learn to communicate with one another. Everyone can offer a perspective on how things are going and suggest new things, rather than sitting on opposite sides of the table in a reopened IEP meeting with an earlier-distributed list of complaints. Teachers often need to learn new things to serve a pupil through inclusion. Parents need to understand that a teacher or outside consultant may have reasons for running her class the way she does for reasons that may not be immediately apparent to them. If everyone (or anyone) suspects the worst of the other, the worst is much more likely to happen.

Teacher Support for the Included Placement. One of the most difficult things for a teacher who, let's assume, wants to teach well, is seeing a child she feels is not learning. Among children with autism who are placed in inclusive settings, there are two basic types—the ones who belong there, and the ones who don't.

It is usually clear in which group a child belongs, but as you near the boundaries, there will be more disagreement.

Putting that aside for a moment, let's focus first on the child who doesn't belong in a general-education classroom. This is the child who, like Louis, shares no overlapping skill sets with his classmates developmentally, and who does not function in any cognitive domain within three years of the level of his age mates. Nothing that is happening in class is accessible to him, and he spends all his time in one-to-one teaching with an aide who is either adapting the curriculum to an extent that it no longer bears resemblance to what others are doing, or he is doing activities separate from the class. In many situations like these, a teacher may try to express her concern that the child is not learning from being in her class. Nevertheless, a teacher may indeed feel quite positively about this child in some ways: For example, she may feel that the child gives more to the class than he gets, that other pupils have learned to be gentle, helpful, altruistic, and more caring because of him (a finding born out by research). But if this teacher also expresses her concern that her class may not be helping the child educationally, she may be right on that too. Especially if the teacher has mainstreamed before, or started out with a very optimistic approach to the inclusion, school administration (and of course parents) should listen carefully.

Some years back, I sat with a sobbing second-grade teacher while her students were out to recess. She told me that she had always wanted to teach, but now was on the verge of giving it up. The previous year, I'd been told, this teacher had won an award for "best new teacher." She'd enthusiastically taken on her inclusion assignment. As the year went on, she'd seen her class repeatedly disrupted by Clare, a child who would grab and crumble the work of others, shout during work times, and kick her neighbors at circle. She'd been criticized by the parents of the child for not doing enough of the inclusion herself, although Clare had two full-time aides. The placement was also under a "stay put" order while Clare's family sued the school district for the right to keep her there. To me, the idea that this teacher might give up teaching was really sad. There are not enough good teachers. Inclusion should not be a burn-out experience.

Successful inclusion takes a certain kind of child and a certain kind of teacher. If both of these ingredients are not there, it's a recipe for failure. I sometimes point out to parents that flogging a dead horse will not bring it back to life. Sometimes there are only dead horses in the barn. In cases where a school fails to provide sufficient supports for inclusion, or where a parent has burned all her bridges by alienating school staff, the best alternative may be another school or other teaching setting.

Working Out Special-Education Supports to Inclusion Aides. The role of aides in relation to the classroom teacher has already been described. It highlights one of the main challenges an aide can face. On the one hand, the teacher is her most readily available expert. On the other hand, a general-education teacher is usually the first to point out that she is no expert on autism. Being an inclusion aide for a child with autism can be isolating and frustrating if there is no one to compliment your successes and no one with whom to share your frustrations or to whom to address your questions. Some inclusion aides are primarily assigned to a special-education class in which the student with autism may be placed part time. If this is the case, the advantage to the child is that the special-education teacher has an opportunity to learn about the child, and then serve as a consultant on the child both to the aide and to the general-education teacher. A further advantage for the aide is that she then has a base (the special-education class) in which techniques can be modeled "live." For an aide, who usually lacks knowledge of theories of autism and development, this can be a much more direct and relevant training experience than reading books or taking courses.

An instructional aide needs access to sources of ongoing training and consultation. An aide should not be expected to deliver the same services as a special-education teacher, as that level of expertise and training is not what is required of the job. Especially when an aide receives an inclusion assignment at a school at which there are no special-education classes and no full-time special educators (like a resource specialist or speech and language pathologist), it may be very difficult to fully carry out responsibilities aimed at meeting a child's IEP goals with just informal or episodic contact. In such cases, the child's IEP should include time for the aide to meet regularly with some special educator who is a dedicated inclusion specialist. The most efficient model I know of is one in which the inclusion aide accompanies the autistic child to his special "pull-out" services. Although this may seem like a perfect time for a coffee break, it is actually the perfect time to watch and get some training. The pull-out therapies can then be imported and incorporated into the inclusion class.

Aide Staffing. In the last several years, "one-to-one" has come to modify the terms "classroom aide" and "shadow." Aides certainly do not have to be one-to-one. While it is wonderfully American to assume that more is better, we should also remember the truth in the words of the architect Mies Van der Rohe—Sometimes less is more.

The purpose of an aide is to help the child with things he cannot fully do or understand on his own. The aide is not a servant. The concept of the "shadow" aide best describes what an aide should be: someone close by who is as unobtrusive as possible. As we discussed in the context of developing peer social skills in chapter 5, the aide is a "facilitor," a "sustainer" of task activity. The aide in the context of instruction in a general education class should seldom if ever be the "initiator" of teaching. For more able children with autism who are placed in the mainstream, there is the temptation to continue the prompt-dependent relationship with the aide that the child might have earlier had in an ABA/DTT program. This scenario is most likely when the aide *is* a one-to-one tutor from the child's ABA/DTT program. It is hard for both the child and the aide to redefine the relationship to become one in which the adult should really be doing as little as possible.

A child with autism, and especially one with both autism and some degree of language disability can be expected to take a bit longer to react to class directives because that child is likely using extra, compensatory processing mechanisms. The aide needs to allow time for this and not always expect her charge to respond as instaneously as classmates.

For many mainstreamed children with an ASD, one or two adaptations might serve as a bridge between needing full-time one-to-one and going to preschool completely independently. The first would be for the preschool to include a couple of special-needs children and for the aide to share her time between them. This would increase the inevitability that sometimes the aide would not be there just at the moment that something was needed, and the child would have to try to do it himself, if it was something he really wanted. Rather than this being a disadvantage, it provides the child with a completely spontaneous and natural problem-solving opportunity. I see such moments as an opportunity for the child to have a self-reinforcing success experience through his own initiative. Sometimes, though, I talk with parents or supervisors of the aide who feel that if the child with autism does not move through an activity as quickly or as completely as the others, he has failed. In a situation such as this, if the aide intervenes before the autistic child has a chance to try, the success belongs to the aide, not the child, and does much less to potentiate independent future success at this task.

The "Obscured" Aide. Another way in which aides can be used to assist more able children in mainstream settings is to have a truly shadow-aide—an aide the child does not know is his aide. This is most easily accomplished if the aide does not work with the child at home or one-to-one at school, does not drive the child to school, and doesn't visit the home regularly for parent or home treatment team meetings. In a mainstream class with more than just a lone teacher, this is particularly easy to accomplish. The aide simply needs to spend time helping other children, and perhaps spend some time consciously not in proximity to the child she is shadowing. In some more integrated classes with multiple special-needs and multiple regular-education pupils, this can be accomplished by having aides trade roles as the "behavior aide" and the "instruction aide" during the day so that during episodes of behavioral or instructional difficulty, it isn't always the same person who intervenes. In the older elementary grades it is important that the shadow-aide is simply known to the other pupils by the same sort of title as the teacher so that pupils are unaware of her focus. To the extent that other pupils, especially in higher grades, are recognized by peers as having an aide, they are stigmatized in a way that may fairly easily create a barrier, rather than increase the likelihood of social contact with classmates.

In the classroom, the aide's role is to increase the child's attention to the teacher, peers, and assignments, not to directly interact with the child. If the aide's responsibility becomes one of pulling the child with autism aside and working with him separately on something of his own, that is not inclusion, and the benefits for that child of being surrounded by typical peers should be reexamined for that part of the instructional day. My model is that the aide should think of herself as Jiminy Cricket who stood on Pinocchio's shoulder and, in a whisper, advised him how to behave. It didn't always work of course, but the function of the aide is to assist the child in internalizing self-generated problem-solving strategies, just like Jiminy Cricket who was the conscience Pinocchio lacked.

Resource Rooms. Increasingly, inclusive education is falling into the purview of resource specialists, and what are coming to be called "inclusion specialists."

Resource specialists are freestanding special-education jacks (and jills)-of-all-trades who often serve groups of children in a separate classroom designed to provided additional services on an as-needed basis. A resource specialist might run a remedial reading group one period and be a math tutor the next. Resource rooms are sometimes like an individualized study hall to which pupils come to work independently at a listening center or on a computer-assisted instruction program. In some schools, resource teaching is all one-to-one. The resource teacher might be designated as a learning disabilities specialist.

From the In-Class Aide to the Resource Room. In the middle school and high school years, a resource room may serve as a homeroom for included pupils with ASDs who simply can't function in a group setting for six hours a day. Sometimes a resource room is a good place for students who are academically at grade level to come at lunchtime or recess so that they don't have to deal with the social overload of other 14-year-olds who can't get enough of one another. For some pupils, the resource specialist is someone who can help to see that the homework assignments are understood and that the pupil has the necessary materials to complete assignments. In other cases, the resource room is a very good place to do homework, especially if there is resistance to parent-supervised homework at home.

For some ASD pupils, the resource room is a place to go while the aide, and the child, takes a break from the classroom routine. The resource room can also be a place for the aide to learn how better to teach her pupil. At an IEP meeting, it may be decided that a given child with autism is ready to try inclusion, but on a limited basis. The placement site for the inclusion (the home school, for example) may be a site with no special day classes appropriate for this pupil to spend even a little bit of his time. Therefore, it can make sense to start inclusion off for part of the day, perhaps with the rest of the time spent in the resource room, increasing overall hours in inclusion as they are well-tolerated. As an adjunct to this procedure, some pupils may benefit from a shorter school day, arriving after a group opening time (for younger pupils), or a homeroom (for older pupils) and step directly into a direct instructional period.

For some pupils, a resource room can be a temporary refuge during times when it is much harder for the child to maintain his equilibrium. When children are going on and off of medications, going through a family crisis, or needing time to separate themselves from a bad classroom incident, they may temporarily become a bit destabilized, and a resource room can provide respite. Being able to increase the time in the resource room temporarily may be critical to needed flexibility for an inclusive placement. The resource teacher can also be an excellent consultative source for the regular-education teacher, especially when the teacher has had no previous experience with children with autism and their responses to the destabilizing circumstances.

Inclusion Specialists. The inclusion specialist often plays a role similar to that of a resource teacher with respect to being a liaison between special-education services and a general-education placement. Her role is to help plan adaptations to the core curriculum and to train and supervise the classroom aide who is carrying out the adaptations on a daily basis. Most inclusion specialists are itinerant former special-education teachers or speech and language pathologists who move from school to school. They attend IEP meetings for about-to-be-included children, visit classrooms to assess the viability of an inclusive placement or to see how such a placement is working out, and may even step in to show the aide how to use a teaching method. There are no formal or additional credentials for inclusion specialists in the way that special-education teachers sometimes have specialized credentials for teaching the "learning handicapped," "emotionally disturbed," or "severely handicapped." As inclusion grows as a methodology in special education, so grows specific expertise in its use.

Autism Specialists. Sometimes the inclusion specialist's role is subsumed under the title of "autism specialist." Some autism specialists may have completed a Master's thesis on autism or spent many years teaching children in the autistic spectrum. Larger school districts or county offices of education in locales in which there are autism-specific classrooms often have autism specialists who are charged with reviewing programs for autistic children, attending their IEPs, and sometimes organizing in-service training on autism for school staff who serve pupils with autism. Autism specialists divide their time between program development and administrative activities like IEPs, and as well as time spent reviewing general education and special education classes. They may oversee implementation of programs teachers have been trained to use, do child-focused observations when a particular pupil has difficulties, or identify specific children who may have further unmet needs.

When a pupil with autism develops a behavioral difficulty in class, the autism specialist may be the first person to analyze the situation, and may then either suggest modifications to the child's behavior plan or recommend hiring a behavioral specialist to conduct a more detailed functional analysis of the child's problem behavior. Autism specialists spend less time in general-education classes than inclusion specialists, but inclusion of children with autism is typically one of many methods of educating a child with an ASD with which an autism specialist will be familiar.

Speech and Language Pathologists and Occupational Therapists. When it is decided at an IEP meeting that an inclusive placement will be appropriate for a child with an ASD, this decision does not affect eligibility for other related special education services. This means that even children who are fully included are entitled to needed speech and language, occupational, and behavior management services. If parents opt to have their child included in a private school of their choice rather than in a public school, the child is still entitled to these services, though they may need to be provided at a public school. When an included child is pulled out of an inclusion class for speech therapy, occupational therapy or adaptive physical education (APE), this provides a good opportunity, as discussed earlier, for the aide to watch a professional work with the child and to learn new strategies that may adapted for the classroom or the playground (in the case of APE). The aide should regard these ancillary therapists as potential consultants who can advise her on the child's development in their respective domains of expertise. It takes a team to teach a child with autism; no one person is the sole expert.

"DEVELOPMENTAL" INCLUSION

The Meaningfully Adapted Curriculum. A term frequently heard in discussions of inclusion is "meaningfully adapted curriculum." One of the underlying principles of the inclusive education movement is that all children, irrespective of physical, mental, or emotional disability, can benefit from the core curriculum taught to all children. This is a very ecumenical principle, but I believe, it bears closer examination. The idea of adapting core curriculum is directly related to the idea that whatever a classroom of typical learners is learning can be changed in a way to constitute a meaningful lesson for the student with a disability. Everyday examples of adaptations of core curriculum include providing books in Braille for blind pupils and allowing untimed tests for students who are slow readers.

Let's examine how an adapted curriculum might look for three pupils with an ASD at different levels of cognitive disability included in a general education second-grade classroom. It's Monday morning and the pupils have received an assignment: "Draw a picture of the most fun thing you did this weekend," "Write a sentence about your picture," and later, at sharing time, "Show your picture, read your caption, and tell us what you did."

The first inclusion scenario: Chaz is a seven-year-old-boy with autism, a mild level of mental retardation, and expressive language at the four-and-a-half-year level. Chaz went to Marine World, and Chaz is an exceptionally good artist for a seven-year-old, so he draws a detailed whale, complete with teeth, waterspout, and dorsal flippers. His handwriting is neat but not his strong suit, so, with his aide's help, he carefully spells "Whale" and "Shamu" under his picture. At sharing time, he is prompted to read the words on his picture, and he answers several questions asked from the teacher about who he went to Marine World with, whether the whale was big, and if his family also went to the Parrot Jungle show. Other second graders comment that Chaz drew a great whale. When other second graders take their turns, they can spontaneously read a complete sentence they have written independently, and some have to have their extended explanations of their weekends terminated by the teacher who interrupts and says, "OK, tell us just one more thing!"

The second inclusion scenario: Zachary is seven and autistic, but he has a moderate degree of developmental disability, meaning his overall functioning is more at the three- to three-and-a-half-year level. When the assignment is announced, Zach's aide, who knows he went to Marine World over the weekend, asks, "Zach, what did you see at Marine World?" Zach does not yet answer open-ended questions so his aide follows up and asks, "Did you see a whale?" "Yes," Zach replies. "OK," says the aide, "Let's draw a whale." She gives him paper and crayons. Zach draws a round blob, and the aide says, "OK, let's write 'whale'—'W-H-A-L-E', good job!" (With letter-by-letter prompting, Zach has independently written "whale.") At sharing time, the teacher asks Zach, "What did you do this weekend?" Again, Zach does not answer this open-ended question, so the teacher rephrases and asks, "What's that?"

pointing to his whale picture. The aide prompts Zach to say "whale" and Zach says, "Whale." Since Zach does not yet speak in spontaneous phrases for expressive functions, this is the end of his turn.

A final inclusion scenario: Garrett is seven and autistic, and functions in the severely impaired range, with a mental age of less than two years. He has no hand preference nor has he developed a pencil grasp, so his one-to-one aide holds the crayon in his hand and with full hand-over-hand assistance, suggests that he make a whale (since she knows he went to Marine World over the weekend). Garrett scribbles for a while, but eventually the crayon is removed after he puts it in his mouth for the third time. The aide announces to him that his whale is "all done." At sharing, he is held in his aide's lap; she holds up his scribbling with him, again, hand over hand. Another second grader asks, "What did Garrett make?" Garrett is nonverbal, so the aide answers, "This is Garrett's whale."

There are general education second grade classes in which each of these three inclusion scenarios might be played out. I would argue that for Chaz, the morning's second-grade curriculum was indeed meaningfully adapted for him. He had an opportunity to exhibit a strength, his drawing skill, which others admired and which served as a social counterbalance to his lesser language abilities. Chaz was able to participate in the activity with minimal assistance because he understood what to do and was motivated to do it. The value of the inclusion experience for Zach was more questionable. He needed much more motoring through the activity. He was not able to meaningfully understand or participate in "sharing"—the oral, final part of the activity. The 20 minutes it took for everyone in the class to share their pictures was basically mental "downtime" for him.

In Garrett's case, there is no doubt in my mind that the experiences were not the best use of his educational time. He still needs to acquire basic fine motor control. He needs work on receptive language. A book about Marine World in which he could receptively identify sea and jungle animals, might have held more intrinsic interest. If Garrett had spent this time looking at such a book with his aide, there would be no resemblance to the activities of the other second graders. In a special day class, a more developmentally appropriate activity might have been to have the teacher present stuffed and plastic Marine World animals in groups of two or three and let pupils take turns coming forward to receptively identify each one from the group. There was neither cognitive nor social benefit to Garrett from this activity in the core second-grade curriculum.

Functional versus Physical Inclusion. The bottom line here is that inclusion makes the most sense when the core curriculum or the adapted version of the core curriculum is within the child's grasp so that it is clear that he is having a learning experience. This means that the activity must link up with existing knowledge structures and build upon them. If a general education class with age mates cannot offer this to a child, it may not be the place to seek an inclusive experience. In any case, academic content probably should not be the focus of an inclusive experience for such a child. Instead, inclusion that promotes an ability to join in with routines and make initial social gains may be developmentally a better fit. Especially in the early elementary grades, inclusive experiences primarily for socialization purposes may be well justified, especially with children with autism for whom this is often the weakest area.

Inclusion with Developmentally Matched Peers. Interestingly, the inclusion movement seems to have hitched its wagon politically to the idea that inclusion implies not only being in the mainstream of typically developing peers, but of peers of the same chronological age. The whole idea of educating children in large, very age-homogeneous classes is actually fairly modern, and until times of suburban living and busing, many children were educated quite locally in mixed-age groups reflecting a neighborhood's demographic. Mixed-aged classes are much less available now, though rural schools and some private schools are more likely to have mixed kindergarten and first grades or to put kindergarten through second grade together. When these classes can still be found, they may be advantageous inclusive placements for the higher-functioning child with autism who may have academic skills at the second-grade level, but language skills at a kindergarten level.

A more readily available variation is inclusion of a child with autism in a class one or two grade levels below chronological age. (In the days before special-education mandates, this *was* special education for many children.) Such inclusion can be done rather seamlessly, especially for a child who is physically average or smaller that others his chronological age. If, as a rule of thumb, meaningful adaptations of curriculum are held at two grade levels, mainstreaming with younger peers can present a great opportunity. By "adaptations of curriculum being held at two grade levels," I mean that a second-grade curriculum can be adapted down to a kindergarten level and still have meaningful essential elements; fifth-grade math can be brought down to a third-grade math level with the use of strong visual augmentation. Stretches greater than that tend to lose any semblance of the core curriculum. The goal is to promote independent learning. It is much better to place a child with younger children if he can function there more independently and with less one-to-one aide time and fewer instructional supports, than to place him at chronological grade level if he will need more one-to-one support there.

This distinction about whether the child can directly participate in the curriculum in the same way as others in the class—but with supports—is sometimes discussed in terms of functional versus physical inclusion. Functional inclusion means that there is a function for the child's being there. There is something he can imitate, something he can attend to and understand, something he can do alongside peers. Sometimes, the main "function" of the inclusive experience is that the child gets an opportunity to be around peers successfully without being disruptive or exhibiting an increased rate of maladaptive behaviors (like increased rocking or flapping). These types of achievements are modest but worthwhile, as it prepares the child for those times when he is out in public, approached by typical peers, or in a restaurant or store in which behavior and activity must be more constrained. However, if the opportunity to be exposed to typical peers and to maintain a behavioral equilibrium comes at the cost of developmentally more appropriate instruction, developmentally appropriate teaching is preferable. Realistically, a range of services and placements can be integrated so that one (like school) can provide education, and another, like a natural extracurricular setting, such as day care or a recreation program, can provide an opportunity for socialization. If school hours are reserved for instruction, and this is best provided in a non-inclusive setting, other times of day can provide inclusive experiences.

EXTRACURRICULAR INCLUSION SETTINGS

Virtually all the literature on outcomes of inclusion focuses on classrooms. However, school is not the only place for a child to experience a meaningful inclusion. Other options are day care, recreation programs, and after school care. Play dates can be an inclusive experience too (as was discussed in chapters 4 and 8). The first consideration when thinking about an inclusive experience is whether the goal is to develop adaptive-social skills, academic skills, or both.

For children for whom academic skills are the main consideration, a classroom setting is probably the right kind of inclusive placement. This is especially true if the child with autism is functioning at or above grade level in a subject like reading or math, as children with Asperger's syndrome sometimes are. However, for children with more challenges academically, or with more serious delays in the development of receptive and/or expressive language, inclusion in a setting emphasizing academics, like an upper elementary or middle school classroom, may only serve to increase the child's sense of insurmountable challenge. All children with autism placed in an inclusive class setting in elementary school are getting dually challenged—once by the rules of classroom life and social interactions, and once by the academics. There are myriad approaches, but it may make sense for children who are substantially less capable than peers in both social and academic domains to work on only one of these areas of difficulty at a time.

Social Inclusion Settings. Day care can be an excellent setting for inclusion because there is usually little academic structure. This affords an opportunity to learn to participate in highly routine, simple activities like snack, lining up, going to the bathroom, and maybe a story time. There are more open-ended opportunities for facilitating one-to-one play than at school, where these opportunities may be limited to recess periods when the children with autism may compete with many agemates for a play partner. Many children have one-to-one aides for classroom time. Fewer receive one-to-one time for recess, as it is often the aide's break time. Facilitating play, especially when it initially can be done one-to-one and especially when there is a lot of "hanging out" time, can be particularly advantageous to the child with autism for whom an inclusive social experience is sought.

A one-to-one aide who attends day care with a child with autism can become the focus of attention for other children which makes including her charge in their play more fluid. In chapter 4 we considered some ideas for how to use this strategy to facilitate social interactions and play. Day care as an inclusive setting is an alterative when the goals being addressed are primarily social and focus on the development of adaptive behaviors related to following the rules and routines of groups.

Peers and Inclusive Placements. Another level of choice provided by day care as an inclusion setting is having an age-heterogeneous group of peers. In classrooms, peers are typically of the same chronological age. In day care, especially in smaller home-based day care arrangements, there are more likely to be mixed-age groups. For many children with autism this presents the dual advantages of access to younger peers, who may have developmentally more similar play interests, and older peers, who have the interest and capacity to play big brother or big sister. This can be an especially relevant consideration when looking for a first inclusive placement for a three- or four-year-old with autism, as typically developing three- and four-year-olds are themselves so egocentric and unable to take another's perspective that they tend to be the least tolerant of a child with autism, who will inevitably be an even more immature "player" than they.

Quality Issues. Any discussion of quality issues with respect to inclusive placements needs to take into account the research literature on outcomes of inclusive placements. First, there is very little "outcomes" research, meaning research that compares groups of children that received inclusion versus those that received a special day class. Of the research that compares these groups, different factors have been explored with respect to the special education child—changes in social initiation skills, changes in behavior problems, and changes in language use. Potential benefits to typical peers who have a special-needs child included in their class have been studied too. Extremely little of this small body of research focuses specifically on autism. Of the research that has been done, much was carried out in model or demonstration programs or in university lab schools at which the master teachers have PhDs in education and the aides are working on Master's degrees. Some of the best results are reported from such studies, but even under such ideal conditions, reported benefits are modest despite the high quality of intervention. In much of the research there are neither benefits nor deficits associated with having been included or having been in special education. In good-quality inclusion programs, elements of needed accommodations can be assumed to have been present. Most of the inclusion outcome studies are of younger children, and children included with typical peers who are one, two, or three years above them developmentally. What the research tells us, not surprisingly, is that the quality of teacher training makes a difference to inclusion outcomes. General education staff need support and help from inclusion specialists who basically provide one-to-one hands-on crash courses on how to teach a child with a given disability.

CHAPTER CONCLUSIONS

Like other methods of intervention for autistic spectrum disorders, inclusion is not for everyone. The principles of inclusive education are grounded in the idea that good models will produce good behavior. If imitation and supports for imitation exist, inclusion may be a viable method. Inclusion also assumes that what is being modeled is developmentally within your grasp. If the autistic spectrum child being included is developmentally comparable to the peers with whom he is to be educated, inclusion may be a viable education method.

In the next chapter, we will attempt to show how all the ideas about how children with autism learn have been brought together in some model programs and exemplary classrooms. This is not to say that these are the best or the only good programs for children with autism. It is not to say that for a program to be good it must be faithful to a tested "model." Rather, the next chapter is meant to show how creative clinicians and educators have succeeded at integrating educational, developmental, and behavioral principles into a range of services that span childhood and the autistic spectrum.

CHAPTER THIRTEEN

Model Programs and Exemplary Classes: What Can We Learn?

KNOWING WHAT'S GOOD

What's the best program in the country for children with autism? The answer, which should be apparent by now, is that there isn't *one*. What makes a program superior is that it has mechanisms that allow it to be individualized according to a child's needs. Some programs accomplish this by applying a specific set of methods to varying curricula. Some programs accomplish this by using a range of methods to teach given content in a variety of ways. Some programs vary both method and curriculum on an individual basis. Given the range of autistic learning disabilities, that is, the way different children with autism learn differently because they have different underlying profiles of weakness and strengths, there are some inherent advantages to flexible use of both curriculum and method. A program that can achieve this can match the needs of a range of children.

As we begin a review of model programs and exemplary classes, we revisit the sorry state of autism treatment research. Today, most of the positive changes in behavior, learning, adaptation, and quality of life that can be effected for children with autistic spectrum disorders comes from behavioral and educational treatments. This is precisely the area of funding for research in autism that gets the fewest dollars. In the last 10 to 15 years, the lion's share of resources has gone to the field of genetics, which promises to help us understand the origins not just of autism but of an array of psychiatric symptoms and disorders. A substantially smaller amount of money targeted for autism issues has been spent on medical research, particularly psychopharmacology, but this is still more money than has been spent on educational and behavioral treatment research.

For those trying to use evidence-based standards to make autism treatment decisions, it would be great if there were more attention to educational and behavioral research. But right now there isn't. (In late 2002, the National Institutes of Health called together a panel of autism treatment experts to define behavioral, educational, and psychosocial autism treatment research gaps and to identify methodologies needed to do such research. Only time will tell what will happen to this initiative.) What this boils down to is that the best way to assess the quality of treatment programs is to relate them to some empirical data on outcomes, some theories about what benefits might be derived if we can tap brain plasticity and transfer of function, some learning theory, and some understanding about neurocognitive development. Clinical experience carries us the rest of the way.

This chapter is a travelogue of visits to programs throughout the United States that are considered models, as well as a description of individual classrooms and programs I've had the privilege to visit that do one or (usually) more things particularly well. The programs described here are not meant to be an exhaustive list of all such programs, nor even a list of the top few. These programs are described so that they can teach by example. More often than not, the best treatment opportunity for a child with autism is when he is paired with a particularly gifted teacher who is both formally educated in her science and skillful at her craft.

Teachers already know this standard is the best that any child can get. Parents more often succumb to thinking that the "best" program is either just a matter of convincing your spouse to sell your house and move across the country or winning whatever you asked for at a due process hearing to resolve IEP disputes. It is so natural to fantasize about the ideal treatment, and then to feel that all that stands between your child and the ideal program is a lawsuit or three thousand miles. Don't be so hard on yourself.

In the next and final chapter we'll discuss how the best education comes from the best collaborations between home and school resources and how to effect "wraparound" treatment. This means that most people and most places can provide a child with autism with substantial educational advantages if resources are well deployed.

There are examples here of each of the three main treatment approaches we have discussed: applied behavior analysis and discrete trial training (chapter 10), the TEACCH curriculum (chapter 11), and inclusion (chapter 12). In the second part of this chapter, we'll cover other treatment models for autism that have been developed to specifically address one domain of development or another and that correspond to the specific learning differences described in chapter 4 as social autistic learning disabilities, in chapters 5, 6, and 7 as communicative autistic learning disabilities, and in chapter 8 as autistic learning disabilities related to relating to the environment. Each of these specific methods, like the more comprehensive methods—ABA/DTT, TEACCH, and inclusion—also lack substantial empirical support (simply because no work has been carried out), but make some sense theoretically, clinically, or educationally.

MODEL APPLIED BEHAVIOR ANALYSIS PROGRAMS

In chapter 10, we thrashed out the various strengths and weaknesses of using the theories of applied behavior analysis in the treatment of children with autism. We distinguished between applied behavior analysis (ABA) as a theoretical field of study, its principles supported by broad and substantial research, and research on the Lovaas's discrete trial training (DTT)-based curriculum for young children with autism. The distinction between ABA as a method, and Lovaas's DTT curriculum as content is important to keep in mind as we examine model ABA programs, not all of which use Lovaas's DTT curriculum, or use DTT as a teaching methodology.

LOVAAS/ LIFE
(LOVAAS INSTITUTE FOR EARLY INTERVENTION)

Clinic and Workshop Models. Lovaas's work in using ABA principles to administer discrete trials of a pre-academic curriculum goes back to the 1970s. In 1981, the first book formalizing this curriculum appeared, and later work has elaborated on it. Research on the effectiveness of this method was based on subjects seen in the Early Autism Project carried out at UCLA. Presently, Lovaas's clinical work continues to be carried out through the Lovaas Institute for Early Intervention (LIFE), which is based in Los Angeles. Over the years, many of Lovaas's former doctoral students from his UCLA program have gone on to found nonpublic agencies that provide very similar services. Some of these agencies continue to maintain close relationships with LIFE; some do not. Some have innovated modifications to the LIFE paradigm either through research or clinical experience, but some more closely replicate the work at LIFE. It is important to understand that replication of Lovaas's original astonishing findings of "normalizing" almost half of autistic children treated with 40 or more hours per week of his ABA/DTT program have still not been replicated at the time of this writing—almost 15 years later. There is also no evidence that a "genuine" Lovaas program produces more positive outcomes than derivative ABA/DTT programs. What the data that have come from the Early Autism Project's attempts to replicate Lovaas's original findings do suggest is that it has been difficult to replicate all the qualities of the original UCLA ABA/DTT "clinic model" in which subjects had weekly checkups/program evaluations from UCLA staff. In particular, there has been some suggestion that the now widely disseminated "workshop" model that was devised to extend provision of these types of services often may not be as powerful.

LIFE follows the curriculum originally described in *The Me Book* (1981), and later elaborated on in *Behavioral Interventions for Young Children with Autism* (1996). Unlike other ABA programs that employ DTT as well as more varied teaching methods, LIFE programs represent the "original" Lovaas method. In the original research-based treatment, all children received the same "clinical" model that was monitored weekly by a core group of experts at UCLA. Presently, however, many children are served using the less intensively monitored "workshop" model just described. In both cases, a hierarchy of junior and senior therapists or tutors provides the bulk of direct intervention with the child. In the clinical model, treatment is carried out in the child's home with two tutors who alternate roles as teacher and data gatherer. When data is not being recorded, the second tutor serves to provide needed levels of prompting of the child's responses to each of the first tutor's requests (discriminative stimuli—or SDs). Weekly team meetings include parents, junior and senior tutors, a case manager (an experienced senior tutor that oversees the training and quality assurance of the more junior and senior tutors), and a program supervisor or director who oversees a number of case managers and their programs and lends a fresh view and a greater breadth of experience to the weekly team meetings which focus on troubleshooting via task analysis and curriculum revision. Weekly revisions can include things like how, when, and how much the child is prompted; changes in materials; addition of new SDs; or the addition of new "programs" (like beginning to teach receptive labels or nonverbal imitation). New programs are added according to a predeveloped flowchart that orders the introduction of skills in roughly developmental sequence. In the original clinical model some years ago, parents were required to participate as tutors and eventually to serve as the most senior therapist for their child's program. This had the advantage of integrating the family into the work with the child and providing a good degree of assurance that goals of the program would be carried into nontreatment hours. Parents are not required to be "senior" therapists in most "workshop" ABA/DTT programs now. However, research that compares and contrasts many different treatments for autism does show that the level of parent involvement is related to positive outcomes. This means that parents as therapists may have been a contributory factor in the originally reported Lovaas ABA/DTT program results.

The Lovaas Model for "Learning to Learn." There are many praiseworthy qualities to the Lovaas model. First, children tend to show an early and robust response to the first programs of the ABA/DTT curriculum, which work on achieving attention and compliance. This means that parents start to see improvements that are easily quantified by data recorded as responses to each SD are noted. Children become more malleable and, as a result, less isolated and unreachable. The tutors are typically young people in, or newly graduated from, college and they tend to be energetic, enthusiastic, and idealistic. A great perk of this approach is the way it brings positive energy into a household that has so recently been depressed by the diagnosis of the child's autism and stressed by the required levels of day-to-day care. In the LIFE workshop model, parents may be responsible for finding and hiring the tutors themselves. Once this is accomplished, there is an initial two- or three-day workshop conducted by a case manager in their home to train the identified tutors as well as the parents themselves, using the child as the training model. This allows the training to be very specific to the learning needs of the child who will be treated. This is a powerful parent intervention, and for many families, provides a special set of rules for addressing the unfamiliar behavioral challenges of autism for the first time.

One potential disadvantage of the workshop model is that tutors recruited by this method may vary a great deal in formal training, commitment, or aptitude. Usually, the tutors are recruited by parents who themselves are not yet trained in the skills the program will require, but who are understandably eager to get enough staff to get treatment as soon as possible. In the workshop model, supervision by a case manager or program manager is much less frequent, often consisting of only two to four hours once or twice month. For some tutors, this may not be enough instruction for them to really understand what they need to do and why. A poor tutor is probably worse for the child than no tutor at all as she may introduce inconsistency in the pattern of expected responses others are trying to develop.

Whether children are served by a clinic or workshop model, the most important factor in an impressive program is that the tutors are talented and able to interact with the children as naturally and as developmentally appropriately as possible. Some of a tutor's success has to do with formal training, but much has to do with the natural gifts of the tutor—many of the best have gone on to get more formal education and become talented special educators.

One aspect of ABA/DTT programs is that parents tend to become involved with other parents who have selected similar programs. Many parents may be unaware of other treatment models (because others may not exist in their area) or because they've been told that ABA/DTT is the only "scientific" model. This is a bit of an overreaching claim, given there's not a lot of science, some of the science that takes ABA beyond Lovaas consists of single-case design studies, and educational models are less often subject to the same rigorous research methodologies as psychological ones. This can leave parents apprehensive about trying other models or modifying their methods. They may feel that other models are a poor substitute for ABA/DTT simply because there are fewer empirical studies to which to turn.

This state of the research is often incorporated into how ABA/DTT programs are marketed. Many parents learn firsthand of ABA/DTT programs from an informational seminar with a videotaped or live demonstration of a child who has responded to treatment particularly well. Although parents can see that their child may differ in key ways from the "demonstration" child, parents can be led to feel that similar results can reasonably be expected. This can be great for getting the customer in the door, but this type of marketing puts people like me in a tough position: I don't want to rain on anyone's parade, and I don't want to curtail chances of improvement for any child, but I also don't want to see already wounded parents disappointed when all the anticipated gains don't materialize. It's really hard not to hope for every kind of improvement when you have a child with autism. However, I think that developing unfounded optimism only makes things harder in the long run.

For children without access to other appropriate zero-to-three services, and children who live in areas in which there are no autism-specific, intensive group-based special-education alternatives, ABA/DTT programs are possibly the best choice as a core program. Even for many children who ultimately will not be high responders, but who might benefit from increased learning readiness, ABA/DTT may be the best starting point.

PRINCETON CHILD DEVELOPMENT INSTITUTE (PCDI)

Many practitioners of ABA see Lovaas and his work in the treatment of children with autism as reflecting the history from which their field has emerged. An excellent example of a program that represents the next generation of ABA treatment applications is PCDI, a private school exclusively for children with autism in Princeton, New Jersey. Dr. Patricia Krantz and Dr. Lynn McClannahan direct PCDI. The goals of PCDI are to teach spontaneous and functional communication skills, develop self-initiated learning skills, and minimize disruptive behaviors to improve the chances that a child will be able to function, to as great an extent as possible, in the mainstream. Each main aspect of curriculum is guided by the idea that interaction and communicative drive will be increased by focusing activity around things in which the child has interest. In other words, making sure that, for each task demand, the autistic child's answer to the "why-should-I-care" question is that the consequences are gratifying or interesting to the child.

How the PCDI Program Is Structured. PCDI is a model program that serves as a training site for teachers from all over the world who come for a period of instruction that includes formal classroom training in behavior theory and autism, as well as hands-on classroom supervision by a training staff member without her own class responsibilities. PCDI also serves as a "residency training program" for directors and teachers at four satellite programs that PCDI coordinates in other parts of New Jersey. The Princeton site serves 50 pupils, a few of whom are toddlers, just under half of whom are school-aged, and the rest of whom are young adults. Classroom staffing is predominantly one-to-one though not all instruction is direct one-to-one instruction, as there is an intentional emphasis on prompt fading and moving the pupil toward functioning both independently and as part of a group. After about a year at PCDI, half of the students transition to inclusive educational programs, and the remaining half continue at PCDI for some additional period. Students who staff believe will potentially transition to inclusion are their priority. Parent training is integral to the PCDI philosophy. Each teacher is assigned one or two home-programming students, and new skills are taught at home as soon as they are mastered at school. Parents must come to toddler classes weekly to observe, and are highly encouraged to come to preschool programs, as well as to programs for older pupils. Parents of toddlers must agree to do 20 hours per week of work with their children and must agree not to hire others to do the work instead.

Activity Schedules. One of the special features of PCDI programs is the use of activity schedules. Similar to picture schedules in a TEACCH program and to other picture communication, the activity schedule is a to-do list that the child constructs for himself at the beginning of each instructional period. Depending on the child's level, the activity schedule might consist of pictures or words. The youngest pupils are motored through its use, and even a toddler was observed to use one with minor assistance. At its simplest, an activity schedule consists of a loose-leaf notebook filled with several laminated cardboard pages with a dot of Velcro on each. Possible work activities are placed on nearby shelves in baskets, with a picture of each activity on both the basket and the shelf. The child constructs a schedule of his activities by choosing one card at a time and attaching each to a successive page in the activities schedule book. When the book is filled, the child returns to the first page, removes the first picture, replaces it on the shelf, removes the corresponding basket, and sits down to the work it contains. The work may be either an interactive activity, such as a discrete trial, or a solitary activity, much as it would be at a TEACCH workstation. When the activity is completed, the child returns the materials to the basket, returns the basket to the shelf, and looks for the next picture of the next task on his activity schedule. This system builds in choice, and therefore motivation, and gives the child a chance to move around while still under the instructional control of the schedule; in this way, it more closely resembles a typical preschool pattern of activity. The oldest children might have a small spiral notebook in which they copy down assignments from the blackboard, making a list of the order in which they intend to complete them. As each assignment is completed, it is crossed off the list.

Language Master. One bit of technology that is used particularly effectively at PCDI is the Language Master. Not a particularly high-tech gadget, the Language Master has been around for a long time and is essentially a computer-card reader cum audiocassette player that digitally reads aloud keypunched words as the card is passed through a slot on the Language Master. The Language Master is used for developing conversational skill, with the child's response initially being prompted by the child's insertion (with a prompt, if needed) of the card that provides the answer or a turn in the conversation. The child then is prompted to echo the Language Master (instead of an adult, who might otherwise have modeled the desired response). As the child becomes fluent with the conversation script, the words on the Language Master card are faded one at a time until a blank card remains (to remind the child that a response is required). The Language Master machine is then faded, and finally so is the card. In this way, the child learns the pragmatics of conversation without the pragmatics becoming convoluted by the conversational partner's verbally modeling responses.

With both the activity schedules and the Language Master, one sees PCDI students taking a more active role in their learning experiences. This active "learning-by-doing" approach is developmentally much more sensitive to the learning style of younger children than the DTT approach of "sit good, look at me" used in a Lovaas program. Through second or third grade, typically developing pupils spend considerable time "doing" as a way of incorporating newly learned concepts and the PCDI model reflects this for older children with autism.

Inclusion Criteria. PCDI works primarily with pupils who they feel may at some point benefit from mainstream curriculum. This doesn't mean that they only work with high-functioning autism and Asperger's; they also serve a number of pupils with mild to moderate disabilities as well. Their guidelines for working with schools to achieve inclusion emphasize selecting a school that is welcoming of a collaborative process and is willing to have a continued behavior-contracting system in place at the new school. Target (severely disruptive) behaviors that interfere with instruction or instructional control are required to be at near-zero levels at school, home, and in the community before inclusion is recommended. Other requirements include the child's being able to work independently on math, reading, and writing tasks, and his being placed according to standardized tests. The child must have some generative (spontaneous, with some novel formulations) language, an ability to follow group instruction, and an ability to tolerate some disruption in class, such as another child's crying. The goal is always to fade the instructional aide over time.

PCDI is a very high-quality program with staff who clearly have exceptional levels of training and skill. Dr. Krantz, who directs program activities on a daily basis, clearly knows each child and the details of each child's learning style. As the research is indicating, this level of pupil individualization amalgamated with teacher training is critical for successful outcomes. While the number of children they serve is relatively small, the outreach and training they provide and the research they carry out on their treatment's effectiveness clearly offers some useful lessons to others hoping to develop and disseminate new skills in working with children with autism.

ALPINE LEARNING CENTER

Alpine Learning Group in Paramus, New Jersey, is both a school and a home-consultation program. It was founded and is directed by Dr. Bridget Taylor, the therapist who worked successfully with the children described in the parent memoir *Let Me Hear Your Voice*. The program is strongly rooted in ABA principles and also reflects a strong basis in high-quality special-educational practices, which are reflected in its curriculum materials and in the highly structured organization of the classrooms.

How the Program Is Structured. The Alpine school site provides day programs for about 30 children between 3 and 17. Children attend the program five days a week (about 24 hours per week). The children are assigned to one of five classrooms, each of which has two teachers and four aides to provide a one-to-one ratio. Parents volunteer three hours per week. Like PCDI, one of the classrooms serves teenagers, focusing on jobs, daily living, and leisure skills. Aides have undergraduate degrees and receive direct and ongoing supervision from Dr. Taylor who, like Dr. Krantz at PCDI, is very "hands-on." The goal of an Alpine placement is transition either to supported inclusion or transition to special education, depending on a child's progress. Criteria for inclusion include a low rate of behavior problems, an ability to follow different kinds of prompts, and an ability to answer questions and to express needs. The developmental "bar" for inclusion using these criteria is a bit lower than PCDI's, but it is similar in its emphases on behavioral control and spontaneous communicative competencies.

The Alpine outreach program serves about half as many families as the day program (about 15). The home outreach uses an initial workshop, like LIFE, and subsequently provides three hours per week of consultation aimed at monitoring the skills of home tutors. Because Alpine's outreach component is smaller than LIFE's workshop component, Alpine's home consultation is provided by a smaller number of very highly trained behavioral-educational specialists. In terms of quality controls, the Alpine outreach is probably providing supervision more comparable to that which was found in Lovaas's original clinical model.

Increasing Independence. Like PCDI, Alpine deemphasizes the use of discrete trials and emphasizes teaching techniques aimed at improving independent task performance. Activity schedules, as well as wide use of visual icons to promote self-initiation of activity and to self-monitor behavior, are key. Choices of reinforcers and a range of token economies, include response cost "warning" systems (in which a child can lose tokens), as well as the usual token economy incentive system, in which good behavior earns tokens. The combined use of positive incentives and response costs for bad behavior promotes independent task completion more powerfully than either system used alone could do. Materials were quite varied, and this cut down on repetitious use of materials, and pupil boredom with them. There was a lot of attention to prompt fading, and great care was taken not to over-prompt. Interestingly, Alpine used a data-tracking method based on independent-observer analysis that allowed for a classroom staff member other than the teacher currently engaged in instruction to record information that could be used for trial-by-trial task analysis. This type of system can reduce the overall amount of data needed to reliably characterize a learner's status and revise instruction. More importantly, such a system frees the teacher for teaching and for maintaining a more instructional and conversational flow with the pupil.

Use of Natural Language. One impressive aspect of the Alpine program was the use of natural language with the children. Many of the school-aged pupils worked in classrooms that looked like those of any small private school, but with a higher staffing ratio. There was an emphasis on engaging children in casual conversation on the spur of the moment, without "setting up" the teaching situation, though the pupils' ability to engage in such conversations had been carefully and systematically taught. There was no "SD talk" (speech in short telegraphic phrases stripped of articles, pronouns, and adverbs) by pupils or staff as is commonly used in a Lovaas-style ABA/DTT program.

Moving High-Quality Behavioral Models into the "Real World." Alpine was an exceptional program, run scientifically by a clinician-researcher who regarded the program as a laboratory for increasing understanding of educational-behavioral programming. What remains to be seen about fine models like Alpine and PCDI is the extent to which their principles and programs can be effective with less well-trained staff, less-excellent supervision, or with higher staffing ratios—all variables that can be empirically tested. It is clear though that, as model programs, they can serve as a training resource for observers or participant-observers, to learn and later disseminate the classroom technology that they have pioneered. The next program we will examine is one that is run by the public schools. It's included here as illustrative of what can be done in a public setting that heretofore had no quality early-intervention services for children with autism.

AUTISM PARTNERSHIP LAS VEGAS

Another program worthy of note is the ABA model preschool for children with autism that has been started within the Las Vegas public schools. (Yes, there are autistic children in Las Vegas too, plenty of them.) It's interesting to consider this program as it is an example of one that tries to take the best practices of a small, private, well-funded, well-supervised program like Alpine or PCDI and move it into the public domain. The initial model classroom was the collaborative project of consultants from Autism Partnership, an ABA/DTT agency originally (though presently less) based on Lovaas's model for early autism treatment, and key school program development staff who had obtained additional specialized training in autism at the Douglass Developmental Center, a model program (that will be described later).

A Promising Training Model. The interesting thing about the Las Vegas model was that its longer-term goal was to put in place *a number* of preschool and early childhood classes for pupils with autism. Acknowledging the need for multiple classrooms was an important step in overall planning for this community (usually not a paragon of planned development). In too many places, resources go into establishing a model class, and when the word gets out, everybody wants in. Typically, the family with the biggest, baddest looming lawsuit gets their child in, whether or not that child is the best fit for the program. Over time, such a program can lose its mission, and the school district is back to square one in developing a way to help the group of kids they initially tried so hard to serve.

In the Las Vegas model, two key district resource specialists, along with about five handpicked instructional aides, initiated the program using ABA/DTT methods and a one-to-one staffing ratio. The plan was that, once the first classroom was running, one of the resource specialists (the new program's "master teachers") would rotate out. This first master teacher would be placed in the classroom of the next preschool special day class teacher designated to be trained in the new program model. The preschool teacher designated for training in the model program was then assigned to the model program classroom for an eight-week internship. During that time, she learned ABA/DTT methods under the supervision of the second master teacher, while the first master teacher remained in the interning teacher's class, reorganizing its physical environment into workstations, introducing children individually to the concept of discrete trials, and, by example, training the aides in that class in ABA/DTT methods. After the eight-week internship in the model program class, the newly trained teacher returned to her reorganized classroom with a new set of skills, pupils with some familiarity in learning via discrete trials, and aides familiar with using discrete trials through their exposure from the master teacher who had been on assignment in their classroom. Next, another preschool special day class teacher was selected to be sent to the model program class, and the master teacher in the model program classroom who had just trained the last interning teacher there switched roles with the other master teacher and moved into the itinerant role, moving into the second interning teacher's classroom. The first master teacher who had just been gone from the model class for eight weeks returned to the model class. There, she trained the second interning teacher for her eight-week rotation in the model program. In this way, each preschool special-education teacher had an opportunity to be exposed to the new model program under the direct supervision of a master teacher. Each classroom got started in using the new model with an experienced master teacher reorganizing things.

The model is definitely an interesting one. It provides a model class that can be used to orient teachers to new methods. A one-way viewing room attached to the model class allowed it to be a site for direct training sessions, either with future teacher-trainees, aide-trainees, or parents. The use of two master teachers with roles that switched every eight weeks ensured there would be no "drift" between the model classroom program and the curriculum being used in the satellite classrooms.

Most of the time, however, schools do not have the resources or numbers of underserved pupils that call for the massive effort that Las Vegas undertook. Rather, in most locales, a gifted, exceptionally well-trained teacher becomes an informal mentor to her peers who face similar challenges. Schools are faced with identifying their best teachers and then trying to figure out how to get what they are doing into other classes.

EXEMPLARY CLASSROOMS

Integrating Early Start (0-3) with Special Preschools (3-5). The special-education landscape has been changing rapidly for young children with autistic spectrum disorders. Increasingly, zero-to-three programs such as Early Start, and preschool-aged special-education programs mandated to serve children under five are confronted with the need to offer specific and intensive services to children with autism.

A big question raised in this regard only a few years ago was whether the intensive ABA/DTT types of programs that were becoming increasingly wide-spread as an early, autism-specific and home-based service could be provided equally well in school as at home. This issue was critical because, while services for children up to three years old are mandated to take place in environments that are natural for an infant and toddler (like home or day care), special-education services for children over three had primarily been established as group- and school-based models with service delivery outside the home.

Several problems presented themselves: First, many children started first interventions just before their third birthday. In most locales, the funding stream for early-intervention services shifts at the third birthday, making for discontinuity between more intensive services that might have started before age three and any services offered to begin at age three. Parents are often reluctant (not to mention displeased and aggravated) to contemplate giving up an ABA/DTT program they just finished working hard to establish. Compounded by the fact that many ABA/DTT children begin showing promising results soon after the program's initiation, the parents' reluctance is quite understandable. Second, schools often offered less intensive services than were available through home-based programs, fewer hours of one-to-one service, and fewer 20- or 25-hour-per-week programs than were increasingly being supported by emerging research. Third, home-based programs offered significant parental support and training, and many school-based programs tended either not to offer parental training, or to offer such training more informally, such as by simply having parents assist in the class.

Orange County, California. An innovative public program in Orange County, California, addressed each of these concerns in rather groundbreaking ways. First, the school system, mandated to serve children over three, contracted with the public developmental-disabilities agency mandated to serve autistic children under three. The developmental-services agency was glad to buy early-intervention services from the schools since they were typically funding home-based programs for their clients with autism from a cottage industry of nonpublic agencies that ranged from excellent to unknown in quality. As soon as the developmental-disabilities agency identified a new case as autistic, the child was referred to the school, which began service immediately and continued it seamlessly through the child's third birthday. The program that children initially entered was intended to provide services comparable to a home-based ABA/DTT program and was overseen by staff originally trained in and around the Lovaas program as well as in later-developed ABA methods. Children attended the program five days a week, five hours a day, which is about as much as an average 32-month-old can stay awake. One day a week, parents watched the class through a one-way mirror with a program staff member who used the classroom activities as live demonstrations of various ABA strategies. One day a week, each parent worked as an aide in the class, preferably not with her own child, practicing, under the teacher's supervision, the techniques she had observed. One day a week, all the parents got together for a session after dropping off their children. The session began with a coffee hour to meet and network, followed by a session led by a program staff member aimed at discussing the child's problems at home, applications of behavioral strategies to solve these problems, and general family-functioning issues. One day a week the classroom teacher would make an hour-long home visit to see how parents were able to work classroom goals into life at home with the child. In the class, children received one-to-one and one-to-two DTT, but also had group time for snack and recess where they could have an opportunity to learn to participate in group routines, a preschool-readiness skill. Recess integrated the children from the autism class with typical peers from a state preschool on the same campus.

Features of Many Classroom-Based ABA/DTT Programs. A number of schools have begun ABA/DTT programs in classrooms. Some of these programs have started in more rural areas, in which homes are too far apart for home-based service providers to get to more than one or two homes a day. Some of these programs have started in areas in which a former ABA/DTT case manager who has obtained an early childhood special-education teaching credential wants to use her behavioral and educational training in a classroom setting.

ABA/DTT classrooms are typically organized into many small carrels containing individual worktables and specific teaching materials. For example, one carrel might contain two- and three-dimensional sets of objects for working on receptive vocabulary, while another carrel might have different sets of blocks for basic block imitation drills. In some such classes, children and an assigned one-to-one aide rotate carrels as they change drills, taking the child's logbook of drills with them.

In other classes, the child remains in his assigned carrel, his own mini-classroom in which individualized picture schedules or token boards might be posted and the teacher retrieves work materials from a central location as needed. With either the activity-specific workstation or the child-specific workstation, advantages include the child's being taught by credentialed teachers, aides being supervised by credentialed teachers, the opportunity for some group-based routines like snack or a morning circle, opportunities for reverse mainstreaming for small group activities, or integration for recess, music, art, or language pragmatics groups. Speech and language pathologists, and occupational therapists are usually on site, so less time is spent transporting children to such services. Disadvantages of these programs can include a lesser emphasis on formal and informal parent training than in many home-based ABA/DTT programs, though not all parents participate in the ABA/DTT program after the initial workshop. (In fact, some (bad) ABA/DTT programs won't even allow parents to remain in the room.) One of the things I really like about school-based ABA/DTT services is that they provide needed access to such services for parents, especially single parents who themselves may not have the sophistication or economic latitude to take the required steps to initiate or maintain a home-based program.

TEACCH MODEL PROGRAMS

In chapter 11, we discussed the TEACCH model for working with pupils with autism. TEACCH's structured teaching methods characterize many special-education programs, and many TEACCH principles about routine, predictability, and task analysis are among the best educational practices for children with a range of disabilities. Because a TEACCH class isn't as strikingly delineated from any other good-quality special education program as an ABA/DTT program, it seemed important, in researching this book, to visit some TEACCH programs at the University of North Carolina (UNC) in Chapel Hill, in which the TEACCH curriculum originated. I had seen many TEACCH programs all over the United States, but wanted to see some of the original programs, just to make sure I wasn't missing anything big. Described here will be the model TEACCH preschool class that is used for observation and training of educators from all over the world.

UNC-CHAPEL HILL TEACCH PRESCHOOL

This classroom was subdivided into many small areas, but each area looked more like a "snapshot" of a typical preschool than the small, contained TEACCH carrels I had often seen elsewhere. The spaces were small enough to help children focus on the specific task in front of them, but not so much so that the alternative to looking at their work was to look at blank walls to the front and sides. These larger spaces (about five-by-five) were designated for individual work, but left enough room for teachers to move in and around the child to help with tasks. There was no single, large open space in the class, so the physical environment suggested channelled rather than open-ended exploration.

How the Program Is Structured. The model class served about five pupils, and staffing was almost one-to-one. Children attended four days per week for half-day sessions. I was told that some children had additional programs or additional structured work times at home in the afternoons, but not all did. All the children appeared to have autism.

Program Intensity. Not all instruction was one-to-one. The rich staffing ratio did however ensure that attention and participation in even group-based instruction was high. One of the impressive things was how, when aides needed to redirect a pupil to a group-based activity (such as a story at circle time), the redirection consisted of requiring a response related to the activity, rather than a more generic behavioral prompt to pay attention or a physical prompt to direct eyes at the speaker. The whole feeling of the class was low-key, rather than high-energy, and I couldn't decide whether this was intended and part of the program, or whether this reflected the more southern flavor of this TEACCH class as compared to the typically high-energy LA feel of many ABA/DTT programs. In any case, the children seemed to be engaged, inattention was minimal, and the program was well-paced for the developmental level of the group.

TEACCH EXEMPLARY CLASSES

TEACCH for Younger and More Retarded Children with Autism. One TEACCH-based early intervention program that serves children up to age five is the Lyn Center in Pittsburgh, California. This program serves children with a range of disabilities, and one class is particularly designated to serve pupils either diagnosed with autism or suspected of autism. About half the children in this class have suspected or confirmed autism, while the rest have other developmental disabilities that do not affect social functioning as much as autism does.

The classroom is very high on structure and routine, with many of the youngest children receiving full motor prompting to move through the highly structured picture schedule for all routinized activities. An initial stage for many of these children is simply learning to be compliant with a routine, learning to recognize a routine as such, and eventually experiencing the sense of independence developed from carrying out routines for themselves. As with the TEACCH preschool at UNC, this TEACCH class gently and consistently insisted on participation in a group routine. Children attended this class two to five mornings per week, and some adjunctively received home-based programs or attended typical preschools.

One of the nicest innovations in this program was the way that icons were used, particularly for interactive tasks. At snack, for instance, samples of the snack item were glued into clear audiocassette boxes, and these were exchanged for the corresponding snack item. The child could see what he would get, but couldn't get at it without an interactive exchange with the teaching adult. It was a very naturally motivating way to smooth the progress of an essentially social exchange.

An Early Elementary TEACCH Class. Another notably excellent TEACCH class for kindergarten, first, and second grades was one I visited in Oxnard, California, a fairly rural area serving a broad catchment area. When I arrived, I noticed a sign above the door in the motif of a needlepoint pillow saying "Welcome to Where My World Makes Sense." Something told me there would be a special teacher here, and there was. This class in many ways demonstrated the most effective utilization of teaching methods that have come to be specifically associated with the TEACCH curriculum.

What made this class so excellent was the way the teacher was able to take advantage of the workstation model to refine the individualization of tasks so that children at different cognitive levels functioned well, side by side. One pupil had a workstation folder that required him to Velcro a cut-out cow from his work basket onto an outline of a cow that was next to another cow, already pasted into the folder, and to repeat this procedure with several more barnyard animals (developmentally, a two-and-a-half-year-old task). Another pupil Velcro-ed the same cow next to the word "cow" in his folder, and then did the same with other barnyard animals (developmentally, a three-and-a-half- to four-year-old task). A third child had three slightly different cows, and had to Velcro each next to the relevant written description like "the big brown-and-white cow" (developmentally a five-year-old task). The ability to accommodate children at different levels well is a great use of workstations.

An Older Elementary TEACCH Class. Another TEACCH class I visited in Compton, California, a rather economically depressed area, reflected, among other things, that you don't need a lot a fancy curriculum materials or classroom equipment to have a good program. These third- through fifth-grade pupils with autism were intended for inclusion into regular-education programs in the next or the following school year. The independence afforded by the TEACCH model was well suited to preparing students for the transition to a general-education class in which one-to-one attention was not available. In this class, many pupils worked on various curriculum areas at or near grade level. As in the Oxnard class, each pupil's workstation tasks were individualized.

The teacher had made a couple of small innovations that were notable: Each workstation had, as expected, three work baskets. Instead of the teacher's assigning icons to the baskets, pupils had prepared icons of their own choosing, much like an employee who works in an otherwise nondescript corporate cubicle who individualizes his workspace. One boy had cut out Winnie the Pooh, Eeyore, and Tigger, which the teacher had then laminated and Velcro-ed to his baskets; another child used other Disney characters.

Most of the 12 or so pupils in this fairly large class did not have individual carrels, something reserved for a few of the more disruptive or distractible pupils. Instead, the teacher had the pupils seated four to a table. This class, described in chapter 11, was the one in which the teacher had used cardboard boxes and duct tape to create increasingly less restrictive workstations. In this way, the teacher had literally prompt faded the cue to mind your own work that is inherent in the workstation concept and had gotten pupils about to enter inclusion settings used to the level of distraction they would face once they were in cooperative work groups in a general education class.

A MODEL CLASSROOM INTEGRATING TEACCH AND ABA/DTT

The early to mid-1990s were probably when the furor over educational methodologies, particularly ABA/DTT versus TEACCH, reached fever pitch. It was during this time that I visited my first classroom that fully integrated the core principles of both ABA/DTT and TEACCH. Admittedly, I was skeptical before the visit. Upon arriving and having a look around at the workstations and DTT one-to-one teaching tables side by side, I conjured up a version of a *Star Wars* movie in which Obi Wan Kenobi and Darth Vader fight it out with their light swords—but with Eric Schopler and Ivar Lovaas in the combatant roles. However, after I watched for a while, it became clear that this integrated model worked really well. DTT areas were a good place to have new skills introduced. Workstations were a good place to practice emerging and more established skills. Since that time, I have seen many such programs, the best of which I'll now describe.

A model for these programs is a public program called PALS, a preschool in Clovis, California (Don't know where Clovis is? It's near Fresno). Great programs are not just to be found in urban centers of learning or culture. PALS serves about 12 pupils, of whom about three are mainstreamed at any one time so that the class functionally has a nearly one-to-one ratio consisting of a teacher, a school psychologist or speech and language pathologist (each of whom are half-time), and five aides. The class served a range of children from preverbal to a couple with near-normal expressive language skills. The class has two activity centers, one of which serves as a snack and lunch table, plus a circle time area, a "go play" center, and four carrels—two for DTT and two for TEACCH workstations. Two staff work one-to-one with children in the DTT carrels while another staff member supervises the children in the TEACCH workstations. One of the two supervisory staff (teacher plus either the psychologist or speech therapist) heads an activity at a work center while the other organizes materials for the next set of activities and oversees children who transition to the "go-play" area as they finish their DTs or workstation tasks. Each child has a visual schedule that, depending upon the child, ranges from photographs to color icons to black-and-white icons with words to words only. A fairly complicated system of groups (the "greens," the "blues," the "reds") indicated by the background color of a child's name card, shows whether the child's next activity is an activity center, DTT, or a TEACCH workstation. This is how they "check schedules," rather than just using an individual picture or word schedule. Depending on the child's level of functioning and IEP goals, different children have different mixes of these. Since one supervisory adult is always free of direct teaching, there is an excellent opportunity for hands-on training of the aides who are, as a result, among the best-trained public school aides that I've seen. Another advantage of having multiple supervisors is that it enables a smooth transition between activities. For example, the teacher started a song in circle as soon as the first child had finished snack and had come to the circle area. This directly attracted other children as they finished snack where another supervising adult oversaw the dawdlers. Some children needed one-to-one supervision at circle, and as they were directed to circle, their respective aides accompanied them. The PALS model, with its structure, strong staffing, and the ability to release a core teaching staff person to train, oversee, and engage in ongoing preparation, demonstrates how intensive teaching can be accomplished in the classroom in a way that exposes the child to learning experiences that are adult-directed (ABA/DTT), self-initiated (TEACCH), and potentially peer-facilitated (as with one-to-two and one-to-three activity-center instruction and "go-play" time).

FULL-INCLUSION MODEL CLASSROOMS

Unlike model programs for ABA/DTT or TEACCH, there are no model full-inclusion programs, but rather very individualized placements with success depending on the pupil's learning characteristics, how well learning style is matched to the placement selected, and the special supports for inclusion in the form of inclusion specialist staff and adaptations to the curriculum. As discussed in chapter 12, this is a complicated set of procedures with success often predicated on the dedication of all parties.

My own clinical experiences of successful inclusion placements very much mirror the literature, with most successful inclusive experiences happening for children who are developmentally least different or who are "protected" by a particularly high level of skill in a specific curricular area like reading or math. I also see inclusion as only working when parents and the general-education teacher all feel the child is in the right place. In addition, the criteria for entering an inclusive placement that I encountered at schools with very individualized instruction, like PCDI and Alpine, are, I believe, a real outline for success in the mainstream for a pupil with autism. Several conditions must be met: First, disruptive behaviors must be very minimal, both for the sake of the included child's time available for learning as well as for that of his classmates. It is not enough for the child with autism to be well liked by classmates, who may regard him more as a younger sibling or a mascot. On some grounds, at least, he must be in striking distance of being an equal in some subject, on the playground, using the computer, or in some other area. Second, in inclusive placements that work, the child must be able to take instruction from the teacher as it is given to the group. The child with autism may need support to carry out work that has been assigned or may need an adapted task, but he should be in "striking range" of what constitutes meaningful instruction for other pupils. The child with autism may only tolerate a shorter day or a shorter class period, or may be better placed in a special day class or resource room for certain types of instruction, but he should be substantially comparable to peers when placed in the inclusive setting.

Integration: Beginnings of Inclusive Education. One potentially beneficial way for inclusion to be introduced to a child with an autistic spectrum disorder is in an integrated class. One effective way in which this can be carried out at the preschool level is with typical peers and with some mildly atypical peers. A balance that works well for children with autism is a small class with perhaps nine to twelve preschoolers of whom three or four are typical, three or four are mildly language or otherwise delayed, and three or four have autistic spectrum disorders. This mix enables formation of a predominant culture in the class that is more social than that of the children with autism, but allows particular emphasis on teaching language with various augmentative strategies that can benefit the majority.

One model program that has done this well is LAUNCH, a public program in Torrance, California, which serves a full range of preschoolers with special-education needs in a separate preschool special-education cluster of buildings on the campus of a regular elementary school. The morning classes serving children with autism operate five days a week and use an integrated model with typical and language-delayed pupils. The staff consists of two co-teachers, or a teacher and a speech therapist plus aides, so that the overall staff-to-child ratio is about one-to-two or -three. The teaching in this program has been so successfully enriched by its extra staff and high-quality curriculum materials that the typical peers are exclusively drawn from families of staff on the special-education and regular elementary parts of the campus. They would let in neighborhood preschoolers, but there's never an opening.

The structure of the program confers several advantages: During circle time, most kids can sing along, even though the autistic children tend to lag on this. It gives the feeling that children mostly have one another to model, rather than just adults, as happens in special day classes in which most of the children are minimally verbal. In group activities, someone always volunteers an answer, and so there is turn-taking that consists not just of teachers calling upon pupils, but of a mix of pupils volunteering information, as well as pupils being asked for responses. During work times, they can create small heterogeneous work groups of two to four children working on the same activity. Older peer tutors can be brought in from elementary classes for specific activities and for adaptive physical education (something the reverse-mainstreamed peer tutors particularly enjoy). The pupils with autism in the class attend this integrated preschool in the morning, and a one-to-one ABA program in the afternoon at the same location after the half-day typical preschoolers and other pupils have gone home. This has allowed access to both integrated, age-appropriate curriculum, as well as to a more intensive curriculum that especially focuses on language learning, and autism-specific teaching.

CONTINUUM OF SERVICES MODELS

Some special-education schools offer a continuum of services designed to meet the needs of autistic spectrum children as they gain skills and can function in successively less restrictive and more mainstreamed environments. One natural facet of such programs is that classes at the different levels share a physical site. This is usually organized with "graduation" criteria for moving from one class to another, with criteria based either on how long the child has been in the program (common for initial "diagnostic" classes), or on when the child reaches certain milestones. Advantages of such programs are several: Teachers who will be teaching a child next can become familiar with him before he is placed in her class. Transitions to new placements can be made gradually, with part of the day still spent in the old class and part in the new class. Teachers are in a common location for after-school in-service training, can readily share materials, and provide social and technical support for one another.

BAUDHUIN SCHOOL

One school for students with autism that offers a continuum of services is the Baudhuin School in Ft. Lauderdale, Florida. The school's primary mission is to serve pupils with autism, but it also serves some children with other learning or language disabilities as well as Head Start pupils, who join classes for pupils with autism once the children with autism can benefit from interacting with peers. Like other model schools for children with autism, there are on-site facilities for ongoing teacher training, case conferencing, and public outreach functions. Each year, each class (two "orienting" classes, two preschool classes, and four kindergartens) start with about five children, and enrollment tends to increase to about twelve per class as the year progresses, with ancillary staff added on an as-needed basis. Children can attend the school until age five, and then may be eligible for the TIP (Therapeutic Intervention Program) between ages five and eight if they are severely handicapped as well as autistic.

How the Program Is Structured. Baudhuin focuses on a continuum of services for pupils with autism who range from higher- to lower-functioning. Admission to the school most often begins with one of the two "orienting" classes, in which children stay for their first six to eight weeks. Orienting class pupils range in age from two-and-a-half- to five-years-old and are divided into two classes, one for the older children and one for the younger ones. This is a place for children to first get used to the routines involved in going to school, and for the school to assess learning readiness, behavioral challenges, and communication competencies. Different methodological approaches are used in the class to see how children respond to each: there are workstations, computer-assisted instruction, verbal language output devices, PECS, and some group-based activities. Each child has a picture schedule, and each child's picture schedule cards are mounted on different colored backgrounds, a nice way to teach the child to relate personally to his schedule. There is a one-way observation room used both for teaching and parent observation. Teachers send home a daily log using PECS of activities the child has done and a comment about each.

After leaving the orienting class, the child may be placed in a contained special day class or in an integrated preschool. One integrated preschool class had eight high-functioning autistic four-year-olds who had started in an orienting class, ten children from Head Start, and three staff, who included a special-education teacher, an early-childhood teacher, and an aide. The class looked like a very good typical preschool, but with very structured teaching that included much attention to breaking tasks into small components, a lot of visual cueing, and intensive eliciting of spoken language by every adult all the time.

There was another preschool class for seven four-year-olds with autism who were verbal, but not yet ready to be included in a general education class. The class had two teachers plus a speech and language therapist, who was often there. These children were slated to attend an inclusion kindergarten the following year, in which each child would be one of only one or two special-needs children in the class, and in which there would be an extra instructional aide for that child (or the two children). Each child in this class had an individually tailored token system and picture schedule to help with transitions. The picture schedules showed each child's play time, sensory time, book time, "basket time" (direct instruction), computer time, and learning-center time (group instruction). Classroom rules were posted as reminders that teachers could use orally or visually as prompts. On another wall there were "scripts" for aides to use in directing behavior such as "sharing," "play organizing," "agreeing," "requesting assistance," and "requesting to share" (for example, "Point to the piece you want.").

Integration of School Day and After-School Services. The TIP program at Baudhuin starts at noon or two, depending on whether the child comes in from a half-day special day kindergarten or from a full-day special-education class. This program serves 42 children in the kindergarten to fourth-grade age range. These are generally more behaviorally challenged children who can't be safely maintained by any family member at home in the afternoon. Some have such marked behavioral challenges that it is very difficult for just a parent, who may have other children at home, to care for the child. The program is oriented toward teaching community and functional skills but also includes time to work on pre-academic skills learned at school in the morning. The staffing ratio is one adult to three children, and a number of children require one-to-one assistance. Such programs are invaluable. Parents of children with autism need day care, just like other parents. Few parents of children with disabilities work outside the home precisely because it is so hard to find day care that can take a child (like a child with autism) and provide an appropriately nurturing environment.

What a model like Baudhuin does best is provide a continuum of services in which a child can move from initial diagnostic placement into one of two kinds of preschools, and from there to one of four slightly different kindergartens. While the kindergartens are not as notably stratified as the preschool classes, being on the same site allows for a good deal of balancing in the composition of each class and a lot of sharing among teachers who used to have some children, who currently have them, and others who might have them next. For a contained site, Baudhuin has been able to do a very good job including Head Start children and children with more minor language disabilities. Along with the provided inclusion supports, integration there works well with the relatively higher-functioning (on average) children that they serve. The TIP program, which largely serves a more severely involved group, struggles to achieve the same degree of coherence. This is apparent in the early-childhood programs, though TIP is providing an incredibly valuable service for a group of children who, largely, develop skills only with much more repetition and structure and learn much more slowly.

DOUGLASS DEVELOPMENTAL CENTER

The Douglass Developmental Center, headed by Dr. Sandra Harris, is on the campus of Rutgers University in New Brunswick, New Jersey. The Douglass model is one that can continually serve children from the early preschool years through young adulthood. The Douglass program sees itself as more developmental in its orientation than other programs that might characterize similar work as more behavioral. Like TEACCH, quality is reflected in the structure of the programs, especially the structure of the preschool classes, which have very highly scheduled programming.

The preschool programs are probably the best recognized of the program's services and consist of three levels. The "Upper School" has four levels—two classes that serve elementary school-aged pupils, and two that serve high school-aged students. Many of the Upper School students attended the early childhood programs but did not "graduate" into inclusive placements, and so the older children served are, on average, more cognitively disabled. Two group home apartments house five young adults each.

How the Program Is Structured. The Douglass program begins with three levels of preschool program. All the preschool classes start using PECS from the beginning, mainly relying on Mayer-Johnson icons. Level 1 serves six children and uses one-to-one DTT programs. Level 2 intersperses one-to-one DTT sessions and work on independent tasks for periods of up to 20 minutes, with 20-minute small group activities. Children are mainly three or four years old, and the overall teaching ratio is one adult to two children. This allows one or more adults to do one-to-one work while one or more adults run a small-group activity. The Level 3 preschool serves 12 older preschool-aged children, half of whom are autistic and are as old as six, and half of whom are typical peers as old as five (including siblings and children of staff). This class has a teacher, three aides, and a speech and language pathologist who work with the children individually in the class. Each child with autism is paired with a typical peer for one-to-two teaching. This is an interesting model because, like the LAUNCH program that was described earlier, the "typical" peers are a somewhat special select group who are exposed to some incidental as well as purposeful coaching to become "study buddies," their role at school. Also, the pairing of one autistic child with one peer helps the additional "information" given by typical peers to be better understood than it is when all are in a larger group containing a number of typical peers, and there is a certain tendency for the typical peers, at times, to attend more to one another than to another child in the class who happens to have autism.

The Upper School at Douglass focuses on functional academics and community contact. The elementary class (Level 1), which serves six or seven six- to nine-year-olds has a teacher and three aides. Most of these children are primarily nonverbal and use PECS for both leisure and work schedules, some with icons and some with words. The elementary class (Level 2) for nine- to thirteen-year-olds is similar. Both elementary classes focus on pre-academic concepts with a functional academic orientation.

Levels 3 and 4 of the Upper School are high school-aged programs. In the early years of high school, the focus is on daily living skills, with a continued focus on functional academics. The teaching space is very functionally organized, with kitchen and laundry facilities. Math and reading tasks are geared to activities related to functioning independently in these spaces. In the later years of the high school program, which provides services until the pupils age out of school services at 21, emphasis is on identifying and acquiring prevocational and vocational skills and on structuring leisure time. There are areas for the high schoolers to learn to socialize, and also solitary activity like listening to music on headphones or watching TV.

Integration of Home and School Services. A large proportion of Douglass preschoolers (about 70 percent) have afternoon home DTT programs supported either by the Douglass Outreach program or by other nonpublic agencies in the area. Because Douglass itself runs some of the home programs, home and school services are well-coordinated. Initially, parents receive two Saturday home-based workshop days (similar to other home-based ABA/DTT programs), along with the specific tutors who are to work with the child. The school runs parent support groups, with separate groups for the preschool parents, Upper School parents, and (much needed, often neglected) sibling groups.

The Douglass Outreach program also provides consultation services to school districts to ensure further integration of services. Most Douglass graduates who enter the mainstream utilize resource-room services. The goal is typically to pull back on the one-to-one aide after one to four years of public school inclusion. After starting at Douglass Center or an outreach program, parents subsequently receive twice-monthly home-based follow-ups to teach generalization of newly emerging skills and to develop targeted behavioral interventions in response to behavior-management difficulties. These services are provided by home behavior consultants who have usually worked in the Douglass school programs and so have a high level of training and a good idea about how to coordinate school and home content.

WHAT DO WE LEARN FROM THE MODEL PROGRAMS?

We've reviewed many model programs here, some public, most private. The private programs are generally incredibly well endowed, with absolutely beautiful physical facilities and more space than any fine public program serving the same number of children would have. Nevertheless, there are both wonderfully innovative public and private models. It is clear that the best programs have a well-thought-out curriculum, high fidelity of implementation, high structure, individualization, and, last and absolutely most importantly, really competent, high-quality, well-trained, creative teaching staff.

After visiting the model private programs, I came away with two strong and conflicting emotional responses. Some of the programs were so wonderful for the children that I wanted to stay all day and just watch. But I realized that the preschool-aged programs in particular, and all the model private programs I saw in general, were serving a selected stratum of the autistic spectrum. It wasn't always the highest of the high functioning that I saw, but in the preschool programs I seldom saw children whom I felt were moderately to severely mentally retarded, though about half the children with a diagnosis of autism are just that. I don't fault the people doing excellent work in running the model programs. Given the chance, I'd likely do the same. As an educator, if you are trying to work out teaching principles, you will need a population with which you can really evaluate the effectiveness of the "tweaks" you make to tune the machinery designed to serve your specific group of children. There is more to be learned from services that can be put in place to serve the upper 50 percent of the autistic spectrum. But that doesn't change the fact that we still know less about what to do for the very, very youngest, and for the most severely impaired children, compared to the higher-functioning ones.

Every parent, every clinician, every teacher hopes that any given preschooler is *not* going to be one of the more severely affected ones—even though, honestly, clinicians and teachers often—quite quickly, have a very good idea of who the more severely affected children are. Maybe this hope that the particular child in front of us at this very moment really is not severely affected has steered us away from treating the real problems these children have, and, instead, we treat them like the children we hope they might be able to be, and they respond less well. Over the years, for me personally, this reality has encouraged me to create more functional, life-skills programs for younger children who are severely impaired.

CHAPTER CONCLUSIONS

The model programs actually served very few children. But what the model programs and exemplary classes make clear is that it is possible to devise excellent programs that make a significant difference. There was a tremendous amount to be learned by getting to know these programs, but the resources they utilized means that in "the real world," educators must select the most powerful features of each of these programs so that they can, one hope, get 90 percent of the bang for 30 to 50 percent of the buck.

I don't think this is impossible. First of all, public education, for better or worse, is mandated to provide "appropriate" education—not necessarily the best education. The private model programs reviewed here are some of the best of the best. However, some of the exemplary public-school classes were just as good. It is not clear from these model programs or exemplary classes or from any outcomes research that currently exists just how much is needed to get the best *outcomes* and how much of what we do is superfluous. Cost effectiveness is a basically untouched, and often taboo, topic in special education, but it has to be broached if all children with autism are truly to have equal access to free and appropriate public educations.

In the next and final chapter, we will discuss taking information about how autistic children learn and combining it with knowledge about treatment models to formulate further suggestions about how program features and teaching methods can be combined and placed in different kinds of learning contexts to permit the child with autism to have active learning experiences as much of the time as possible.

CHAPTER FOURTEEN

Putting the "I" Back in IEP: Creating Individualized, Meaningful Learning Experiences

"IN THE IDEAL WORLD"

What's the best kind of program to have? Where does ABA/DTT fit in? Where does TEACCH fit in? Where does integration and inclusion fit in? ABA/ DTT, TEACCH, integrative education, and inclusion are all methods of education. What about content once the method is selected? By now, it should be clear that the autistic spectrum disorders are not one-size-fits-all—not with respect to cause, not with respect to learning differences among children with autism, and so it follows, not with respect to treatment. How then can guidelines be developed to provide a range of services (methods, numbers of hours of treatment, curriculum content) that different children within the autistic spectrum will need? After initial services are in place, how can procedures be developed to ensure that the child is actually getting what is promised? Too often, lack of hoped-for progress is taken as evidence that promised services are not being delivered.

When asked about services for pupils with autism, many school administrators start by saying, "We have a TEACCH class, do we need to support an ABA/ DTT program too?" Parents will say, "I need a home ABA/DTT program because my school only has a TEACCH class." Schools that provide both ABA/

DTT and TEACCH methods are often concerned about how children should transition from one to another, or whether they should receive some of both, and, if so, how to adjust the mix.

Parents often ask, "If I could do either ABA/DTT or TEACCH for my child, which is best?" Or "Should he be in full inclusion instead of a special-education class?" Good questions, but complicated. There is just not enough data on outcomes from the different kinds of special-education methods used for children with autism to say that one method is consistently going to be more effective than another. The method has to be best fitted to who the child is right now and then individualized in terms of treatment content. Then, later on (and this can be a really underappreciated point), this child is likely to become someone different, educationally speaking. This means that the best fit will change.

Establishing Instructional Control. One way to think of the different methods for teaching children with autism is to place the different treatment approaches along some sort of continuum of services the child may need as his learning needs change. ABA/DTT has strong advantages in the "learning-to-learn" phase of instruction. The use of high levels of direct reinforcement, shaping, and prompting whip into shape a basic repertoire of learning prerequisites like attention, compliance, and imitation. These skills constitute the fundamentals of instructional control. However, instructional control can be developed in a TEACCH class too, when sufficient intensity is employed. Remember, TEACCH also uses principles of applied behavior analysis; it just doesn't use the method of discrete trial training: You must initially prompt and shape a child to use picture schedules and workstations, just as you must initially prompt a child to respond to each discriminative stimulus before instruction can proceed.

TEACCH utilizes strong visuals from day one, with the introduction of picture schedules—much more copasetic for a highly visual, nonverbal autistic child with no solid receptive language. Usually in ABA/DTT, the child needs to demonstrate he's *not* an "auditory" learner, before a shift is made (if it is made at all) to picture-based icons for communication. But an ABA/DTT program could use visual icons from the beginning too. Although TEACCH or ABA/DTT could be a first treatment, for most children with autism, ABA/DTT will usually produce quicker initial results (especially in the first 6 to 12 weeks), though often with more protest than in early stages of a TEACCH program.

While no one likes to upset little kids, the protests associated with the early stages of an ABA/DTT program only last until the child figures out and accepts the system of "I need to do something to get something." This is arguably no better or no worse that letting infants and toddlers "cry it out" until they learn to sleep through the night.

More substantive is the issue of what children initially learn, in terms of content, in early stages of an ABA/DTT program compared to the early stages of a TEACCH program. The accomplishments in attention, compliance, and instructional control often seen in an ABA/DTT program can be impressive. However, I, personally, am not wowed by the rote recitations of colors, numbers, shapes, body parts, and other classificatory nouns that children learn as part of compliance training and that, for some, passes as receptive, and even expressive, language. I am frankly embarrassed and don't know what to say when I am introduced to a four-year-old child with autism who never spontaneously uttered more than a single word at a time, but who has been trained to emit what I am told is: "My name is Jeremy Hunter. I live in Costa Mesa, California" in a single exhale. Of course, as we discussed in chapter 10, ABA/DTT techniques do not have to be used this way; instead, the discrete-trial methodology can be used to teach skills using multiple SDs simultaneously and more developmentally. In this case, the child can make quick *and* developmentally meaningful progress.

In TEACCH programs, on the other hand, progress is, from the beginning, usually slow but steady. Progress has to do with learning to function as part of a group, to follow routines, and to organize pro-social behaviors independently. The same pre-academic content is taught in TEACCH as in an ABA/DTT program, but it is taught in a way that is more a hybrid of the direct, focused instruction we associate with DTT and the "learning through doing" we see in typically developing preschool-aged children. Compared to the rote recitations that a Lovaas-style ABA/DTT program can produce in the first four months, it seems much more age-appropriate when a language-limited four-year-old takes his work basket off the shelf on his own, opens the folder in it, and matches eight mommy animals to their baby animals.

Weighing ABA/DTT and TEACCH for Earliest Programs. Since both ABA/DTT and TEACCH can confer slightly different advantages, the question is how to get the best of both worlds. All things, like program availability, program quality, and cost being equal (which they never are), children need access to both

ABA/DTT and TEACCH programs. Ideally, access to a good-quality ABA/DTT program to establish instructional control, nonverbal, and, if possible, verbal imitation would be a great place to start. The ABA/DTT program providers would not rigidly adhere to ABA/DTT as the only viable methodology, but would gladly work cooperatively with TEACCH teachers to enrich the child's experience with a complementary component of classroom-based TEACCH, giving the child an opportunity to be with developmentally comparable peers to practice new skills. The child would continue to receive DTT at home or school each day, with special emphasis on introducing new concepts in a developmentally structured way. Then the child would have time to work with these emerging concepts at his TEACCH work station, going at his own pace, and under his own initiative, taking the necessary time for "inside out," more self-initiated learning. The TEACCH class would serve both ASD and other developmentally disabled children, including children with language disabilities, so that the child with autism would have peers with similar developmental capacities, but who had more social interest than other children with autism. In this way, group time would hold greater potential for social engagement and would serve to prompt imitation of more advanced social models.

Reexamining Truisms. Life is not one-to-one. More is not always better. Learning something new faster or sooner is not necessarily better. In a child with autism, learning certainly needs to be supported, scaffolded. The ability to learn spontaneously and independently—a key to learning throughout life—can easily be quashed by too much adult-led teaching. TEACCH offers a very strong alternative in terms of an ALD-specific program that also nurtures the develop- ment of self-guided learning. ABA/DTT offers a way to introduce the child to new ideas that he is unlikely to discover (that is, observe, choose to read about, experiment with) on his own. Because he is autistic, the child likely prefers the familiar to the novel, and ABA/DTT programs are well suited to help such a child move past that proclivity and gain exposure to new ideas.

DEVELOPMENT AND UTILIZATION OF HYBRID PROGRAMS

It should be apparent at this point that I see no one method that is perfectly suited to all children with autism, nor do I see where one method can confer all the learning advantages that any one child needs. This means considering ways that methods for teaching children with autism can be combined so that synergies are formed, and individual children can have their educational needs met. From this perspective, treatment is a dynamic, ever-changing process that will need constant reconsideration with the mix of formal and more natural educational opportunities changing as the child acquires more skills and can learn in more diverse ways from different kinds of experiences. This means more focused, direct, repetitive teaching for the youngest children who initially just need to develop learning-readiness skills. As these skills emerge, it is important that the child has opportunities to use them in a variety of settings to see that learning can occur anywhere. Once a child has some ability to comply, for example, compliance should not just be confined to complying while at school, but should be expected at home, when the child needs to "come here." Once the child can pay attention to an activity set in front of him at a work table, he should be given opportunities to use that skill to pay attention to what he's eating, and systematically feed himself the way he can systematically finish a multi-piece puzzle. This means constructing less formal learning opportunities in a variety of settings using all of the teaching approaches we have talked about in this book.

BALANCING ADULT-LED TEACHING AND CHILD-INITIATED LEARNING

A Continuum of Teaching Methods. One major dimension of providing children with diverse learning opportunities is to balance the time spent in direct or adult-led instruction with time spent in child-initiated activity: Traditional "Lovaas" ABA/DTT programs are very much adult-led and represent one end of the continuum. Other methods of teaching that use ABA principles but do not use DTT, such as pivotal response training and incidental teaching methods that use prompting, prompt-fading, and chained approximations of behaviors, fall next on the continuum. Methods that give direction via visual means, such as VIA (introduced in chapters 5 and 6) and PECS, come next, although these methods focus primarily on communication training. In the more comprehensive TEACCH curriculum, or in using activity schedules (as discussed in the last chapter), the child is under constant control of a command, but that command is embedded in a picture or word rather than a person telling the child what to do, even though the adult is still present for needed prompting. Next on the continuum come choice paradigms, in which the child is still following some set of instructions, but has chosen the task for himself. Included here is the use of strategies such as "Activity Schedules." Finally, more child-directed treatments like Floor Time (discussed in chapter 4) allow the child to be the initiator of the topic for engagement.

The need to develop more hybrid treatment opportunities for children with autism is predicated on two assumptions about the continuum of methods that has just been described: First, more highly adult-directed programs serve (among other things) to expose children with autism to information they would not likely have sought on their own. Second, more child self-initiated programs help the child build a sense that self-selecting meaningful activities can be rewarding, and so the tendency to learn about new things is promoted. Third, the mix of adult-led and child-led activities is governed by how well established the child's basic abilities to learn are. The child still without basic learning-readiness skills will need more adult-directed teaching. The child being exposed to new and unfamiliar ideas, materials, and vocabulary will need more adult-directed teaching. As the child develops learning readiness and learns to use those skills in different situations, he is ready for some more child-initiated learning experiences. Increasingly, self-initiation is associated with self-motivation, which is, in turn, associated with the learning experience's being perceived as rewarding.

Rewarding experiences may be associated with neurochemical events that potentiate more powerful plastic responses in the brain. This means that the ultimate goal of teaching is to change the child's brain in a way that supports increased functionality. The challenge, then, is in devising learning experiences in which the child is motivated by the experience itself to do or learn more. In this way, he is more likely enabling positive changes to his own brain function. It is then that the learning process can become self-sustaining. If the child is not interested in the learning activity for its own sake, but is simply completing a task to receive an external reward, the response of the brain to the learning experience may be qualitatively less enriching. It is for this reason that it is important to teach the child using materials and contexts he cares about. Shaping an ability to learn with an external reward (like a food) is OK to start out. It's just that in the long run, dependence on external rewards is less likely to lead to self-perpetuated learning.

Therefore, one should not choose teaching methods using the Chinese-menu-lunch-special method, in which the educator suggests that the parent simply select whatever she finds "tasty." Instead, the mix of teaching strategies should be based on information about the child's learning readiness, capacity to generalize learning-readiness skills to more independent settings, and mastery of the curriculum content. Developmentally appropriate and meaningful curriculum content has a much better chance of engendering self-perpetuated learning in the future. Said more succinctly, the child needs to be taught things he finds interesting.

INTEGRATING METHODOLOGIES

By way of example, we will now briefly review some ways in which key curriculum models can be integrated. Some of these strategies have been mentioned earlier when the methods themselves were described, but they are presented here to illustrate what is meant by the development of hybrid treatment programs for children with autism.

Bringing Picture Communication into ABA/DTT Programs. A key addition to the way in which many young children with autism are initially taught is using picture-communication methods in the beginning stages of ABA/DTT programs for preverbal or markedly language-delayed children. The picture-communication method could be the Visual Interaction Augmentation (VIA) method or the Picture Exchange Communication System (PECS) discussed in chapter 6. (My preference, as I stated, is for more literal icons, like actual but inaccessible objects, or photographs of objects. These are more congruent with the "thinking-in-pictures" cognitive style of preverbal children and nonverbal children with ASDs, and are more motivational because recognition of the icon is likely to be more immediate.)

Neither developmental theory, the scant existing research, nor what we know about autistic learning styles supports the contention that if a child with autism is taught a picture system to communicate, verbal development will be delayed. Rather, developmental theory suggests that normal infants and preverbal toddlers think in pictures and develop receptive labels well in advance of speaking. A picture-communication system bridges nonverbal language pragmatics with a visual-icon system that can later segue to a verbal communication system. What we know about autistic learning styles is that the autistic child looks for the path of least resistance in getting his needs met—getting things for himself when he can, and only resorting to hand-leading or tantrumming when he can't. If the child is made to exchange a picture for a wanted object, he will do so, especially if hand-leading and tantrumming become ineffective. If the child can say the word instead of exchanging an icon, he will if he comes to see that as a quicker way to get his request fulfilled. VIA or PECS make verbalizing functional and thereby useful to the child with autism. Rotely learned vocabulary is not likely to be self-reinforcing in the same way, and such teaching takes the child down the wrong path in early priming of self-initiated learning skills. By pairing VIA or PECS with ABA/DTT vocabulary teaching, the emphasis switches from a randomly selected set of preschool "words" (like animals, colors, shapes) to things the child cares about (preferred foods, toys, activities). This not only motivates communication more effectively, it teaches vocabulary in a sequence more like lexical acquisition patterns seen in typically developing kids.

More importantly, children with autism should not have to fail before they succeed. Many language-delayed, preverbal, or nonverbal children with autism who are not developmentally at the stage for spoken language to emerge (or never get there), will be quite frustrated when verbal expression is requested, especially in the form of prompts for specific sounds with no intrinsic communicative link to the subsequent reinforcer. (This means that saying "e-e-e" or "a-a-a" to get a desired Fruit Loop as a reinforcer does not reinforce specific communicative intent the way handing over a picture of a pile of Fruit Loops and saying "f-f-f" does.) By integrating picture-exchange strategies with early ABA/DTT programs, use of communicative efforts for specific intents is started from the beginning, which is how typically developing children learn to talk.

Combining ABA/DTT and TEACCH. In reviewing model programs in the last chapter, we included illustrations of exemplary classes using both TEACCH methods and ABA/DTT. Visual scheduling of the day's activities helps keep instruction organized, even in a class with all ABA/DTT teaching. Activity schedules, as developed in a model ABA program, are essentially a choice-based use of the TEACCH picture-schedule concept.

In other classes, moving from one-to-one DTT to one-to-two DTT is a prime method for ABA programs to introduce brief opportunities to learn from a model and to benefit incidentally from instruction not directed to the child himself. TEACCH workstations can serve a similar purpose, with the child moving away from direct one-to-one instruction and moving more toward the instructional control of visual directions (like a work basket task). Assigning teachers to two or even three pupils using workstations, depending on the age and competencies of the pupils, and their familiarity with the materials, similarly allows more opportunities for the child to keep himself on task. A particularly synergistic arrangement can be to use DTT to introduce new materials and then use TEACCH workstation materials to practice and generalize concepts that first have been directly taught.

Developing Play and Leisure Skills. A final example shows how more child-directed activity can be used to complement the time the child is under instructional control of one-to-one teaching (ABA/DTT), specific materials (TEACCH), or group-based instruction. Both ABA/DTT and TEACCH curricula provide semi-structured "go-play" break areas, or, for older pupils, "recreation centers." For ABA/DTT programs, access to these break areas is more frequent for younger children and less frequent for older children, with the younger group using them about every 5 to 15 minutes for 3 to 5 minutes. In TEACCH programs, children earn time in the play center after completing a series of three workstation tasks. In many ABA/DTT and TEACCH programs, the teacher uses the child's break time as an opportunity to take data or to reorganize materials for the next teaching session. In a class setting with sufficient staff, this time can be used for an adult to engage in guided participation in the child's play activity, letting the child choose his toy and activity, but pressing the activity into the shape of an interactive exchange lead by the child's choice of materials and functions. The teacher in such an instance would generally be following the principles of the Floor Time model, in which the child's interest in social interaction can develop through having his chosen activity made more interesting for him. In any case, time in the break or leisure center of a classroom should be overseen by an adult for several reasons: to prevent mental downtime, which can be quite self-sustaining, to allow a period of child-initiated activity that is still guided to incorporate recently taught vocabulary or other skills, to demonstrate more imaginative use of the toys, and to facilitate mutual peer activity if two children are in the play area at the same time.

Integration of Home and School. In addition to the many considerations of how various educational methods can be hybridized to provide very individualized treatment, there is the question of how a balanced mix of learning experiences can be continued into the child's life beyond the treatment program or classroom. How parents can become integral to the educational process? In the next section, we will examine roles for parents both in and outside of their child's formal educational experiences. This is really important because research increasingly demonstrates links between parent participation and positive outcomes. A variety of model programs and classes make access to the program contingent on parent involvement for this reason.

THE IMPORTANCE OF PARENTS

Parents as Teachers

How much difference can parents make in the outcome of their child's treatment? Research consistently points to parent involvement in a child's treatments as a critical factor in quality. Model programs virtually always include parent training or support. What other roles are there for parents? So far in this chapter, we have emphasized just how important it is to individualize a child's learning experiences. This may mean combining aspects of different kinds of programs, having the child spend different parts of the day in different classes or even in different schools. It means combining different methods of teaching and different sites for the teaching as part of the child's overall experience. Who does this? Many parents express the need for a third parent who would do nothing but make all the things around the care of the child with autism work right! But, is being an autism secretary the most valuable contribution parents can make to their child's progress?

Parents as Micromanagers and "Micro-Stimulators" of Development. A good way to think about the important role of parents is to compare your ideal of a parent of a typical child to a parent of a child with autism. The role of a typical child's parent includes many things that a child with autism's parent does too, like selecting a school, learning what special resources a school has, and signing their child up for the school they feel might be most beneficial. Parents of typically developing children plan extracurricular activities like being on a soccer team and going to a camp for part of the summer. Parents also try to actualize their child's potential by helping them with homework so they can better understand what the child is studying, and try to spark a deeper interest or appreciation of certain topics. Parents are also the guardians of the child's social and moral development, and develop rules, set limits, and give rewards for fine accomplishments. Parents of children with autism essentially do all these things too.

Some parents of typically developing children also do a lot of what might be called micro-stimulating their child's development. What does this mean? For example, coming out of the grocery store, I encountered a father with what looked like his three-and-a-half-year-old, five-year-old, and six-year-old. The four-year-old asked why the ice cream they had just bought had a cow on it. The father explained that it was Ben and Jerry's ice cream and that it was made in Vermont. Then, he asked the six-year-old if he knew the capital of Vermont, and the six-year-old replied, "Montpelier." The five-year-old asked if she had ever been to Vermont. The father said, "No, but if we went to Vermont now it would be very cold with lots of snow. What do we do with lots of snow?" he asked the three-and-a-half-year-old. "Ski!" she said. There was a whole civics and geography lesson going on as this family loaded groceries into their trunk. Many parents would not be talking to their children at a time like that, or might just be giving directions, like telling the six-year-old to hold his little sister's hand while he put the groceries in the car. Some parents, though, make a trip to the market into a bit of a field trip. I would call this "micro-stimulation" of children's development. This is admirable, energetic, and probably good for kids' minds, though perhaps a bit obsessive, as parenting styles go.

There are some parents of children with autism who are "micro-stimulators" too. Every moment becomes a teaching opportunity. They are constantly in touch with when, where, and what to teach. They know just how hard to push (just enough, but not too much), so that learning and a lesson are not the same thing. These are parents of children with autism who can exquisitely sense an opportunity to teach or reinforce a lesson, and know just when to jump on it. This is an art, not a science. It's more instinctive than intentional. If you do it a second too late, the topic is no longer of as great interest and the intrinsic reinforcement value of having your curiosity requited is lost. If the answer is made into a lesson, the child does not experience the pleasure of getting information on that quick, contingent, "need-to-know" basis: If the father in the last example had responded to the question about why the cow was on the ice cream by telling the child to wait until the groceries were in the car, and they were all in their car seats, it would have been boring for him to say, "Well, back in the parking lot a few minutes ago, Stacey asked why there was a cow on the ice cream. Does anyone have an answer?"

Children with autism may not express curiosity in things around them the way four-year-old Stacey asked about the cow on the ice cream, but very responsive parents of children with autism are able to tune into a much fainter signal. A parent might notice the child looking at the ice cream with the cow on it, and take the pint and say, "Is that a horse?" or "Do you see a cow? What color are the cow's spots?" A parent of a bright six-year-old with autism with a well-known interest in state capitals might entice him to move from the observation of the cow, to learning that lots of cows live in Vermont, to ice cream's being made in Vermont from cow's milk, to Vermont's being a state— so what's the capital?

Occasionally, I meet exceptional parents who naturally pick up these faint signals that their child with autism emits and amplify them in the way I've just described. Others learn to pick up on such signals quickly with just a little guidance. A third group tries just as hard, but remains mired in talking to their child in "SD" talk (as if life were a discrete trial) and gives many on-the-spot lessons that they insist the child complete, whether he wants to respond or not. Most parents, however, do recognize their special role of "amp-ing" up their child's often-faint signal from the natural learning opportunities in the world around him.

What is not always acknowledged is how important this micro-stimulating role likely is. In a study we did of very high responders to very intensive early interventions, a common characteristic of the "most-improved" kids was that they had parents who wouldn't leave them alone. This type of cognitive and social micro-stimulation was accompanied by micromanaging the child's education. In the earlier years, these parents would choose therapists very carefully, replacing ones who were not quite right, visiting every possible inclusion-preschool site, and figuring out exactly which children were there at which times of day, and therefore which session would be the best fit for their child. In later years, these parents carefully cultivated peer buddies in any inclusion setting, and pre-taught school assignments at home themselves. By high school, some of these moms were still interviewing every English teacher to see how he felt about making adaptations to the core curriculum. Many were reluctant to give up the autism "label," even after the children did not meet diagnostic criteria anymore (which did make them very happy), because *they* still saw work to be done and wanted the leverage of the diagnosis to recruit ongoing help. These moms can be annoying to school personnel and therapists, but they are uniformly respected. From what I can see, time put into directly enhancing the child's awareness of his world is far more valuable to the child than time spent mounting the fifth IEP of the year trying to get just three more months of this, or two more hours of that.

WAYS OF TRAINING PARENTS

Many micromanaging moms seem to be born and not made. How do you make them? One fantasy I've had is to bottle some essence of the best of these moms and sprinkle it over those who need the most help. One such mother appeared on the television show *20/20* discussing her daughter's dramatic improvements, crediting her child's ABA agency—which indeed had been wonderful. The TV people had interviewed me, too, and I told them that if they only quoted one thing I had to say, please say that this mother was at least as important to her daughter's improvement as the treatment program she received. They didn't, and I think it was because the mother herself did not give herself the credit she was due.)

Special Components of Parenting a Child with Autism. We have to work harder to identify the components of the talents of the best parents: What might these components be?

First, it looks like these parents have given themselves permission to really love being with their child. Yes, they are worried about their child's future. Yes, they are concerned they might do the wrong thing. Yes, they get concerned that the child is not getting enough. These worries do not, however, stand in the way of just having a good time with the child. Worry itself does not make things better, but can make things worse by setting up a barrier between child and parent. Parents need to follow their intuition and be as silly with their children with autism as they are with their typical child. A playful atmosphere makes learning a desirable experience.

Second, parents can work as their child's teacher, but must not give up the role of parent—because there are many people who can be the child's teacher, but only one who can be his mother and one who can be his father. Parents need to become educated about what autism is and how children with autism learn.

Finding yourself immersed in any singular treatment focus (like nutrition, diet, or the immune system) should be a warning that anxiety is taking over and naturally causing a desire to reduce all the scary feelings to one or two simple things that can be controlled. This is a natural response to fighting autism—a problem of the brain, which you have learned is different in some way no one can really see.

Parents Need to Help Themselves First. It is incredibly stressful to parent a child with autism. The stress and anxiety comes from observing current deficits, fear of future deficits, and the day-to-day strain of the additional and unusually demanding care. I had the honor of participating on a panel of speakers that included the mother of an eight-year-old lower-functioning boy with autism. In her address to this audience, infant educators who were dealing with parents just as their children were being diagnosed, she had one theme: to tell, convince, support, cajole, insist that the mothers of their charges get psychotherapeutic support for themselves. She spoke of how this can be so hard to do when a family is pressed with new expenses related to the care of the autistic child. She talked about the guilt of diverting to oneself any resources that could possibly be used for the child. It is, however, absolutely necessary, she argued. "It saved me," she told them. As a mother who had been involved in autism self-help groups, it was her solid impression (and there are some data on this too) that the first two years after diagnosis pass in a haze of depression for most of the parents she had gotten to know.

The diagnosis of autism is definitely a major life stressor, up there with getting divorced, having a child die, or being left permanently crippled by a car accident. For most life stressors, it is well accepted that at least brief psychotherapy can be very helpful in assisting a person to get back to normal or establish a new norm. There is no psychotherapy content specific to parents of a disabled child the way there is for breast cancer patients or veterans with posttraumatic stress disorder. A good psychotherapist who perhaps knew the parent prior to the child's birth, or one recommended by the child's diagnostician as having a special interest in families with a child with a disability, would be a good place to start investigating a therapist, if you are the parent of a newly diagnosed child with autism. Burying grief does not work. It burns like acid into the personality. Many parents who have not addressed their grief convert the negative energy into anger, not at the child, but at those who do not make the child well, because if the child was well, the grief would disappear. Since most children with autism get better, but do not get well, there is, for many, a lot of unresolved grief.

Parents as Co-Therapists. Although parents are the child's only parents, they can be excellently suited to be therapists as well. It's not for everyone, but can be an important contribution for the parent who has the predilection to do the work. Working with one's own child therapeutically obviously does require specialized additional training, and this means the parent's working as a pupil of the training therapist, while still retaining the executive control of being the child's parent. This can be a bit of a sensitive position, but certainly can be done well with ABA home-based workshops being a particularly well-developed model for bringing the parent in as a co-therapist. One strategy to recommend for parents functioning as a therapist or a tutor for their child is to delimit those activities by conducting them in a specific part of the house, wearing a smock or other garment that delineates the parent's teaching time as separate from their parenting time. In chapter 10, when we talked about ABA/DTT programs, we discussed how the UCLA Early Autism Project used to require parents to become senior therapists for their child.

As special-education rights have come to the fore, and more services have become available, there are unfortunately some parents who view their recruitment as therapist or co-therapist as nothing but a ploy to save the special-education system money. This is a sad, cynical idea that potentially hurts no one but the child. Depending on the child's age, the intensity of treatment he can use, his functioning, and the coordination among existing available services, there is often an important and integrative role that only the parent can play if that parent gets training that is congruent with other therapies and education the child is receiving.

Parents as Interpreters. A critical role that parents can serve for their children with autism is as the child's interpreter. It is well understood that because children with autism have specific motivation problems, they do as little as is absolutely necessary to get what they want they tend to use many context-specific, and idiosyncratic, cues, so it may be hard for anyone other than a parent or teacher who knows the child well to know what he likely means by what he says or does.

While the purpose of education is to make that communication less idiosyncratic and less in need of an interpreter, the parent or teacher experienced with the child is often needed to let others know what all is going on in that little head. To the extent that parents, therapists, and teachers have opportunities to watch one another work and interact with the child, there is an opportunity to form a bridge of understanding how the child does things, what causes misunderstandings, and how better to teach the child.

Being an interpreter in this manner is a delicate job. It involves understanding the child, and especially understanding those things that may not be apparent to others, but also being able to work with the child's misapprehensions and misunderstandings and correct them in a way that introduces new and more efficient compensations for the kinds of understandings the child currently holds. This can involve parents watching speech and language therapy sessions and working collaboratively with the speech and language therapist afterward to share things she may have missed or to understand how it was she got the child to do something new, or something that only happens inconsistently. The more the parent can tell the various professionals working with the child what works, the better. The more the parent can learn new ways of understanding how the child learns, the better.

Parents as Head Hunters. A unique role that parents fulfill in putting together their child's treatment plan is to find the best people to work with their child. This is another part of micromanaging the child's life. Many parents visit all possible class placements, interview several speech therapists, and relentlessly lobby the ABA agency they feel will work best for their child. Advocacy of this sort has advantages, including the education received by talking to many different professionals and learning the rationales behind their approaches. Some parents have more of a knack for this than others. What mostly interferes is either availability of choices or an anxiety that drives justification to select the first option that happens to come along. Parents who head hunt well will often choose an eclectic mix of services, intuitively appreciating the need for the child to have some direct one-to-one service, some inclusive experiences, some adult-led teaching, and some child self-initiated learning, for example. Most impressive are parents who, initially unsure of what will work and how to make sense of rather antithetical theoretical rhetoric heard from different providers, will try all sorts of services, but quickly and systematically cull the services that seem ineffective. Susceptibility to placebo effects can be a big problem in selecting effective services over ineffective but well-marketed ones.

Another aspect of good parenting of a child with autism is knowing when to switch. Services that may be perfect for a child at one stage of development may not offer the right kinds of stimulation later. A preschool that was a fabulous experience for a typical older sibling may not be as good for the later-born sibling if parents have just learned he has autism. It can be hard to make unanticipated changes of service. It can seem disloyal and untrusting. Understandably, parents do, and should, form alliances and sometimes even close personal friendships with therapists and teachers who provide them with service. A difficulty can arise when it is time to move the child from that person's services to whatever the next step is. For example, I often encounter this in day-care arrangements. Take the case of Sergio, a three-year-old newly diagnosed with autism who has been going to the same day-care center at his mother's place of employment since he was six weeks old. Sergio has moved from the infant to toddler to preschooler rooms. The family knows the staff well, and the staff know this child well. The child, however, participates in none of the three-year-old activities, and in fact has become aggressive toward his peers as they have become more active, noisy, and verbal. On one hand, the parents don't want to pull Sergio from a place he's known all his life, especially when he's just starting to get help for his autism. On the other hand, Sergio's parents agree that a small family day care they have visited as a potential after-school program might be a better place for a teen tutor to facilitate one-to-one play with younger children. In situations like these, parents are often wary of hurting the feelings of caregivers who have been of major importance in their lives and that of the child. Often, though, the care providers or teachers know when a child is not, or is no longer, getting the benefit they might hope from their services or program, but they hesitate to tell the parent because *they* don't want to be seen as disloyal or less interested in the child now that it is known that the child has a disability. In these cases, acting in the benefit of the child is really best.

PARENT-TEACHER RELATIONSHIPS

Building a Trusting Collaboration. The parent-teacher relationship is critical to any child's successful treatment. There are many things that can be done to help this relationship be one of two-way communication and mutual learning, but first there must be trust. On behalf of their children, parents really should feel obliged to start out on the right foot when they first meet with people to treat their child.

I truly believe that even the best teachers cannot do their best job for a child who has a parent who is constantly criticizing and back-biting. Many parents of newly diagnosed children start off on the wrong foot. As soon as their child is diagnosed, they hook up with parent-support groups or advocates who tell them they need to be prepared to fight. I have never seen a situation in which the child is best served by having parents start off with schools and therapists with a clearly displayed lack of trust. Even in cases in which treatment providers are not the sharpest tacks in the drawer, education, discussion, and negotiation can only help the child. Even when parents are well justified in making unilateral decisions not recommended by the school, it is not in the child's long-term interest to come out swinging. Sometimes I feel that parents have been further aggrieved by other parents—the very folks who should be giving emotional comfort.

There are excellent providers of interventions for autism, and there are some not-so-great providers of interventions for autism. There are very, very few bad apples. No one goes into special education to become rich or famous. People who select this profession are natural altruists and feel they can make a difference somewhere that it will count. If I seem exasperated about parents who approach getting services for their child angrily, I am. You attract more bees with sugar than vinegar. Parents who think that being angry is the way to get help are making it harder to form the necessary working relationships with helping professionals. Parents who do not think twice about alienating everyone in their school in order to get a home-based program for their three-year-old need to take a good hard look at what they are doing. Think of the possible repercussions of alienating the folks that will be in the child's educational picture when the child is six or sixteen. In the end, a parent who cannot be on speaking terms with people who care for their child is not doing the best they can for their child.

It's not that there aren't special educators out there who don't even know what they don't know. There are nonpublic agencies and schools that also don't even know what they don't know. Not that it keeps them from being confident about what they think they do know. Even when dealing with people like these, being respectful in speech and extending common courtesies like being on time to meetings, responding to correspondence, and not bringing a lawyer or advocate to initial IFSP or IEP meetings can help.

Parents and teachers should have regular contact. These should be daily notes or weekly home visits when children are youngest. Opportunities to meet for coffee after school, for parent-teacher lecture nights, or for potlucks in the classroom in addition to meeting at the IEP meetings are important ways of having something other than a very formal relationship. With typically developing children, parents volunteer in the classroom and expect to be told what to do when they show up. At least the same expectations for volunteerism should apply to parents of children with autism. Being a small part of the educational process gives the parents an opportunity to earn the respect of the teacher and to make themselves subject to the teacher's training, acknowledging her expertise. In-service training opportunities, special speakers, and autism society meetings provide opportunities for parents and teachers all to be part of the process.

Clearly, parents are critical in the treatment and education their child receives. The parents are the grout that holds the mosaic of the "tiles" of treatment together. For many parents this "holding it all together" function means school pickups and drop-offs in the middle of the day, hours of reading magazines in a speech and language pathologist or occupational therapist's office, advertising for tutors, and calling long lists of respite-care providers in order to attend a weekend event at a sibling's school. Coordinating the child's treatments takes hours, leaving the rest of the parent's life to be scheduled around it. I am amazed at how some people manage this: One California father drives between programs much of the day and stays up half the night to run his business in Asia by teleconference—11 time zones away. Mothers of children with disabilities are underrepresented in the workforce, irrespective of the jobs they had before their child with autism was born. This change in lifestyle is part of the stress. Is there any way around this? Realistic compromises are sometimes worthwhile. Everything in life is trade-offs. Maybe the speech and language therapist two miles from home who seems 80 percent as good as the one ten miles away will be fine. Letting the child ride the bus for 70 minutes each way may be worth the two-and-a-half-hour chunk out of mom's day that it would take to drive to the school and back, especially if it means compromising another child's activities. This is what the parents' therapy is for— to work these things out and feel OK about such decisions.

FORMAL VERSUS NATURAL EDUCATIONAL ENVIRONMENTS

Intensity

Descriptions of model programs, programs reporting positive outcomes, and some of the limited outcome research all agree that "intensity" is important.

What exactly constitutes intensity of treatment? There isn't agreement. There are many ways to index intensity—number of hours of one-to-one instruction, how dense the number of interactions per hour are, how many responses are elicited, number of hours of overall participation in paid treatments or planned activities, or number of hours the child does not engage in repetitive or nonfunctional activities. All these definitions have relevance. Measures of these definitions are usually correlated. What these definitions all reflect is agreement on diverse ways to provide learning experiences.

In one study we did, we explored different definitions of intensity. Under the broadest definitions, parents typically reported 50 to 60 hours per week in which things were planned for the child. One mother, with a son who had shown remarkable improvements, insisted that she had delivered about twice the hours others reported. When we checked on this, it turned out she was reporting that she had seen herself intervening every waking hour of the child's life for the previous 12 years. While there might be a little hyperbole in that, her point is well-taken. In children who do very well, there is little opportunity for them to experience the regressive comfort of repetitious activity, staring into space, or mental downtime of any sort. Of course, there is a relationship between children with the capacity to do well and their ability to utilize or even tolerate this level of stimulation.

Intensity of intervention accrues through all the meaningfully engaged activities a child experiences, not just those with paid therapists or those that take place within the walls of a school or in a little schoolroom made from a bedroom or family room. This is important because, without an understanding that it is the activeness of the child's mind that is important, pasting together a meaningful mosaic of the child's day can seem like an even more impossible task.

Defining Meaningful Engagement. It often seems unappreciated that learning is something that all children, including all autistic children, can be doing all the time. The goal in planning a comprehensive and individualized set of interventions for a child with autism is to fill the day with a variety of meaningful experiences. This certainly must consist of the use of formal instructional and other therapeutic strategies, but it should also consist of other activities. A broad and diverse experience of the world, of different places, different learning modalities, and both formal and informal learning experiences, form the texture of a mentally stimulating life. With typically developing children, there is the ability on the part of the child to provide many informal experiences and conduct many informal experiments for himself. These are usually key learning experiences in the first five years of life. The problem for children with autism is that they tend not to fill "free" time very constructively, and so intentional teaching situations need to be contrived to create the texture of a diverse and mentally stimulating life. What this means is developing some guidelines for what constitutes meaningful engagement.

Defining Natural Education. Creating opportunities for meaningful engagement does not mean ramping up a 30-hour-per-week ABA/DTT program to 40 hours per week. On the contrary, a diversity of learning experiences is more beneficial for a child than repeated activity of a similar sort in a similar setting. Interestingly, some parents will tell me they have gone from a 30- to a 40-hour-a-week ABA/DTT program, and then tell me that the additional ten hours is not "table work" but field trips to the park, a library hour, trips to the market to get ingredients to make cookies, and so on. This is great, and exactly on track for what a child with 30 hours per week of one type of intervention needs. It's not DTT, but it is likely to be incrementally beneficial to the child because it provides opportunities to practice vocabulary and use observations he has been taught formally, but while using new skills in a more natural setting.

Sustaining Engagement. During direct instruction, a child is meaningfully engaged when trying to problem solve, being motored through a partial response, or watching a model. As we talked about in chapter 10, even intensive ABA/DTT programs have times when the child is not meaningfully engaged, when he stares off into space, waiting for the next SD, or permission to "go play." In chapter 11, we talked about children in TEACCH classes in which their independent work is not monitored, and who can spend long periods just staring off into space, having learned that remaining quiet in the cubicle can feel better than active problem solving, and that they can do it as long as no one notices.

We have already talked about disengagement in the context of instruction, but it can occur, and maybe occurs more often outside of classroom and therapy hours than inside. How can this be minimized? Natural education can be thought to include all those micromanaged moments of opportunistic informal conversation and play. The autistic child's natural educational opportunities can also include taking time that typical children spend in free play, and making the same activity a more meaningful form of engagement for the child with autism by having someone there (parent, relative, babysitter, older sibling, or neighbor) scaffolding the play with toys as we discussed in chapter 8. Natural education can occur by keeping the child meaningfully engaged while he watches a video—learning how to act out the scenes with corresponding action figures as we discussed in chapter 4.

How Does It All Add Up? So far in this chapter, we have looked at ways to integrate different teaching approaches so that they can be put together in complementary ways that afford a continuum of learning experiences that can flexibly change as the child develops. We have also looked at the role of parents, both in working with schools and mustering resources for their child, as well as in terms of the unique cohesion parents can provide to a child who is meaningfully engaged in myriad experiences. The next and final issue that will be addressed in this book is where years of education and treatment take a child with an autistic spectrum disorder. The purpose of this section is to give parents and treating professionals a broad sense of where the child can be expected to go, and what will happen along the way. This is meant not so much as a "crystal ball" session—no one has one for children with autism, but a meter for judging whether a child is on a generally expected course so that those around the child know whether their actions are doing well by that child.

LIKELY TREATMENT OUTCOMES

The big question is what kinds of treatment outcomes are there for autism? Are any children ever "normal" after having received a diagnosis of autism? Of PDD,NOS? Of Asperger's? If so, what does it take to get there? What happens to most children with autism when they grow up? Parents, naturally, have no way of knowing the answer to this when they find themselves thrust into the world of learning about autism. Surprisingly, many special-education professionals don't really know either because they increasingly lose track of the children they have worked with in the years after the child leaves their class or therapy. Parents usually start by asking: Will my child ever be able to get married? Will he drive a car? Will he live independently? Educators more often ask: What percentage lives at home and in group homes? What percentage can work in supported employment? In sheltered workshops? As adults, do they get less autistic and more social; but more like others with similar degrees of mental retardation?

There are two key concepts to keep in mind as one thinks about treatment outcomes in the autistic spectrum disorders: The first is that some percentage of the variability in outcome comes from treatment—all the things that have been talked about in this book. The second is that some percentage of variability in outcomes comes from who the child is. The child is not a blank slate that can be created in the parents' image. The child can only meet his own potential. Parents and professionals can actualize that potential, but it is very likely they cannot change it completely. As we discussed in chapter 1, you probably can't make a child with the talent to be a baseball player into a violinist if he has no talent for the latter. As far as treatment outcomes go, the child brings some of the pieces of the puzzle to the table, while the parents and professionals bring the rest.

In recent years, there has been a tremendous emphasis on early intervention for autism, based largely on our understanding that the brain is more malleable early on. Intensive early interventions have proceeded willy-nilly, driven more by ideology than by data. There is an absence of long-term empirical follow-up results on comparative merits of types of treatments, responders' characteristics, and the role of treatment intensity. This state of affairs leaves us reliant on preliminary impressions that can be drawn by those who have been involved in autism treatment for a number of years. In my clinical research, we have begun to follow a group of toddlers, now high school students who were among the first to have receive ABA/DTT treatments in the late 1980s and early 1990s.

Many other clinicians who work specifically with older individuals with autistic spectrum disorders have impressions of long-term outcomes too. These impressions are based on retrospective looks at the types of interventions adults in their programs may have received as children. Retrospective and prospective reports will vary a great deal depending on whether you talk to professionals who specialize in higher-functioning children, or others who work primarily with the most behaviorally difficult-to-manage lower-functioning individuals. For clinicians in the former group, outcomes are rosier. For clinicians in the latter group, outcomes may seem overall rather dismal. The section that follows is a synthesis of the fairly sparse existing outcome literature, my own research, and clinical experience with over three thousand children with autistic spectrum disorders, some of whom have been followed for more than ten years.

THE LOWER 15 PERCENT OF TREATMENT RESPONDERS

The Most Mentally Retarded of Children with Autism. A small proportion of children in the autistic spectrum also have at least moderate to severe mental retardation. This means that developmental age is 70 to 90 percent below chronological age. For these children, mental retardation—as much or more than the autism—limits the rate at which the child can learn. At this level of disability, teaching strategies and content are very similar for both autistic and mentally retarded children without autism. These children are among those considered for placement in severely handicapped classes (though severely handicapped classes often also serve children in the lower half of the "medium-functioning" group of children with autism too). At the time of diagnosis, these children are usually seen as mentally retarded, though the degree of mental retardation may be estimated as "moderate" or even "mild" and sometimes is more fairly described as "unspecified"—meaning that it's clearly there, but how much is not yet certain. Initially, it can be hard to accurately characterize just what constitutes apparent cognitive impairment, as we have already discussed. However, with the most severely affected children, some significant degree of impairment is evident right away.

This can be the most poignantly sad group of parents with whom a professional may deal. It's one thing to grasp that your child has a disorder, another to grasp that your toddler or preschooler is not likely ever to talk, live independently, or perhaps ever be completely independent in life skills. Amazingly, some parents handle all of this pretty well. In some ways, it may be easier not to have the ambiguity about how normal or independent the child can become. Compared to parents of higher-functioning children, these parents have less of a psychological burden in some ways. They don't live in apprehension that if, as the parent, you do not act adequately, it may make the difference between an adult who can lead a basically independent life, and one who can't.

Range of Treatments for the Lowest 15 Percent. Children in this lower-functioning group are not as likely to be good candidates for initial ABA/DTT because they learn quite slowly, may not be at a level at which direct instruction is developmentally appropriate (like under a mental age of nine months). Such children may understand so little or come to understand new things so slowly that a very intensive treatment process is unduly arduous, resulting in a very frustrated, unhappy child who cannot figure out the rules of instruction. When ABA/DTT is tried, there may be small (and worthwhile) gains in compliance and attention, though few gains in pre-academic program content. Many of the lower-functioning children with autism, as well as some of the children in this lower half of the medium-functioning group, may develop iatrogenic side effects of ABA/DTT when it is used. These can include problems with aggression, self-injury, agitation, and running away. With the lowest-functioning children, these problems may start quite soon after initiation of an ABA/DTT program, and, for the low- to medium-functioning children, after a couple years of ABA/DTT, especially when an oral-only language approach continues to be used for a child who is still largely nonverbal. In both cases, these maladaptive behaviors arise when the child has no other way of venting his frustration at not being able to make sense of how to respond. These maladaptive patterns of behavior are essentially a "tertiary" effect of the child's failing to accommodate successfully to his limitations (as discussed in chapter 2) and occur when the child has been taught with methods he cannot readily utilize. Not all lower-functioning children develop negative behaviors when over-challenged. Some become highly passive as the result of a training program that may inadvertently reward passivity (sitting nicely or giving a response—any response) at least as frequently as it rewards success.

A group-based TEACCH class that emphasizes visuals, routines, repetition, predictability, and functional skills is ideal. This is what might be referred to as a TEACCH class for "lower-functioning" children. For these children, the transition from ABA/DTT to such a TEACCH class would probably be best after no more than a year of a part-time ABA/DTT program, or after a year to two years of an eclectic class that, from the beginning, emphasized group and one-to-one (possibly including ABA/DTT) teaching, with a strong visually augmentative and functional emphasis all along.

Quality of Life for the Lowest 15 Percent. Lower-functioning people with autism face the greatest limitations as adults. "Institutionalization" is largely a thing of the past. Legislation in the United States that favors community-based treatment of both the mentally ill and developmentally disabled has created a major cultural shift in the care of our most disabled adults. Similar to somewhat more capable people with autism, lower-functioning individuals with autism often reside in group homes. Typically, a higher level of care is required, often one-to-one or one-to-two care. Individuals who lack hygiene skills or exhibit disruptive or self-injurious behaviors typically qualify for one-to-one aides.

Home activities focus on increasing independence at tasks of daily living, like dressing, eating, grooming, and leisure skills. Meaningful work activities are harder to identify or can only be tolerated for small parts of the day, so day treatment, rather than sheltered workshops or supported employment, is typically used. Day treatment can focus on going into the community, taking walks to get exercise, developing leisure skills, and generalizing adaptive behaviors taught at home to new settings. Increased independence at routines of daily living is a major focus.

Lowering-functioning individuals with autism often leave home sooner than the less severely impaired. Typically, years of managing an increasingly large individual with limited receptive language who continues to march to the beat of his own drummer takes its toll on caregivers. No one parent (and no two parents) can keep up with the behavior management needed to keep an active (and often persistent) young adult with autism from getting what he wants for himself. This may include doing things that endanger himself or others, like leaving the house unescorted, playing with plumbing, electricity, or electronics in undesirable ways, or being outright physically aggressive toward whoever might try to stop him. My position is that no "home team" can duplicate the efforts of three eight-hour shifts of behaviorally trained staff in the specially structured environment of a group home. There comes a point at which the individual with autism may be happier and less of a danger to himself and others if he can live somewhere that he is not an accident waiting to happen. Placement out of the home should also happen before family members who can provide the parents with their best social support are alienated. It should happen before typical siblings (who may be expected to oversee their brother or sister's care after parents no longer can) are alienated. It is a decision that is inevitable within this group of individuals and should be made when there is an opportunity to consider the alternatives, not in the midst of a crisis brought on by the individual's not being able to function according to someone else's expectations.

THE MIDDLE 70 PERCENT OF TREATMENT RESPONDERS

Medium-Functioning Autism. Most children with autism end up as "medium-functioning." There is no real way to draw a line with respect to such a classification, but it is widely recognized that some children in this group do particularly well, and some children—those on the low end who are limited by maladaptive behavioral patterns and moderate mental retardation—generally do more poorly. At the time of diagnosis it can be easiest (though certainly not perfectly easy) to detect which children are likely in the top and bottom 15 percentiles of the autistic spectrum, but it is relatively more difficult to tell whether a child in the middle 70 percent is likely in the higher or lower half of that group.

What distinguishes those in the higher and lower subgroups is how much spontaneous functional verbal language they are able to develop by age six or seven. The higher half of the middle 70 percent is composed of those who have at least some capacity for spontaneous language use. The lower half of the middle 70 percent is composed of those who remain nonverbal, or what some describe as "speaking" (speaking when prompted, having a limited though functional expressive verbal vocabulary understandable primarily to caregivers).

Range of Treatments for the Middle 70 Percent. What difference do various methods of instruction make for children in this group? Let's go back to the idea that treatment outcome is partly due to the child's traits, partly to treatments received. My impression is that for children with traits that would initially place them in the bottom half of this middle group, intense treatment moves them, prognostically, into the top half of this middle group. Conversely, children with traits that would initially place them in the top half of this middle group probably move to the bottom half if they do not receive sufficiently intense early treatments. Given that the ABA/DTT approach is clearly good at delivering early intensity and makes the child receptive to tolerating a greater and a more intense range of future teaching experiences, it is likely to be important early on to this group.

As the child is able to make sense of routines, participating in some group-based activities, developing semi-independent working skills, and working in a one-to-two group with a peer model, provides ways intensity can be maintained in a greater variety of ways but moving toward functional independence.

Developmental Practice Standards. The upper half of this group of children who begin talking (albeit in a slow and limited manner—but as a primary mode of communicating), I believe, can benefit from a transition from sole ABA/DTT treatment into a special day class that may continue to offer ABA/DTT, but will also offer other learning/teaching modalities as a next developmental step, as long as overall treatment intensity is maintained.

For children in this upper half of the 70 percent group, a TEACCH class with more pre-academic content, content that utilizes skills that may have initially been acquired via ABA/DTT training and applies it to new materials and situations, enables them to gain skills in self-guided learning, self-initiative, and group functioning that will be crucial for success in a mainstream setting. These children are ones who can start the year in a pure TEACCH class and by the end of the year be doing quite well in a class that more closely resembles a preschool. This type of class is the ideal place from which to launch a partial-inclusion experience—a preschool on the same site with an aide or an integrated "50/50" preschool. In an "ideal world", these children would likely have had to have started with about 6 to 12 months of home-based ABA/DTT, a year or so of an eclectic class providing DTT and TEACCH curriculum components, and a year of TEACCH faded to a more integrated typical-preschool model program. A substantially similar experience can be achieved by combining elements of a TEACCH class and a home-based ABA/DTT program, a TEACCH class and an inclusion preschool, or a combination of ABA/DTT and inclusion preschool.

The Role for Inclusive Education. The move from one-to-one to inclusive group-based education can include placement in a special day class as an incremental step. Some children with autism in the upper half of this middle group make the additional transition into inclusive educational settings. Many children in this middle group benefit from the learning advantages of integrated and inclusive preschool, kindergarten, and, for the most able of this group, some early elementary classes. By third or fourth grade, the focus on independent work, language-arts abilities, and more abstract reasoning tends to widen the educational gap between work that is done by the higher medium-functioning child with autism and typical peers. Some of these medium-functioning autistic children return (or go for the first time) to special day classes in the upper elementary grades. At this point, the advantages of learning to take group-based instruction, model peers to the extent possible, and follow group routines has usually been achieved to the extent that it can. Subsequent placement of medium-functioning children with autism at later elementary grades into learning-handicapped special day classes can be a good way to continue to provide peer models who are more socially typical, while continuing instruction at the child's developmental level

When a "medium-functioning" child with autism is in a special day class at school, it is understandable that parents still want that child to have time in the mainstream. An alternative to educational integration for medium-functioning pupils with autism may be inclusion with developmentally comparable peers in a non-academic setting such as an after-school, a tutoring or resource program, or extracurricular activities. This may be a small group of typical peers, those who are a bit younger, or an age-mixed group in which some peers are developmentally similar (the younger ones) and some are helpers or "scaffolders" (the older ones). The group size should be small so as to gradually add challenge to the task of tolerating and understanding how to function as part of a group.

Most children in the medium-functioning group who have had early, intensive one-to-one programs do well to transition first (or permanently) into a special day class, as this can provide a gradual transition to more self-initiated learning, but in a setting with lots of support. In these cases, when a special day class is selected, the best fit is often a TEACCH class, a class mainly for communicatively impaired children, or a learning-handicapped class in which others are developmentally comparable.

Special Day Classes or Inclusive Settings? This suggested set of developmentally based practice guidelines is differently reasoned from what parents sometimes hear from ABA/DTT providers. These providers, speaking from a behavioral (and non-developmental) perspective maintain that the child with autism needs age-appropriate models—so he can copy whatever he sees—so it might as well be the behaviors of someone his own age. (This is the problem of children "skipping" developmental stages, discussed in chapter 12.) Unfortunately, these assertions tend to dovetail with parental hopes that all the hard work put into the ABA/DTT approach has "worked" and that the bulk of their special work on behalf of the child is over because the child is deemed ready for an age-appropriate class. Especially for parents who do not have other children in addition to their child with autism, or who only have younger children, what is really required to be a kindergartener or first grader may not be intuitive. Parents are in a precarious position emotionally when it comes to the desire to have their child in a mainstreamed class. For educational specialists, it can be worrisome when it looks like the "marketing" of normalcy in the form of an inclusive placement may have a winning appeal that a carefully developmentally stratified special-education class does not.

One more emotional factor works on parents when they are faced with deciding on a special day class or an inclusive setting, especially parents who have sidestepped special day classes in favor of a home-based program for the first three, four, or five years of life: Someone else's developmentally disabled child will always look more disabled to you than your own child, and this can make it disturbing for parents to visit their first special day classes. But, everybody is somebody's baby! It is virtually impossible to know how "your" child (here I include both parents and ABA tutors) looks to others, because you have made so many unconscious dispensations, and adaptations and have such in-depth knowledge of what the child means by what he says—or doesn't say. Your child might, in fact, look just as handicapped to others as these children do to you. You just don't know them. Being dysmorphic ("looking retarded") or having a physical handicap says nothing about your level of mental capacity. Many, however, including parents of other disabled children, may stigmatize other people's children based on physical appearance and decide they are unsuitable classmates.

For many children in the lower half of the medium-functioning group, placement in a special day class, or transition to a special day class from an ABA/DTT program, is an easier, more obvious decision. It is likely the best place in which developmentally comparable peers will be of nearly the same chronological age. (A five-year-old child with autism with eighteen-month-old social skills cannot be "included" in a program for 18-month-olds the way a two-and-a-half-year-old can.) These are typically the children who have developed no, (or only non-spontaneous,) verbal communication, sometimes after two, three, or more years of ABA/DTT programs. Often, parents of these children have been through multiple ABA/DTT providers, hoping with each switch that maybe doing the program just a little differently will make the critical difference. When one examines where these children are at developmentally—much more visual than verbal, with verbal comprehension below the three-year level—these children are the ones who can likely be helped earliest by a switch to a high-quality, high-intensity TEACCH or other special day class in which the emphasis is on visually augmentative communication and development of functional and adaptive skills rather than on development of verbal and pre-academic skills. Many times, unfortunately, parents of children in this group see the transition to a TEACCH class, as an example, as a defeat, as if expectations for the child have somehow been lowered so the child is not worthy to be given as much. Parents are often, understandably, concerned that if one-to-one learning is laborious, small group instruction and instruction in which the child is expected to perform independently will result in even slower learning. We don't have much in the way of comparative research to look at this question in detail, but from a pragmatic and developmental point of view, there is much to be gained by giving the child an opportunity to function as part of a group, learn through routines, and adapt to a visually augmented communication world. Since parents fear regression, it is a good idea, and a low-risk one if the child is placed in a good special day class, to monitor the child's first months in the special day class so that absence of regression, and progress—both according to predetermined parameters—-can be gauged. While educators may feel certain that regression won't happen and progress will, they need to be sensitive to the fact that changing to a special day class from a home program can feel, to some parents, like jumping off a cliff. Demonstrating a satisfactory transition will help ally parents with the special day class and allow them to be more supportive of the work being done there.

Parents, on the other hand, sometimes think that somehow learning only happens in the ABA/DTT program, and so if that program continues at home on a partial basis, that any learning must only be coming from that setting, because that is how the child has learned in the past. (This is problematic because it is logical to attribute benefits to an intervention you see rather than to one you don't see.) It may help for the parent to have guided observations or guided participation in their child's class so they can understand the possible learning opportunities in that setting as well as in the ABA/DTT program.

Longer-Term Outcomes for the Middle 70 Percent. Most medium-functioning individuals with autism continue to need support through their adult years. This means that such individuals either continue to live with family or live in group homes. Group homes, typically licensed, staffed, and overseen by public developmental disabilities agencies, are houses or apartments in which residents either have their own room or share a room with a roommate. For the medium-functioning individuals with some language, staffing is usually one-to-two or one-to-three in these residences, and eight-hour shifts keep the facility staffed around the clock, or whenever residents are at home. Staff teach the residents and assist in preparing meals, doing household chores, and organizing and supervising leisure activities. Individuals with autism often (though not always) live with some more socially skilled, developmentally disabled young people to create a culture in the group home that is more social and includes group activities and trips. Individuals who develop severe behavioral problems are usually moved to a higher level of care with more intensive, sometimes one-to-one staffing—which can benefit that individual as well as prevent disruption to the rest of the residents.

Many individuals in the medium-functioning group work in sheltered workshop settings. Sheltered workshops can be run by well-known agencies, like the Salvation Army or St. Vincent De Paul, and provide on-site job training and supervision as well as coordinate transportation to and from the workers' residence. Sheltered workshop activities tend to be piecework, involving common items that we all use, like packages containing airline headphones; shrink-wrapped foods; stapled boxes; or lightbulbs packed two to a box, six boxes to a carton, six cartons to a crate. Sometimes community facilities like public cafeterias, parks, recreation areas, or recycling centers employ people with autism who come to work with job coaches. People with autism make really good workers for highly repetitive tasks that others might find boring. This is where eschewing novelty and preferring familiarity can be a rather adaptive trait.

It is not possible for parents of a preschool- or even elementary school-aged child with autism to think of their child living away from home in a group home and working in supported employment. In the early years, it is not even really possible to imagine what a child with autism (or any child) will be like as an adult. Parents of young children most often say to me, "He'll always live with me!" Letting go is a developmental process for parents of autistic children that they can no more envision for their school-aged child with autism than they can for his typical sibling. There is no real value in dwelling on possible adulthood scenarios for a seven-year-old, and there is no point in thinking you can really make a fully informed decision about where he will or will not live—all that will unfold. For many families, leaving home for the medium-functioning child with autism comes about naturally when he graduates from high school and moves into a different service-delivery system, or comes when the nest otherwise becomes empty.

THE TOP 10 TO 15 PERCENT OF TREATMENT RESPONDERS

High-Functioning Autism and Asperger's Syndrome. The designation of high-functioning autism is usually reserved for those with normal verbal and performance IQs, with performance IQ usually notably higher than verbal ability . Most children meeting these criteria in the later elementary grades when IQ has stabilized are part of the top 10 to 15 percent of autism-treatment responders. Asperger's syndrome is seldom detectable; though it may be suspected in a three-year-old, is virtually never part of a diagnosis for a child under three. By middle school, this diagnosis is apparent, if present, and these children, too, contribute to the higher end of outcomes associated with the autistic spectrum.

A small number (maybe 10 to 15 percent) of children who start on an ABA/DTT programs (and also other intensive treatment plans) seem able to shift from first gear to second, and then to overdrive. They cruise without having to be taught everything in between repeatedly, or taught step by step. These are the children with autism who often initially tested with normal nonverbal IQs and had some verbal communication prior to treatment. These children showed more curiosity and resulting exploration of their worlds prior to treatment, even if the exploration consisted of intense autistic play.

There is a real question as to how much treatment response in such children is specific to the type of treatment received or to the fact that a concerted, intense effort was applied to stimulate development. It is also not clear with this group whether some had developmental lags that were consistent with autism at ages one, two, and even three, that became less consistent with autism at least partly as a result of maturation—an observation that seems clinically supported in my experience and has also been suggested by the literature for some time. All had started out as higher functioning.

"Normalization" Criteria. Among the top 10 to 15 percent, perhaps half come to meet what might be referred to as "normalization" criteria. In our clinic, normalization is defined as a verbal and performance IQ in the normal range (above 70), all Vineland Adaptive Behavior Scales in the normal range, not meeting criteria for autism or PDD on the Autism Diagnostic Interview (a standardized structured interview for autism used in research), and attendance at a public or private school in a general education class without any individualized instructional assistance in class.

In retrospect, about a third of those meeting normalization criteria may have been those we now consider to have been showing early developmental lags that were consistent with autism between ages one and three and perhaps later would have been seen more like the language-disordered sibling phenotype that was first described when early research began to identify ways that autism seemed to run in families in which some individuals would show some but not all traits of autism. (This doesn't mean that such children did not benefit from early intensive treatments, indeed, by some standards, they may have benefited most.) Of the normalized children, most reached this status by second or third grade. Some, while no longer meeting criteria for an autistic spectrum disorder, still have repetitive motor movements that they have learned to keep private or have more obvious symptoms consistent with possible obsessive compulsive disorder. Some are doing well in school because they are particularly mathematically gifted, but continue to be weaker in language-based reasoning, and so have difficulty extracting themes from readings in English class, or abstract concepts from history class. While parents tend to be acutely aware of such things, these pupils are in many respects no different from other students who excel in one subject but are only average, or even below average, in others. Most of the normalized children have a few good friends but are largely not socially gregarious. Some have graduated from high school. Teachers, often uninformed of their earlier diagnoses, tend to see them as shy, or even as awfully well behaved. There are some children that certain clinicians might be tempted to categorize as having Asperger's syndrome because of a certain shyness and rigidity, but these teens lack the pedantic speech and odd interests and can truly talk about such things as their own feelings and those of others. Among children we have followed who have come to meet normalization criteria, a marginal majority are those who received early ABA/DTT programs, though there is a significant minority who received TEACCH or other eclectic early treatments. What was common to all of the strongest treatment responders was the role that parents and other informal supports played in making the child's life full and active.

Longer-Term Outcomes. At this point, one of the ways that we know about longer-term outcomes for higher-functioning children with autism is by looking at our young adult population with autism and retrospectively considering the services they received and how they may have affected what they have been able to achieve. The very highest-functioning two to three percent of young adults live more or less independently, meaning with an adult sibling, in a shared apartment organized by parents, or, sometimes, alone. The best occupational outcomes involve finding "ecological" niches, in which the work activities complement the individual's particular interests and talents. Work productivity is usually lower for others in the same job, which can translate into working fewer hours per day and/or fewer hours per week. Most work in small businesses or family businesses in which there is a willingness to accommodate eccentricities. Work that is fairly repetitive (like sorting mail, preparing flowers for a floral shop, or changing movie reels) tends to be preferred by those who are successfully employed, as do jobs that don't involve a great deal of interaction with co-workers and certainly don't involve unpredictable changes in job responsibilities.

Higher-functioning adults usually establish satisfying life routines and interests, but very, very rarely marry (and largely don't feel too badly about this), seldom drive cars or drive much beyond habitual routes. Most have a self-satisfied level of independence, and when company is wanted, most find it in organized groups (including high-functioning autism groups), activity-oriented clubs (like a chess club), or increasingly, the Internet.

The rate of co-morbid (co-occurring) psychiatric disorders in this top 15 percent has been estimated to be as high as one in three, with most cases being anxiety, depression, or obsessive compulsive symptoms, or, in rarer cases, psychoses. These are individuals who are smart enough to know that others see them as different and to feel badly about that, but often lack the insight either to identify what is not liked or how to change. An ongoing supportive psychotherapeutic relationship using a cognitive behavioral model makes a lot of sense, and in coming years, one hopes, its efficacy with this group will be studied.

What we don't know is whether those with HFA or AS who are currently in their twenties and thirties represent what the young adult lives of the current high-responders to more recently introduced intensive interventions will be like. Even in the early 1970s when some of today's high-functioning adults were young, some parents intuitively provided high levels of intensity, even before there was mandatory special education. Temple Grandin, definitely in the top half of the top one percent, can readily recall how her mother provided her with intensity in the 1950s.

CHAPTER CONCLUSIONS

In this chapter, we have tried to pull together all the information from earlier ones on how children with autism learn and, in particular, how that information translates into individualizing educational and other treatment plans. Hybrid programs that afford children the opportunity to benefit from multiple methodologies were emphasized, as was the important role of parents in bringing cohesiveness to the myriad experiences that comprise any child's formal and informal, natural education. All of these experiences become part of meaningful engagement in the world around the child. Finally, we concluded with a brief overview of the longer-term picture of development for different groups of children within the autistic spectrum, beginning with those also having the most marked degrees of cognitive impairment, more medium-functioning individuals who comprise the bulk of the autistic spectrum, and finally those with high-functioning autism or Asperger's syndrome.

Every child with an autistic spectrum disorder is different. Each in his own way has weaknesses in social understanding. Most have deficits in communicating fully and effectively. It is likely that no one way is best for one particular child. There are more likely many ways things can be done that will lead to similar results.

Many parents, clinicians, educators, and therapists would agree that the more you know about autism treatment, the more there seems to be differences rather than similarities in what each individual needs. The information here is meant to emphasize both individuality and general treatment principles—important so we don't lose track of the fact that each child with autism is an individual first.

FURTHER READINGS

PART I
The Fundamentals of Autistic Learning Styles

CHAPTER ONE

Understanding the Origins of Autism and Its Meaning for Development

• **TECHNICAL REFERENCES FOR TEACHERS AND OTHER PROFESSIONALS**

Bryson, S. E. (1997). "Epidemiology of Autism: Overview and Issues Outstanding." In D. J. Cohen and F. R. Volkmar (Eds.), *Handbook of Autism and Pervasive Developmental Disorders* (2d ed.; 41-46). New York: John Wiley and Sons, Inc.

Folstein, S. E., and Santangelo, S. L. (2000). "Does Asperger Syndrome Aggregate in Families?" In A. Klin, F. R. Volkmar, and S. S. Sparrow (Eds.), *Asperger Syndrome* (159-171). New York: Guilford Press.

Piven, J. (2000). "The Broad Autism Phenotype." In P. J. Accardo, C. Magnusen, and A. J. Capute (Eds.), *Autism: Clinical and Research Issues* (214-224). Baltimore, MD: York Press.

Szatmari, P., and Goldberg, J. (2000). "Epidemiology of Autism and Other Pervasive Developmental Disorders: Current Controversies." In P. J. Accardo, C. Magnusen, and A. J. Capute (Eds.), *Autism: Clinical and Research Issues* (25-36). Baltimore, MD: York Press.

• **FURTHER READINGS FOR PARENTS AND TEACHERS**

Ratey, J. J., and Johnson, C. (1997). *Shadow Syndromes.* New York: Pantheon Books.

Wing, L. (1996). *The Autistic Spectrum: A Guide for Parents and Professionals.* London: Constable and Company Limited. (Especially Chapters 5, 6, and 7)

CHAPTER TWO

When Atypical Development and Typical Development Cross Paths

• **TECHNICAL REFERENCES FOR TEACHERS AND OTHER PROFESSIONALS:**

Aram, D. M., and Healy, J. M. (1988). "Hyperplexia: A Review of Extraordinary Word Recognition." In L. K. Obler and D. Fein (Eds.), *The Exceptional Brain: Neuropsychology of Talent and Special Abilities* (70-102). New York: The Guilford Press.

Gardner, H. (1985). *Frame of Mind: The Theory of Multiple Intelligences.* New York: Basic Books, Inc.

Siegel, B. (1991). Toward DSM-IV: "A Developmental Approach to Autistic Disorder." *Psychiatric Clinics of North America* 14: 53-68.

- **FURTHER READINGS FOR PARENTS AND TEACHERS:**

Wing, L. (1996). *The Autistic Spectrum: A Guide for Parents and Professionals.* London: Constable and Company Limited. (Especially Chapters 1 and 2)

CHAPTER THREE

Autistic Learning Disabilities Defined:
How Strengths Compensate for Weaknesses and Form Autism

- **TECHNICAL REFERENCES FOR TEACHERS AND OTHER PROFESSIONALS:**

Ozonoff, S. (1997). "Causal Mechanisms of Autism: Unifying Perspectives from and Information-Processing Framework." In D. J. Cohen and F. R. Volkmar (Eds.), *Handbook of Autism and Pervasive Developmental Disorders* (2d ed.; 868-879). New York: John Wiley and Sons, Inc.

Rourke, B. P., and Tsatsanis, K. D. (2000). "Nonverbal Learning Disabilities and Asperger Syndrome." In A. Klin, F. R. Volkmar, and S. S. Sparrow (Eds.), *Asperger Syndrome* (231-253). New York: Guilford Press.

Siegel, B. (1996). "Atypical Ontogeny: Atypical Development from a Developmental Perspective." In J. H. Beitchman, N. J. Cohen, M. M. Konstantareas, and R. Tannock (Eds.), *Language, Learning, and Behavior Disorders: Developmental, Biological, and Clinical Perspectives* (38-58). New York: Cambridge University Press.

Siegel, B. (1999). "Autistic Learning Disabilities and Individualizing Treatment for Autistic Spectrum Disorders." *Infants and Young Children* 12: 27-36.

Treffert, D. A. (2000). "The Savant Syndrome in Autism." In P. J. Accardo, C. Magnusen, and A. J. Capute (Eds.), *Autism: Clinical and Research Issues* (193-214). Baltimore, MD: York Press.

PART II

Autistic Learning Disabilities and Autistic Learning Styles:
What Makes the World of the Autistic Child Different?

CHAPTER FOUR

Social Autistic Learning Disabilities: Description and Treatment

- **TECHNICAL REFERENCES FOR TEACHERS AND OTHER PROFESSIONALS:**

Baron-Cohen, S. (1995). *Mindblindness: An Essay on Autism and Theory of Mind.* Cambridge, MA: MIT Press.

Golding, M. M. (1998). "Beyond Compliance: The Importance of Group Work in the Education of Children and Young People with Autism." In S. Powell and R. Jordan (Eds.) *Autism and Learning* (46-60). London: David Fulton Publishers.

Happe, F. (1995). *Autism: An Introduction to Psychological Theory.* Cambridge, MA: Harvard University Press.

Hobson, R. P. (1993). *Autism and the Development of Mind.* Hove, UK: Lawrence Erlbaum Associates.

Jordan, R. and Libby, S. (1998). "Developing and Using Play in the Curriculum." In S. Powell and R. Jordan (Eds.) *Autism and Learning* (28-45). London: David Fulton Publishers.

Klin, A.; Volmar, F. R.; and Sparrow, S. S. (2000). *Asperger Syndrome.* New York: Guilford Press.

Lord, C. (1993). "Early Social Development in Autism." In E. Schopler, M. E. Van Bourgondien, and M. M. Bristol (Eds.) *Preschool Issues in Autism* (61-94). New York: Plenum Press.

Mundy, P., and Stella, J. (2000). "Joint Attention, Social Orienting, and Communication in Autism." In A. M. Wetherby and B. M. Prizant (Eds.), *Autism Spectrum Disorders: A Transactional Development Perspective* (Vol. 9; 31-54). Baltimore, MD: Paul H. Brookes Publishing Co.

Murray, D. K. C. (1998). "Autism and Information Technology: Therapy With Computers." In S. Powell and R. Jordan (Eds.) *Autism and Learning* (100-117). London: David Fulton Publishers.

Rogers, S. J., and Bennetto, L. (2000). "Intersubjectivity in Autism: The Roles of Imitation and Executive Function." In A. M. Wetherby and B. M. Prizant (Eds.), *Autism Spectrum Disorders: A Transactional Development Perspective* (Vol. 9; 79-108). Baltimore, MD: Paul H. Brookes Publishing Co.

Schreibman, L.; Stahmer, A. C.; and Price, K. L. (1996). "Alternative Applications of Pivotal Response Training: Teaching Symbolic Play and Social Interaction Skills." In L. K. Koegel, R. L. Koegel, and G. Dunlap (Eds.), *Positive Behavioral Support Including People with Difficult Behavior in the Community* (353-371). Baltimore, MD: Paul H. Brookes Publishing Co.

Schuler, A. L., and Wolfberg, P. J. (2000). "Promoting Peer Play and Socialization: The Art of Scaffolding." In A. M. Wetherby and B. M. Prizant (Eds.), *Autism Spectrum Disorders: A Transactional Development Perspective* (Vol. 9; 251-278). Baltimore, MD: Paul H. Brookes Publishing Co.

Volkmar, F. R.; Carter, A.; Grossman, J., and Klin, A. (1997). "Social Development in Autism." In D. J. Cohen and F. R. Volkmar (Eds.), *Handbook of Autism and Pervasive Developmental Disorders* (2d ed.; 173-94). New York: John Wiley and Sons, Inc.

• **FURTHER READINGS FOR PARENTS AND TEACHERS**

Park, C. C. (2001). *Exiting Nirvana: A Daughter's Life with Autism.* New York: Little, Brown, and Company.

Quill, K. A. (2000). *Do-Watch-Listen-Say: Social and Communication Intervention for Children with Autism.* Baltimore, MD: Paul H. Brookes Publishing Co.

CHAPTER FIVE

Autistic Learning Disabilities of Communication: Identifying the Components of Communication

• **TECHNICAL REFERENCES FOR TEACHERS AND OTHER PROFESSIONALS:**

Haber, R. N., and Haber, L. R. (1988). "The Characteristics of Eidetic Imagery." In L. K. Obler and D. Fein (Eds.), *The Exceptional Brain: Neuropsychology of Talent and Special Abilities* (218-41). New York: The Guilford Press.

Klin, A.; Volmar, F. R.; and Sparrow, S. S. (2000). *Asperger Syndrome.* New York: Guilford Press.

Lord, C. and Paul, R. (1997). "Language and Communication in Autism." In D. J. Cohen and F. R. Volkmar (Eds.), *Handbook of Autism and Pervasive Developmental Disorders* (2nd ed.; 95-225). New York: John Wiley and Sons, Inc.

Waterhouse, L. (1988). "Extraordinary Visual Memory and Pattern Perception in an Autistic Boy." In L. K. Obler and D. Fein (Eds.), *The Exceptional Brain: Neuropsychology of Talent and Special Abilities* (325-40). New York: The Guilford Press.

Wetherby, A. M.; Prizant, B. M.; and Schuler, A. L. (2000). "Understanding the Nature of Communication and Language Impairments." In A. M. Wetherby and B. M. Prizant (Eds.), *Autism Spectrum Disorders: A Transactional Development Perspective* (Vol. 9; 109-42). Baltimore, MD: Paul H. Brookes Publishing Co.

- **FURTHER READINGS FOR PARENTS AND TEACHERS:**

Quill, K. A. (2000). *Do-Watch-Listen-Say: Social and Communication Intervention for Children with Autism.* Baltimore, MD: Paul H. Brookes Publishing Co.

CHAPTER SIX

Autistic Learning Disabilities of Communication: Treatments for the Preverbal and Nonverbal Child

- **TECHNICAL REFERENCES FOR TEACHERS AND OTHER PROFESSIONALS:**

Klin, A.; Volmar, F. R.; and Sparrow, S. S. (2000). *Asperger Syndrome.* New York: Guilford Press.

Schuler, A. L.; Prizant, B. M.; and Wetherby, A. M. (1997). "Enhances Language and Communication Development: Prelinguistic Approaches." In D. J. Cohen and F. R. Volkmar (Eds.), *Handbook of Autism and Pervasive Developmental Disorders* (2d ed.; 539-71). New York: John Wiley and Sons, Inc.

Wetherby, A. M.; Warren, S. F.; and Reichle, J. (1998). *Transitions in Prelinguistic Communication* (Vol. 7). Baltimore, MD: Paul H. Brookes Publishing Co. (Especially, Chapters 1-6, and Chapter 17 regarding visual augmentative communication)

- **FURTHER READINGS FOR PARENTS AND TEACHERS:**

Bondy, A. and Frost, L. (2001). *A Picture's Worth: PECS and Other Visual Communication Strategies in Autism.* Bethesda: Woodbine House.

Simpson, R. L., and Kregel, J. (2001). *Focus on Autism and Other Developmental Disabilities* (Vol. 16). Austin, TX: PRO-ED, Inc.

Grandin, T. (1995). *Thinking in Pictures: and Other Reports of My Life with Autism.* New York: Bantam.

CHAPTER SEVEN

Autistic Learning Disabilities of Communication: Treatments for the Verbal Child

- **TECHNICAL REFERENCES FOR TEACHERS AND OTHER PROFESSIONALS:**

Klin, A.; Volmar, F. R.; and Sparrow, S. S. (2000). *Asperger Syndrome.* New York: Guilford Press.

Prizant, B. M.; Schuler, A. L.; Wetherby, A.; and Rydell, P. (1997). "Enhancing Language and Communication Development: Language Approaches." In D. J. Cohen and F. R. Volkmar (Eds.), *Handbook of Autism and Pervasive Developmental Disorders* (2d ed.; 572-605). New York: John Wiley and Sons, Inc.

Wilcox, M. J., and Shannon, M. S. (1998). "Facilitating the Transition from Prelinguistic to Linguistic Communication." In A. M. Wetherby; S. Warren; and J. Reichle (Eds.), *Transitions in Prelinguistic Communication* (Vol. 7; 385-416). Baltimore, MD: Paul H. Brookes Publishing Co.

- **FURTHER READINGS FOR PARENTS AND TEACHERS:**

Bell, N. (1997). *Seeing Stars.* San Luis Obispo, CA: Gander Publishing.

CHAPTER EIGHT

Autistic Learning Disabilities in Relating to the World of Objects: Description and Treatment

- **TECHNICAL REFERENCES FOR TEACHERS AND OTHER PROFESSIONALS:**

Anzalone, M. E., and Williamson, G. G. (2000). "Sensory Processing and Motor Performance in Autism Spectrum Disorders." In A. M. Wetherby and B. M. Prizant (Eds.), *Autism Spectrum Disorders: A Transactional Development Perspective* (Vol. 9; 143-66). Baltimore, MD: Paul H. Brookes Publishing Co.

Grados, M. A., and McCarthy, D. (2000). "Stereotypies and Repetitive Behaviors in Autism." In P. J. Accardo; C. Magnusen; and A. J. Capute (Eds.), *Autism: Clinical and Research Issues* (77-101). Baltimore, MD: York Press.

CHAPTER NINE

Autistic Learning Disabilities and the Skills of Daily Living

- **TECHNICAL REFERENCES FOR TEACHERS AND OTHER PROFESSIONALS:**

Dunlap, G., and Fox, L. (1996). "Early Intervention and Serious Problem Behaviors: A Comprehensive ApproaChapter" In L. K. Koegel, R. L. Koegel, and G. Dunlap (Eds.), *Positive Behavioral Support Including People with Difficult Behavior in the Community.* (31-50). Baltimore, MD: Paul H. Brookes Publishing Co.

Fox, L.; Dunlap, G.; and Buschbacher, P. (2000). "Understanding and Intervening with Children's Challenging Behavior: A Comprehensive Approach." In A. M. Wetherby and B. M. Prizant (Eds.), *Autism Spectrum Disorders: A Transactional Development Perspective* (Vol. 9; 307-32). Baltimore, MD: Paul H. Brookes Publishing Co.

Koegel, L. K.; Koegel, R. L.; Kellegrew, D.; and Mullen, K. (1996). "Parent Education for Prevention and Reduction of Severe Problem Behaviors." In L. K. Koegel, R. L. Koegel, and G. Dunlap (Eds.), *Positive Behavioral Support Including People with Difficult Behavior in the Community.* (3-30). Baltimore, MD: Paul H. Brookes Publishing Co.

- **FURTHER READINGS FOR PARENTS AND TEACHERS:**

Baker, B. L., and Brightman, A. J. (1997). *Steps to Independence: Teaching Everyday Skills to Children with Special Needs* (3d ed.). Baltimore, MD: Paul H. Brookes Publishing Co.

Durand, V. M. (1998). *Sleep Better: A Guide to Improving Sleep for Children with Special Needs.* Baltimore, MD: Paul H. Brookes Publishing Co.

Wing, L. (1996). *The Autistic Spectrum: A Guide for Parents and Professionals.* London: Constable and Company Limited. (Especially Chapter 10)

PART III

Methods of Teaching Children with Autism: How they Address Autistic Learning Disabilities and Autistic Learning Styles

---

- **TECHNICAL REFERENCES FOR TEACHERS AND OTHER PROFESSIONALS:**

Schopler, E.; Mesibov, G. B.; and Kunce, L. J. (1998). *Asperger Syndrome or High-Functioning Autism?* New York: Plenum Press.

Quill, K.A. (Ed.) (1995). *Teaching Children with Autism: Strategies to Enhance Communication and Socialization.* New York: Delmar Publishing.

- **FURTHER READINGS FOR PARENTS AND TEACHERS:**

Ozonoff, S.; Dawson, G.; and McPartland, J. (2002). *A Parent's Guide to Asperger Syndrome and High Functioning Autism.* New York: Guilford Press.

- **FURTHER READINGS FOR PARENTS AND TEACHERS:**

Ayres, A. J. (1998). *Sensory Integration and the Child.* Los Angeles: Western Psychological Services.

Greenspan, S., and Wieder, S. (1998). *The Child with Special Needs: Encouraging Intellectual and Emotional Growth.* Reading, MA: Addison-Wesley Longman, Inc.

Kaufman, B. N. (1994). *Son-Rise: The Miracle Continues.* Tiburon, CA: H. J. Kramer Inc.

Tomatis, A. (1990). *L'Oreille et la Vie.* Paris: Laffont.

CHAPTER TEN

Applied Behavior Analysis and Discrete Trial Training: Separating Methods from Curriculum

- **TECHNICAL REFERENCES FOR TEACHERS AND OTHER PROFESSIONALS:**

Handleman, J. S., and Harris, S. (1994). "The Douglass Developmental Disabilities Center." In S. L. Harris and J. S. Handleman (Eds.), *Preschool Education Programs for Children with Autism* (71-86). Austin, TX: PRO-ED, Inc.

Lord, C. (Chair; 2001). *A Report of the National Research Council: Educating Children with Autism.* Washington, D.C.: National Academy Press.

McClannahan, L. E., and Krantz, P. J. (1994). The Princeton Child Development Institute. In S. L. Harris and J. S. Handleman (Eds.), *Preschool Education Programs for Children with Autism* (107-26). Austin, TX: PRO-ED, Inc.

Schreibman, L. (1997). "Theoretical Perspectives on Behavioral Intervention for Individuals with Autism." In D. J. Cohen and F. R. Volkmar (Eds.), *Handbook of Autism and*

Pervasive Developmental Disorders (2d ed.; 920-33). New York: John Wiley and Sons, Inc.

- **FURTHER READINGS FOR PARENTS AND TEACHERS:**

Harris, S. L., and Weiss, M. (1998). *Right from the Start: Behavioral Intervention for Young Children with Autism.* Bethesda, MD: Woodbine House, Inc.

Leaf, R., and McEachin, J. (Eds.) (1999). *A Work in Progress: Behavior Management Strategies and A Curriculum for Intensive Behavioral Treatment of Autism.* New York: DRL Books.

Lovaas, I.O. (2002). *Teaching Individuals with Developmental Delays: Basic Intervention Techniques.* Austin, TX: PRO-ED, Inc.

Maurice, C.; Green, G.; and Luce, S. C. (1996). *Behavioral Intervention for Young Children with Autism: A Manual for Parents and Professionals.* Austin, TX: PRO-ED, Inc.

CHAPTER ELEVEN

The TEACCH Curriculum

- **TECHNICAL REFERENCES FOR TEACHERS AND OTHER PROFESSIONALS:**

Lord, C. (Chair; 2001). *A Report of the National Research Council: Educating Children with Autism.* Washington, D.C.: National Academy Press.

Lord, C., and Schopler, E. (1994). "TEACCH Services for Preschool Children." In S. L. Harris and J. S. Handleman (Eds.), *Preschool Education Programs for Children with Autism* (87-106). Austin, TX: PRO-ED, Inc.

Schopler, E. (1994). "A Statewide Program for the Treatment and Education of Autistic and Related Communication Handicapped Children (TEACCH)." In F. R. Volkmar (Ed.), *Child and Adolescent Psychiatric Clinics of North America* (Vol. 3; 91-104). Philadelphia: W.B. Saunders Company.

Schopler, E. (1997). "Implementation of TEACCH Philosophy." In D. J. Cohen and F. R. Volkmar (Eds.), *Handbook of Autism and Pervasive Developmental Disorders* (2d ed.; 767-95). New York: John Wiley and Sons, Inc.

CHAPTER TWELVE

Mainstreaming that Works: Too Accommodating or Really Including?

- **TECHNICAL REFERENCES FOR TEACHERS AND OTHER PROFESSIONALS:**

Burack, J. A.; Root, R.; and Zigler, E. (1997). "Inclusive Education for Students with Autism: Reviewing Ideological, Empirical, and Community Considerations." In D. J. Cohen and F. R. Volkmar (Eds.), *Handbook of Autism and Pervasive Developmental Disorders* (2d ed.; 796-807). New York: John Wiley and Sons, Inc.

Kauffman, J. M., and Hallahan, D. P. (1995). *The Illusion of Full Inclusion: A Comprehensive Critique of a Current Special Education Bandwagon.* Austin, TX: PRO-ED, Inc.

Kohler, F. W.; Strain, P. S.; and Shearer, D. D. (1996). "Examining Levels of Social Inclusion within an Integrated Preschool for Children with Autism." In L. K. Koegel, R. L. Koegel, and G. Dunlap (Eds.), *Positive Behavioral Support Including People with Difficult Behavior in the Community.* (31-50). Baltimore, MD: Paul H. Brookes Publishing Co.

Lord, C. (Chair; 2001). *A Report of the National Research Council: Educating Children with Autism*. Washington, D.C.: National Academy Press.

Strain, P. S., and Cordisco, L. K. (1994). "LEAP Preschool." In S. L. Harris and J. S. Handleman (Eds.), *Preschool Education Programs for Children with Autism* (225-44). Austin, TX: PRO-ED, Inc.

CHAPTER THIRTEEN

Model Programs and Exemplary Classes: What Can We Learn?

There are no specific references for this chapter because it consists entirely of case illustrations.

CHAPTER FOURTEEN

Putting the 'I' Back in IEP: Creating Individualized, Meaningful Learning Experiences

• **TECHNICAL REFERENCES FOR TEACHERS AND OTHER PROFESSIONALS:**

Klin, A., and Volmar, F. R. (2000). "Treatment and Intervention Guidelines for Individuals with Asperger Syndrome." In A. Klin, F. R. Volkmar, and S. S. Sparrow (Eds.), *Asperger Syndrome* (340-66). New York: Guilford Press.

Lord, C. (Chair; 2001). *A Report of the National Research Council: Educating Children with Autism*. Washington, D.C.: National Academy Press.

Autistic Learning Disabilities Inventory

The Autistic Learning Disabilities Inventory (ALDI) is a list of the various autistic learning differences discussed in this book as "autistic learning disabilities" and "autistic learning styles." It is intended as a way of collecting and organizing information about the way in which a particular child with an autistic spectrum disorder may or may not be able to receive information, understand it, or use it. The ALDI can be a first step in making a psychoeducational assessment, in identifying and prioritizing areas of learning handicaps needing intervention, and in individualizing treatment strategies within a comprehensive program designed for autistic spectrum children. It can be used to organize a discussion or interview about a child's strengths and weaknesses between parents and potential treatment providers. The ALDI has no formal scoring, but rather is designed to help identify areas of learning that have been most heavily affected by the child's ASD. Each area of learning is covered in this book in terms of specific and comprehensive treatment strategies that may improve competencies.

AUTISTIC LEARNING DISABILITIES INVENTORY

Please answer the following questions using a 1-5 scale. There are no 'right' or 'wrong' answers. This is an inventory of your child's learning strengths and weaknesses to help plan intervention approaches.

Child's Name_____ Date of Birth_____ Date_____

	SOCIAL AUTISTIC LEARNING DISABILITIES	Awareness	Reciprocity	Imitation
	Give the response that shows, on average, what is true: (Mark answer in box.) 5= **Very definitely true**, all or almost all the time 4= Between a '5" and a '3' 3= **Can be true**, be is not consistently the case 2= Between a '2' and a '1' 1= This is **never or very seldom** the case			
1	Acts as if in own little world.			
2	Foremost motivation is to please self.			
3	More readily learns things that result in meeting own needs.			
4	Fails to notice certain things that others this age usually notice.			
5	May behave as if unaware that caregivers are in the same room.			
6	Seems to lack a desire to do things just to please others.			
7	Modifies actions if some else is made sad/ pretends to be sad by his actions.			
8	Becomes more quiet or reserved if someone else gets sad, upset, or cries.			
9	Offers comfort to others when they appear sad, upset, or are crying.			
10	Looks around to see who is noticing when he/she cries.			
11	Smiles and looks pleased in response to verbal praise (like "Great job!").			
12	Can be counted upon to repeat an activity that has been verbally praised.			
13	Can be counted on to repeat an activity that has been reprimanded.			
14	Apparent lack of concern about the effect of his behavior on others.			
15	Uninterested in trying to do new things just to earn approval of others.			
16	Does not seem to be motivated to copy actions or attitudes of others.			
17	Does not readily learn by being shown by others; must figure it out on own.			
18	Doesn't copy others just to be to be 'cool', or appear more grown up.			
19	Low level of interest in peers.			
20	Acts as though other children (aside from siblings) are not even there.			
21	Only engages with older children who act like/ are 'big sister' or 'big brother'.			
22	Show more interest in younger children than those his own age.			
23	Shows more interest in older children than those his own age.			
24	No interest in participating in group games with other children the same age.			

COMMUNICATIVE AUTISTIC LEARNING DISABILITIES	Receptive Gesture & BL	Expressive Gesture & BL.	Comprehension of Spoken Lang.	Use of Spoken Language
Give the response that shows, on average, what is true:(Mark answer in box.) **5=** Very definitely true, all or almost all the time **4=** Between a '5" and a '3" **3=** Can be true, be is not consistently the case **2=** Between a '2' and a '1' **1=** This is never or very seldom the case **0=** Doesn't talk yet. (For items marked "*")				
1 Doesn't look to where something is pointed out.				
2 Doesn't look back after seeing something to see if you've seen it, too.				
3 Stops an action when you shake your head 'no'				
4 Stops an action when you shake your head 'no' *and* look stern.				
5 Stops an action just when receiving a stern look.				
6 Stops an action after hearing a strict, serious tone of voice saying 'No!'.				
7 Knows that a nod of the head 'yes' means that what s/he's doing is OK.				
8 Points with index finger at things he wants.				
9 Points with index finger at things that are interesting, but not wanted.				
10 Points at something and then looks to see if you've seen it, too.				
11 Smiles in response when someone else smiles at him or her.				
12 Looks unhappy or worried if someone on TV cries, is sad or is hurt.				
13 Looks happy if others act happy, like after a happy ending on TV.				
14 Waves bye-bye either when he wants to leave, is leaving, or afterward.				
15 Can clearly read the emotion of 'shame' on child's face.				
16 Can clearly read the emotion of 'guilt' on child's face.				
17 Can clearly see when child feels proud.				
18 Difficult to tell if child is not understanding or not complying.				
19 Child understands only when he wants to understand.				
20 Understands names of things (nouns) better than action words(verbs).*				
21 May figure out what is meant by context in which the words are said.				
22 Uses words only when useful to get immediate needs met.*				
23 Doesn't use words just to comment on interesting things.*				
24 Does not 'chit-chat' or 'converse', even with babbling.				
25 Makes sure you are looking before s/he communicates in any way.				
26 Echoes some of your speech to show you he's 'with' the conversation.*				
27 Uses echolalic (exact, repeated speech) to re-enact play from videos.*				
28 Uses odd, not-quite-right, but understandable phrasing in speech.*				

AUTISTIC LEARNING DISABILITIES RELATING TO THE PHYSICAL WORLD Give the response that shows, on average, what is true:(Mark answer in box.) 5= **Very definitely true**, all or almost all the time 4= Between a '5" and a '3' 3= **Can be true**, be is not consistently the case 2= Between a '2' and a '1' 1= This is never or very seldom the case	Sensory Processing	Repetitions/ Novelty	Play
1	Seems actually not to hear (not just ignores) some sounds/ speech.			
2	Seem over-sensitive to some sounds, as if too loud.			
3	Very positive response to movement—like swinging or bouncing.			
4	Very negative about tactile irritations—like shirt labels, tight sleeves.			
5	Puts non-food items in mouth, as if this helps to learn about them.			
6	Picky about textures in mouth, and what is chewed or swallowed.			
7	Prefers old familiar toys to new toys.			
8	Initially fearful of something he now loves, e.g., vacuum, carousel.			
9	Once something is done one way, it's always done the same way.			
10	Has odd little rituals—like only drinking from one cup, for no reason.			
11	Prefers certain toys—because they spin, make certain noises, etc.			
12	Very focused in play with one thing, showing good concentration.			
13	Toy play is one action at a time—like a car crashes, a plane flies.			
14	Plays with toys, but without acting out a scene or story.			
15	Copies actions of people or videos with dolls, figures, or animals.			
16	Uses sounds to narrate play, like driving, crashing, or animal noises.			
17	Uses words to narrate play.			

INDEX

A

ABA/DTT (applied behavior analysis/ discrete trial training), 9, 311–51, 439, 467
  burnout from, 336–37
  cause and effect understanding and, 316–17
  child's capacity in, 318, 337, 344
  considerations in setting up, 325–30
  data collection for, 320, 339
  developmental aspects of, 312–13, 320–21, 345–47, 348–49
  discriminative stimulus in, 180–81
  early intervention and, 348–50, 461
  in exemplary classrooms, 418–21, 424–25
  features of, 330–39
  history of, 313–14
  home *vs.* school-based, 321–25, 328–29
  hours/week required, 314–15
  imitation concept for, 318–20, 340–41, 379
  inclusion programs and, 344–45, 377
  intensity in, 334–35, 418
  as learning to learn, 315–25
  medium-functioning autism and, 462, 463–64, 465
  mental retardation and, 337–38, 458–59
  methods *vs.* curriculum, 312
  in model programs, 408–9, 417
  motor prompting in, 318, 330–31, 341
  origins of, 407–11
  overview of, 311–15
  parents and, 321, 322, 323–24, 409, 410, 418–21
  picture communication in, 441–42
  PRT and, 334, 349–50
  reinforcement in, 53, 331–34
  special education and, 323, 325, 329
  for specific skills, 339–45
  task analysis in, 338–39
  TEACCH and, 354–57, 373, 374–75, 376, 436–38, 442–43
  tutor training for, 326–27, 328, 329–30
  workshop model, 409–10
ABCs of behavior analysis, 70–72, 321–22, 338
abdominal X-rays, 31
ability/disability matrix, 4, 49–50, 73, 112
  deficit profile and, 44–48
  perseveration and, 58–59
  reinforcers and, 53
  secondary deficits and, 66–67
  See also strengths and weaknesses
abstract thinking, 134, 192, 193, 243
accommodations
  failed, 48–49
  imitation and, 112, 114, 115
  See also self-accommodations
accompanied time-out, 217, 279
acquired deficits, 66
  See also secondary deficits/disabilities
activity schedules, 412, 440, 442
adaptive behavior skills, 272, 284
  See also daily living skills
adolescents
  independence of, 299–300
  sexual interest and, 297–99
  socialization of, 264–67
  teen expert player, 144–46
adult-initiated teaching, 39, 439, 440
adults, limit-setting by, 200–201
adults, play activity and, 134–43, 302, 443
  as followers, 136–37
  as interpreters, 135–36
  as leaders, 137–38
  as shadows, 138–43
  See also parents; teachers
adults, TEACCH programs for, 369–72, 376
affiliative orientation, 63–64, 65, 152, 155, 265
  imitation and, 109, 113, 116
  See also social ALDs
AFP (alpha-fetal protein) screen, 26
after-school services, 430
  See also day care
age-appropriate play, 249
  See also developmental age
age of initiation of treatment, 307
aggression, 69
aides. *See* one-to-one aides; teaching aides
ALDs. *See* autistic learning disabilities (ALDs)
Alpine Learning Center, 414–16
amniocentesis, 26
amygdala, in brain, 54
antecedents of behavior, 71, 72, 338
Anthropologist on Mars (Sacks), 35
aphasia, 155, 174
Appendix A, 168, 239, 245, 479–82